Obesity and Associated Eating Disorders: A Guide for Mental Health Professionals

Guest Editors

THOMAS A. WADDEN, PhD
G. TERENCE WILSON, PhD
ALBERT J. STUNKARD, MD
ROBERT I. BERKOWITZ, MD

PSYCHIATRIC CLINICS OF NORTH AMERICA

www.psych.theclinics.com

December 2011 • Volume 34 • Number 4

SAUNDERS an imprint of ELSEVIER, Inc.

W.B. SAUNDERS COMPANY
A Division of Elsevier Inc.

1600 John F. Kennedy Boulevard • Suite 1800 • Philadelphia, PA 19103-2899

http://www.theclinics.com

PSYCHIATRIC CLINICS OF NORTH AMERICA Volume 34, Number 4
December 2011 ISSN 0193-953X, ISBN-13: 978-1-4557-1163-5

Editor: Sarah E. Barth

Psychiatric Clinics of North America (ISSN 0193-953X) is published quarterly by Elsevier Inc., 360 Park Avenue South, New York, NY 10010-1710. Months of issue are March, June, September, and December. Business and Editorial Offices: 1600 John F. Kennedy Blvd., Suite 1800, Philadelphia, PA 19103-2899. Periodicals postage paid at New York, NY and additional mailing offices. Subscription prices are $286.00 per year (US individuals), $504.00 per year (US institutions), $141.00 per year (US students/residents), $347.00 per year (Canadian individuals), $627.00 per year (Canadian Institutions), $431.00 per year (foreign individuals), $627.00 per year (foreign institutions), and $210.00 per year (international & Canadian students/residents). Foreign air speed delivery is included in all *Clinics'* subscription prices. All prices are subject to change without notice. **POSTMASTER:** Send address changes to *Psychiatric Clinics of North America,* Elsevier Health Sciences Division, Subscription Customer Service, 3251 Riverport Lane, Maryland Heights, MO 63043. Customer Service: 1-800-654-2452 (US). From outside the United States, call 1-314-447-8871. Fax: 1-314-447-8029. E-mail: journalscustomerservice-usa@elsevier.com (for print support) and journalsonlinesupport-usa@elsevier.com (for online support).

Reprints. For copies of 100 or more, of articles in this publication, please contact the Commercial Reprints Department, Elsevier Inc., 360 Park Avenue South, New York, New York 10010-1710. Tel.: (212) 633-3813, Fax: (212) 462-1935, E-mail: reprints@elsevier.com.

Psychiatric Clinics of North America is covered in *MEDLINE/PubMed (Index Medicus), Current Contents/Social and Behavioral Sciences, Social Science Citation Index, Embase/Excerpta Medica,* and PsycINFO.

Printed and bound by CPI Group (UK) Ltd, Croydon, CR0 4YY

Transferred to Digital Print 2011

Contributors

GUEST EDITORS

THOMAS A. WADDEN, PhD
Professor of Psychology, Center for Weight and Eating Disorders, Department of Psychiatry, Perelman School of Medicine at the University of Pennsylvania, Philadelphia, Pennsylvania

G. TERENCE WILSON, PhD
Oscar K. Buros Professor of Psychology, Rutgers–The State University of New Jersey, Graduate School of Applied and Professional Psychology, Piscataway, New Jersey

ALBERT J. STUNKARD, MD
Professor of Psychiatry, Center for Weight and Eating Disorders, Department of Psychiatry, Perelman School of Medicine at the University of Pennsylvania, Philadelphia, Pennsylvania

ROBERT I. BERKOWITZ, MD
Professor of Psychiatry, Children's Hospital of Philadelphia, and Center for Weight and Eating Disorders, Department of Psychiatry, Perelman School of Medicine at the University of Pennsylvania, Philadelphia, Pennsylvania

AUTHORS

KELLY C. ALLISON, PhD
Assistant Professor, Department of Psychiatry, Perelman School of Medicine at the University of Pennsylvania, Philadelphia, Pennsylvania

ROBERT I. BERKOWITZ, MD
Professor of Psychiatry, Children's Hospital of Philadelphia, and Center for Weight and Eating Disorders, Department of Psychiatry, Perelman School of Medicine at the University of Pennsylvania, Philadelphia, Pennsylvania

GEORGE A. BRAY, MD, MACP
Pennington Biomedical Research Center, Louisiana State University System, Baton Rouge, Louisiana

KELLY D. BROWNELL, PhD
Professor of Psychology, Epidemiology and Public Health; Director, Rudd Center for Food Policy and Obesity, Yale University, New Haven, Connecticut

MEGHAN L. BUTRYN, PhD
Department of Psychology, Drexel University, Philadelphia, Pennsylvania

VICTORIA A. CATENACCI, MD
Assistant Professor, Endocrinology, Anschutz Health and Wellness Center, University of Colorado Anschutz Medical Campus, Aurora, Colorado

KELLIANN K. DAVIS, PhD
Department of Health and Physical Activity, University of Pittsburgh, Physical Activity and Weight Management Research Center, Pittsburgh, Pennsylvania

VICKI DILILLO, PhD
Associate Professor, Department of Psychology, Ohio Wesleyan University, Delaware, Ohio

KRISTOFFEL DUMON, MD
Assistant Professor of Surgery, Department of Surgery, Perelman School of Medicine at the University of Pennsylvania, Philadelphia, Pennsylvania

ANTHONY N. FABRICATORE, PhD
Assistant Professor of Psychology in Psychiatry, Perelman School of Medicine at the University of Pennsylvania, Philadelphia; Senior Director, Research and Development, Nutrisystem, Inc., Fort Washington, Pennsylvania

LUCY F. FAULCONBRIDGE, PhD
Center for Weight and Eating Disorders, Department of Psychiatry, Perelman School of Medicine at the University of Pennsylvania, Philadelphia, Pennsylvania

GARY D. FOSTER, PhD
Laura H. Carnell Professor of Medicine, Public Health and Psychology; Director, Center for Obesity Research and Education, Temple University, Philadelphia, Pennsylvania

MATTHEW R. HAYES, PhD
Translational Neuroscience Program, Department of Psychiatry, Perelman School of Medicine at the University of Pennsylvania, Philadelphia, Pennsylvania

JAMES O. HILL, PhD
Professor, Pediatrics, Anschutz Health and Wellness Center, University of Colorado Anschutz Medical Campus, Aurora, Colorado

JOHN M. JAKICIC, PhD
Department of Health and Physical Activity, University of Pittsburgh, Physical Activity and Weight Management Research Center, Pittsburgh, Pennsylvania

ROBERT F. KUSHNER, MD
Professor of Medicine and Clinical Director, Northwestern Comprehensive Center on Obesity, Feinberg School of Medicine, Northwestern University, Chicago, Illinois

ANGELA MAKRIS, PhD, RD
Assistant Professor, Center for Obesity Research and Education, Temple University, Philadelphia, Pennsylvania

NIA S. MITCHELL, MD, MPH
Assistant Professor, General Internal Medicine, Anschutz Health and Wellness Center, University of Colorado Anschutz Medical Campus, Aurora, Colorado

NICOLE L. NOVAK, MSc
Research Associate, Department of Psychology, Rudd Center for Food Policy and Obesity, Yale University, New Haven, Connecticut

DONNA H. RYAN, MD, FACP
Pennington Biomedical Research Center, Louisiana State University System, Baton Rouge, Louisiana

DAVID B. SARWER, PhD
Associate Professor of Psychology, Departments of Psychiatry and Surgery; Director of Clinical Services, Center for Weight and Eating Disorders, Perelman School of Medicine at the University of Pennsylvania, Philadelphia, Pennsylvania

ALBERT J. STUNKARD, MD
Professor of Psychiatry, Center for Weight and Eating Disorders, Department of Psychiatry, Perelman School of Medicine at the University of Pennsylvania, Philadelphia, Pennsylvania

ELLEN P. TARVES, MA
Doctoral Candidate, Department of Psychology, LaSalle University, Philadelphia, Pennsylvania

MARION L. VETTER, MD, RD
Assistant Professor of Medicine, Department of Medicine, Perelman School of Medicine at the University of Pennsylvania, Philadelphia, Pennsylvania

THOMAS A. WADDEN, PhD
Professor of Psychology, Center for Weight and Eating Disorders, Department of Psychiatry, Perelman School of Medicine at the University of Pennsylvania, Philadelphia, Pennsylvania

VICTORIA WEBB, BA
Center for Weight and Eating Disorders, University of Pennsylvania, Philadelphia, Pennsylvania

DELIA SMITH WEST, PhD
Professor, Department of Health Behavior, Fay W. Boozman College of Public Health, University of Arkansas for Medical Sciences, Little Rock, Arkansas

NOEL N. WILLIAMS, MBBCh, MCh
Associate Professor of Surgery, Department of Surgery, Perelman School of Medicine at the University of Pennsylvania, Philadelphia, Pennsylvania

G. TERENCE WILSON, PhD
Oscar K. Buros Professor of Psychology, Rutgers–The State University of New Jersey, Graduate School of Applied and Professional Psychology, Piscataway, New Jersey

HOLLY R. WYATT, MD
Associate Professor, Endocrinology, Anschutz Health and Wellness Center, University of Colorado Anschutz Medical Campus, Aurora, Colorado

Contents

> Despite growing recognition of the problem, the obesity epidemic continues in the United States, affecting every segment of the population and increasing the risk of many chronic diseases. Obesity rates are also increasing around the world. Approximately 34% of U.S. adults and 15% to 20% of children and adolescents are obese. The obesity epidemic arose gradually, apparently from a small, consistent degree of positive energy balance. Substantial public health efforts are being directed toward addressing obesity, but without clear evidence of success yet, and it may be one of the most difficult public health issues our society has faced.

> The central nervous system control of energy balance is a multideter-mined process involving a distributed network of communication between various brain regions and the body. The brain continuously receives and processes internal signals of energy availability and in turn issues autonomic and behavioral output commands. Environmental, emotional, rewarding, and learned factors influence the brain's perception of these signals and ultimately promote behaviors that drive the system to conserve energy and ingest energy-dense foods in excess. This article discusses the energy balance system under normal physiologic conditions and the processes that have evolutionarily developed to promote energy surplus.

> The nature of the relationship between obesity and psychopathology has become the focus of increasingly sophisticated empirical investigation. This article summarizes data from epidemiologic studies and clinical trials related to five key questions: (1) How are obesity and psychopathology related cross-sectionally? (2) How are these characteristics associated in longitudinal observations? (3) How common are psychiatric disorders among obese persons seeking weight loss

therapy? (4) How does intentional weight loss affect psychopathology (and vice versa)? and (5) How can psychotropic agents that induce weight gain be managed in patients who require such medication?

Obesity is characterized by an excessive amount of fat, which is estimated by body mass index (BMI). Persons with a BMI of 30 kg/m² or greater are considered obese. In the past, obesity was been considered an eating disorder. We have learned that most overweight and obese persons do not overeat in any distinctive pattern. For a smaller number, however, 2 clear patterns of overeating have been identified: Binge eating disorder and night eating syndrome. Both are more prevalent among overweight and obese persons than among persons of normal weight, and they contribute to the overweight of such persons.

Cognitive–behavioral therapy and interpersonal psychotherapy are currently the most effective treatments for binge eating disorder in terms of cessation of binge eating, reduction of specific eating disorder psychopathology, and associated forms of psychopathology and psychosocial functioning. Treatment effects are generally well-maintained at follow-up. These specialty psychological treatments do not produce clinically significant weight loss, however. Guided self-help is a brief, cost-effective, and readily disseminable alternative to specialty treatments that require significantly more time and resources. Behavioral weight loss treatment produces short-term weight loss that is typically regained over follow-up. Pharmacotherapy is unsupported by available evidence.

This article reviews the research published to date for treatment of night eating syndrome. These results include trials of selective serotonin reuptake inhibitors, cognitive behavior therapy, behavior therapy, abbreviated progressive muscle relaxation, and light therapy. Case examples are included to illustrate the clinical features and response patterns of those who present for treatment of night eating syndrome.

physical activity, and combining lifestyle modification with pharmacotherapy. Finally, innovative programs that can be used to disseminate behavioral approaches beyond traditional academic settings are discussed.

Motivational interviewing (MI) is a patient-centered counseling strategy designed to help individuals explore and enhance motivation to change behaviors in a collaborative fashion in a context that supports autonomy and emphasizes self-efficacy. MI has been implemented in a range of settings targeting a variety of health-related behaviors. Emerging evidence suggests that MI and MI-based strategies show promise for facilitating weight loss and enhancing treatment engagement among overweight and obese individuals. This article provides a brief introduction to MI and reviews the literature on MI in the context of weight management.

As we develop new drugs to treat obesity, we need a descriptive framework. This framework divides them into 3 groups: Those that reduce food intake, those that alter metabolism, and those that increase thermogenesis. Medications for obesity treatment should be viewed as useful adjuncts to diet and physical activity and may help selected patients achieve and maintain weight loss. Thus, physicians must be knowledgeable regarding the efficacy and safety profiles of currently available medications.

Bariatric surgery is the most effective and durable treatment for extreme obesity. Restrictive procedures limit gastric capacity and, thus, food intake while leaving the gastrointestinal tract intact. Malabsorptive procedures shorten the length of the intestine to decrease nutrient absorption. Combined procedures include restriction and gastrointestinal rearrangement. Procedures that bypass segments of the gut are associated with greater weight loss and greater improvements in comorbid conditions than gastric banding. High-quality, long-term, randomized, controlled trials are currently underway to compare the efficacy, safety, and cost-effectiveness of the various bariatric surgery procedures, and with intensive, nonsurgical weight loss interventions.

Considerable evidence illustrates that the current obesity epidemic has social, economic, and political causes and that effective responses to obesity must take place on a population level. Viewing obesity as a medical problem is an advance over simply blaming individuals for being overweight, but there is a strong need to view this issue from a public health perspective that emphasizes changes in the environmental drivers of the problem. This article compares medical and public health models and ends by proposing public policy changes the authors believe may help advance the field.

THE CLINICS ARE NOW AVAILABLE ONLINE!

Access your subscription at:
www.theclinics.com

Preface

Obesity and Associated Eating Disorders: A Guide for Mental Health Professionals

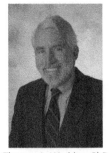 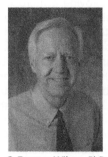 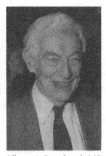 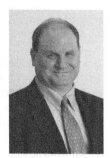

Thomas A. Wadden, PhD   G. Terence Wilson, PhD   Albert J. Stunkard, MD   Robert I. Berkowitz, MD
Guest Editors

The epidemic of obesity is well known to readers of this issue, as it is to just about anyone who reads a newspaper, watches television, or scrolls the Internet. Most recent data from the National Health and Nutrition Examination Survey (2007–2008) indicate that 34% of US adults are obese, as defined by a body mass index (BMI) of 30 kg/m^2 or greater. An additional 34% are overweight, characterized by a BMI of 25.0 to 29.9 kg/m^2. Perhaps the most encouraging news from the recent survey is that the prevalence of obesity and overweight appears to have stopped increasing. However, there is still cause for great concern. Obesity contributes to hundreds of thousands of deaths per year, through its association with cardiovascular disease, type 2 diabetes, several cancers, and other conditions. The physical and emotional consequences of obesity, for those afflicted, are accompanied by direct and indirect costs to our nation of more than $100 billion a year.

This edited issue joins others in providing an overview of the etiology, consequences, prevention, and treatment of obesity in adults. This issue, however, differs in its intended audience, which is principally psychiatrists, psychologists, social workers, and primary care providers, who are accustomed to assessing and treating psychiatric disorders. The present issue updates our 2005 issue of *Psychiatric Clinics of North America* and provides several new articles that address topics of particular interest to mental health providers. We are grateful to our outstanding group of contributors, all of whom are experts in their fields of study and have a wealth of clinical and research experience.

The articles are not formally divided into sections but fall into seven parts: (1) overview of the prevalence, etiology, and physical consequences of obesity;

Psychiatr Clin N Am 34 (2011) xiii–xvi
doi:10.1016/j.psc.2011.09.001
0193-953X/11/$ – see front matter

(2) psychiatric complications and eating disorders associated with obesity; (3) the management of psychiatric disorders, including binge eating and night eating; (4) medical and behavioral assessment of the obese patient; (5) behavioral interventions for overweight/obese adults, including diet, exercise, behavior therapy, and motivational interviewing; (6) pharmacologic and surgical interventions; and (7) the prevention of obesity through public policy. The articles are briefly introduced according to these sections.

Nia Mitchell, James Hill, and colleagues provide a thorough introduction to the epidemic of obesity. They describe the prevalence and complications of this disorder, as well as the relative contributions of genetic and environmental factors to obesity. They underscore how ancient genes that promoted survival in times of scarcity make losing weight so difficult in times of abundance and what can be done to close the excess "energy gap." In the article that follows, Lucy Faulconbridge and Matthew Hayes illuminate the basic mechanisms of body weight regulation. Seminal discoveries in this area over the past 20 years have revealed that energy intake and expenditure are regulated by an elaborate neuroendocrine system that has multiple targets in the hypothalamus, as well as the hindbrain. Mental health practitioners will be familiar with the important role that the hypothalamus plays in the regulation of emotion, sleep, and other basic functions.

Part 2 of the issue begins with Robert Berkowitz and Anthony Fabricatore's examination of the psychosocial status of obese individuals. They describe the high prevalence of mood and anxiety disorders observed in individuals with extreme obesity (ie, BMI >40 kg/m^2), who often are encountered by mental health practitioners during evaluation for bariatric surgery. The authors also examine the bidirectional relationship between obesity and depression (ie, each can contribute to the other) and address the critically important topic of weight gain associated with the use of psychiatric medications. In the article that follows, Albert Stunkard introduces two eating disorders that are frequently encountered in obese individuals---binge eating and night eating. With each, he provides an overview of the key behavioral features, as well as the etiology and the prevalence of the conditions, and distinguishes them from bulimia nervosa. Binge eating disorder and night eating syndrome are found in only a small minority of obese individuals but are associated with significant emotional distress, as compared with the presence of obesity alone.

Part 3 of the issue is devoted to the treatment of these two eating disorders. Terence Wilson thoroughly reviews the results of randomized trials that have addressed the problem of binge eating disorder. The evidence leads him to conclude that cognitive behavioral therapy is superior to both pharmacologic intervention and traditional behavioral weight control for the long-term amelioration of binge eating disorder. In the article that follows, Kelly Allison and Ellen Tarves's examination of treatments for the night eating syndrome reveals that there have been fewer trials on this condition than on binge eating disorder. Nonetheless, practitioners will likely find useful the description of the cognitive behavioral intervention developed for night eating syndrome, as well as findings for the antidepressant medication, sertraline.

Robert Kushner and David Sarwer's article on the medical and behavioral evaluation of patients with obesity is the fourth part of the issue and covers two principal issues. Before undertaking significant weight loss, obese individuals should complete a medical evaluation to identify possible contraindications to treatment, as well as to fully assess physical complications of excess weight. Psychiatrists are unlikely to perform the physical examination but should be aware of frequently overlooked complications, including obstructive sleep apnea, polycystic ovarian syndrome, and nonalcoholic fatty liver disease. Mental health professionals will welcome the guidance the authors provide for assessing possible behavioral complications of obesity, taking a weight (and weight loss) history, and determining the contribution of eating and activity habits to the patient's weight problem.

The four articles that comprise part 5 of the issue introduce behavioral interventions for obesity (ie, nonpharmacologic or nonsurgical approaches). Algorithms developed by the National Heart, Lung, and Blood Institute, as well as the World Health Organization, recommend that obese individuals initially be treated by a comprehensive program of diet, exercise, and behavior therapy—an approach often referred to as lifestyle modification. In their article on dietary management, Angie Makris and Gary Foster review principles of sound nutrition for weight loss and examine nearly a decade's worth of research on the effect of macronutrient composition on weight loss. Readers will recognize controversies concerning the purported benefits of low-carbohydrate versus traditional low-fat diets for weight loss, as well as the possible benefits of higher protein diets or those with a low glycemic index. The review reveals that, when level of energy restriction is held constant, the macronutrient composition of the diet does not appear to affect weight loss but may influence the control of comorbid conditions. In the article that follows, John Jakicic and Kelliann Davis examine the importance of regular physical activity for improving cardiovascular health and for facilitating the maintenance of lost weight. Studies increasingly suggest that successful weight losers (ie, those who have lost 10% or more of initial weight) need to engage in the equivalent of approximately 275–300 minutes of brisk walking per week. This is a tall order but can be met by methods that include exercising in multiple short bouts (ie, 10 minutes). Meghan Butryn and colleagues review principles of behavior therapy that are used to facilitate patients' adoption of new eating and activity habits. Behavioral treatment can be provided in either group or individual sessions and induces a loss of approximately 8% to 10% of initial weight in 4 to 6 months. Much of the article is devoted to describing efforts to disseminate behavioral treatment, using the Internet or community-based interventions. The final article in this section, by Vicki DiLillo and Delia West, describes the use of motivational interviewing as an adjunct to comprehensive lifestyle modification. Readers who work in the area of substance abuse will be familiar with motivational interviewing, an approach designed to help patients identify and resolve ambivalence they have about changing their behavior. Results of randomized trials suggest that motivational interviewing holds promise in strengthening traditional behavioral interventions for obesity.

Part 6 of the issue examines pharmacotherapy, which is an option for patients with a BMI of 30 kg/m^2 or more (or >27 kg/m^2 in the presence of comorbid conditions) who are unable to achieve a 10% weight loss with lifestyle modification alone. George Bray and Donna Ryan examine current FDA-approved medications for obesity, as well as those on the horizon. Two combination therapies, which combine medications already approved for other indications (ie, phentermine plus topirimate, as well as bupropion plus naltrexone), were not approved by FDA on the first review, but the sponsors are continuing to seek approval. Marion Vetter and colleagues complete the examination of obesity therapies with their review of surgical options, which are appropriate for persons with a BMI of 40 kg/m^2 or more (and ≥35 kg/m^2 in the presence of comorbid conditions). The authors review weight losses, as well as risks and benefits, of the most common procedures, including the Roux-en-Y gastric bypass, laparoscopic adjustable gastric banding, and sleeve gastrectomy.

Space limitations prevented us from addressing the management of obesity in children and adolescents. However, in the last part of the issue, Nicole Novak and Kelly Brownell argue cogently that treatment alone is not the answer to the epidemic of obesity, in either children or adults. Instead, in their view, far greater attention must be devoted to the prevention of obesity by tackling the toxic environment that lies at the heart of the epidemic. Such efforts call for public health campaigns and bold policy initiatives, as used to address cigarette smoking, drunk driving, and the AIDs epidemic. We agree fully. While we must improve treatments for individuals who already are obese, the greater need is to prevent the development of this disorder.

We hope that this updated and expanded edition of our prior publication in *Psychiatric Clinics of North America* will help mental health professionals do their part in caring for individuals who suffer from obesity and its associated eating disorders. We thank Sarah Barth of Elsevier, for her able assistance in guiding the development of this issue, as well as Caroline Moran and Victoria Webb, for their outstanding editorial assistance. Finally, we thank again our distinguished group of contributors, many of whom are among our closest friends and colleagues.

Thomas A. Wadden, PhD
Center for Weight and Eating Disorders
Department of Psychiatry
Perelman School of Medicine
at the University of Pennsylvania
3535 Market Street, Suite 3029
Philadelphia, PA 19104, USA

G. Terence Wilson, PhD
Rutgers–The State University of New Jersey
Graduate School of Applied and Professional Psychology
152 Frelinghuysen Road
Piscataway, NJ 08854, USA

Albert J. Stunkard, MD
Center for Weight and Eating Disorders
Department of Psychiatry
Perelman School of Medicine
at the University of Pennsylvania
3535 Market Street, Suite 3029
Philadelphia, PA 19104, USA

Robert I. Berkowitz, MD
Children's Hospital of Philadelphia, and
Center for Weight and Eating Disorders
Department of Psychiatry
Perelman School of Medicine
at the University of Pennsylvania
3535 Market Street, Suite 3029
Philadelphia, PA 19104, USA

E-mail addresses:
wadden@mail.med.upenn.edu (T.A. Wadden)
tewilson@rci.rutger.edu (G.T. Wilson)
stunkard@mail.med.upenn.edu (A.J. Stunkard)
Rberk@mail.med.upenn.edu (R.I. Berkowitz)

Obesity: Overview of an Epidemic

Nia S. Mitchell, MD, MPH*, Victoria A. Catenacci, MD,
Holly R. Wyatt, MD, James O. Hill, PhD

KEYWORDS

• Obesity • Epidemic • Body mass index • Health risks

The obesity epidemic in the United States continues. In the last few years, obesity rates have not increased significantly in some US subpopulations, but it is too soon to tell whether this means that the epidemic has reached maximum levels in these populations.[1,2] There is clear evidence that obesity rates are increasing in much of the rest of the world.[3,4] A large amount of research is now directed toward better understanding and treatment of obesity, and substantial public health efforts are directed toward reducing obesity rates. To date, however, there is little evidence of success in reversing the epidemic in the United States.

PREVALENCE OF OBESITY

In adults, overweight and obesity are defined based on body mass index (BMI), which is determined as weight (kg) divided by height^2 (m). **Table 1** shows the categories of BMI. A healthy BMI range is 18.5 to 24.9 kg/m^2. Overweight is defined as a BMI from 25 to 29.9 kg/m^2, and obesity is defined as BMI of 30 kg/m^2 or greater.[5] Obesity can be further subdivided based on subclasses of BMI as shown in **Table 1**. Waist circumference can be used in combination with a BMI value to evaluate health risk for individuals.

The strongest data on obesity prevalence rates over time in the United States come from results of the National Health and Nutrition Examination Surveys (NHANES). NHANES periodically collect measured heights and weights in representative samples of the population. The most recent NHANES data were collected during 2007–2008.[1]

As shown in **Fig. 1**, obesity rates for adults have been gradually increasing over the past 3+ decades, with the latest statistics showing that in 2007–2008, approximately 68% were overweight or obese, and approximately 34% were obese.[1]

This work was supported by grants DK02703, DK42549, and DK48520 from the National Institutes of Health.
Anschutz Health and Wellness Center, University of Colorado Anschutz Medical Campus, 13001 East 17th Place, Aurora, CO 80045, USA
* Corresponding author.
E-mail address: Nia.mitchell@ucdenver.edu

Psychiatr Clin N Am 34 (2011) 717–732
doi:10.1016/j.psc.2011.08.005
0193-953X/11/$ – see front matter © 2011 Elsevier Inc. All rights reserved.

Table 1
Categories of BMI and disease risk[a] relative to normal weight and waist circumference

	BMI (kg/m²)	Obesity Class	Men ≤102 cm (≤40 in) Women ≤88 cm (≤35 in)	>102 cm (>40 in) >88 cm (>35 in)
Underweight	<18.5		—	—
Normal[b]	18.5–24.9		—	—
Overweight	25.0–29.9		Increased	High
Obesity	30.0–34.9	I	High	Very high
	35.0–39.9	II	Very high	Very high
Extreme obesity	≥40	III	Extremely high	Extremely high

[a] Disease risk for type 2 diabetes, hypertension, and CVD.
[b] Increased waist circumference can also be a marker for increased risk even in persons of normal weight.
Data from Expert Panel on the Identification, Evaluation, and Treatment of Overweight in Adults. Clinical guidelines on the identification, evaluation, and treatment of overweight and obesity in adults: executive summary. Am J Clin Nutr 1998;68:899–917.

Since the 1970s, the prevalence of obesity has increased throughout the U.S. adult population—among men and women of all ethnic groups, ages, and educational and socioeconomic levels.[6] Although the entire population seems to be getting heavier each year, there is evidence that obesity affects some subgroups in the population to a greater extent than others. For example, African American and Mexican American women have a higher prevalence of obesity (BMI >30 kg/m²) than Caucasian women or than men of any ethnic background (**Table 2**). Note that obesity prevalence rates increased over time in all gender–ethnic groups (**Fig. 2**). Obesity rates are increasing

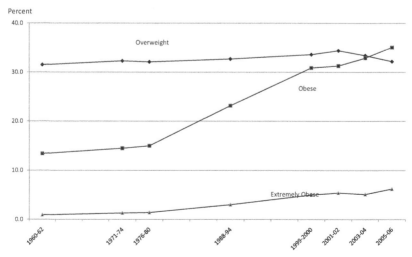

Fig. 1. Trends in overweight, obesity, and extreme obesity, ages 20–74 years. Note: Age-adjusted by the direct method to the year 2000 US Bureau of the Census using age groups 20–39, 40–59, and 60–74 years. Pregnant females excluded. Overweight defined as BMI ≥25 but < 30; obesity defined as BMI ≥30; extreme obesity defined as BMI ≥40.

Table 2
Prevalence of obesity by race and gender

Race	Males	Females
Caucasian	31.9	33.0
African American	37.3	49.6
Mexican American	35.9	45.1

Reprinted from Prevalence of overweight, obesity, and extreme obesity among adults: United States trends 1976–1980 through 2007–2008. Available at: http://www.cdc.gov/NCHS/data/hestat/obesity_adult_07_08/obesity_adult_07_08.pdf.

among people in all income and educational levels (**Figs. 3** and **4**), but absolute rates are higher in those with low incomes and low education levels.[7–9] This suggests that the gap among socioeconomic strata for obesity rates may be closing.[6]

The finding that minority and low-income individuals are disproportionately affected by obesity is not surprising. The most inexpensive foods are those containing high levels of fat and sugar.[10] Thus, the way to get the most calories for the least money is to eat a diet that is high in fat and sugar. This interaction of biology and economics thus supports the obesity epidemic. Foods for which we have a high biological preference (ie, foods high in sugar and high in energy density), and that contribute to overeating, are currently the cheapest and most accessible.[10,11] Further, minority and low-income individuals may engage in less physical activity than other sectors of the population.[12,13] One reason for this disparity may be because problems with neighborhood safety in low income areas may prevent adults and children from engaging in outdoor physical activities. People who have more financial resources combat these circumstances more easily and, consequently, are more physically active and less obese than those with fewer resources.

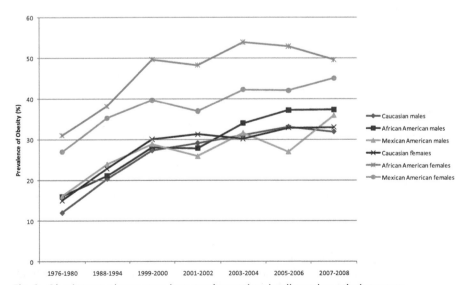

Fig. 2. Obesity prevalence rates increased over time in all gender–ethnic groups.

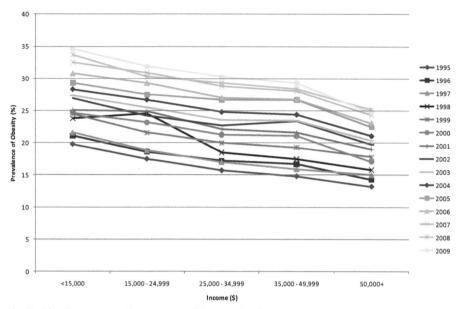

Fig. 3. Obesity rates are the same at all income levels.

In children, overweight is defined as 85th to 95th percentile for age and gender, and obesity is defined as 95th percentile or greater for age and gender.[14] As shown in **Fig. 5**, obesity rates in children and adolescents have continued to increase over the past 3+ decades.[2] According to NHANES 2007–2008, 17% of US children and adolescents between the ages of 2 and 19 years were at or above the 95th percentile for weight. Among children and adolescents, Mexican American males and African American females are more likely to have a higher BMI (**Fig. 6**).[2]

HEALTH RISKS ASSOCIATED WITH OBESITY

Obesity negatively affects most bodily systems. It is linked to the most prevalent and costly medical problems seen in our country, including type 2 diabetes, hypertension, coronary artery disease, many forms of cancer, and cognitive dysfunction.

Type 2 Diabetes and Prediabetes

BMI, abdominal fat distribution, and weight gain are important risk factors for the development of type 2 diabetes. It is estimated that 90% of individuals with type 2 diabetes are obese.[15] It is further estimated that 30% of US adults have prediabetes.[16]

Dyslipidemia

Visceral obesity is associated with elevated triglycerides; low high-density lipoprotein (HDL) cholesterol; and increased small, dense low-density lipoprotein (LDL) particles.[17]

Coronary Artery Disease

Obese persons, particularly those with abdominal fat distribution, are at increased risk for coronary artery disease (CAD). The American Heart Association added obesity to its list of major risk factors for CAD in 1998.[18]

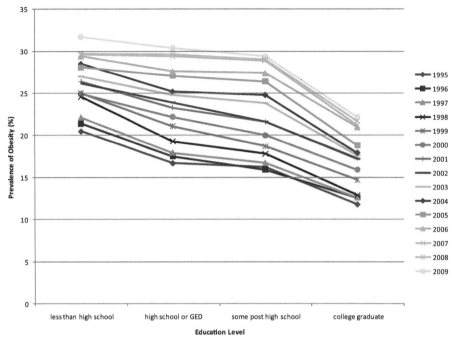

Fig. 4. Obesity rates are the same at all education levels.

Sleep Apnea

Obese men and women are also at high risk for sleep apnea, in which partial or complete upper airway obstruction during sleep leads to episodes of apnea or hypopnea. The interruption in nighttime sleep and repeated episodes of hypoxemia lead to daytime somnolence, morning headache, systemic hypertension, and can eventually result in pulmonary hypertension and right heart failure.

Cognitive Dysfunction

Data about the link between obesity and cognitive dysfunction are mixed. Numerous studies have shown an association between obesity and cognitive dysfunction, including worse executive function[19–21] and memory deficits.[22] Although obesity is linked with many diseases that are associated with cognitive dysfunction, some imaging studies have shown lower overall brain volume[23] and gray[24,25] and white matter[26] in obese versus normal weight individuals without weight-related comorbidities. Lower brain volumes have also been found in obese individuals with mild cognitive impairment and Alzheimer disease.[27] One study found that obesity in middle age may be associated with developing dementia later in life, but may be protective in older-aged adults.[28] Another study found overweight and obesity to be protective against cognitive decline associated with mild cognitive impairment, Alzheimer disease, and vascular dementia.[29] A meta-analysis[30] of prospective studies that looked at BMI in midlife and dementia showed underweight, overweight, and obesity were all associated with developing dementia later in life. A systematic review of longitudinal population-based studies concluded that higher BMI is likely a risk factor for developing dementia.[31]

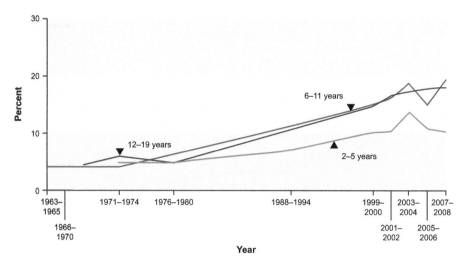

Fig. 5. Obesity rates in children and adolescents have continued to increase over the past 3 decades. NOTE: Obesity is defined as body mass index (BMI) greater than or equal to sex- and age-specific 95th percentile from the 2000 CDC Growth Charts. SOURCES: CDC/NCHS, National Health Examination Survey II (ages 6–1), III (ages 12–17), and National Health and Nutrition Examination Surveys (NHANES) I-III, and NHANES 1999–2000, 2001–2002, 2003–2004, 2005–2006, and 2007–2008.

Nonalcoholic Fatty Liver Disease

Obesity is associated with a spectrum of liver disease known as nonalcoholic fatty liver disease (NAFLD) or nonalcoholic steatohepatitis (NASH). Manifestations of this disorder include hepatomegaly, abnormal liver function tests, and abnormal liver histology including macrovesicular steatosis, steatohepatitis, fibrosis, and cirrhosis.[32,33]

Cancer

Overweight and obesity are associated with increased risk of endometrial, esophageal, renal cell, pancreatic, ovarian, breast, colorectal, thyroid, and gallbladder cancers. They also are associated with leukemia, multiple myeloma, non-Hodgkin's lymphoma, and malignant melanoma.[34,35]

Health Risks of Obesity in Children and Adolescents

As more and more children and adolescents are becoming obese, they are beginning to develop risk factors for chronic diseases usually seen much later in life, such as dyslipidemia, hypertension, and hyperinsulinemia.[36] For example, an increased number of obese children and adolescents are now being diagnosed with type 2 diabetes,[37] a disease that was virtually nonexistent in this population a few generations ago. Similarly, there is evidence that obesity in children and adolescents facilitates progression of cardiovascular disease.[36,38]

HOW DID THE EPIDEMIC ARISE?

To understand how the obesity epidemic arose, it is helpful to examine how body weight is regulated. The key to understanding body weight regulation is understanding

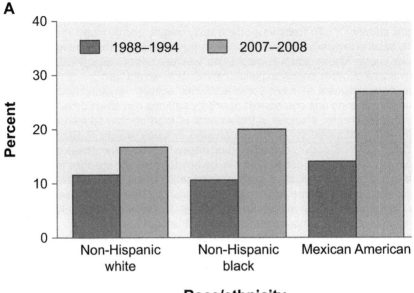

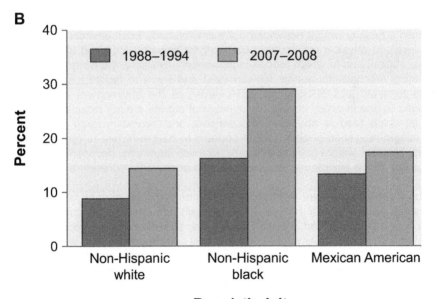

Fig. 6. (*A, B*) Among children and adolescents, Mexican American males and African American females are more likely to have a higher BMI. NOTE: Obesity is defined as body mass index (BMI) greater than or equal to sex- and age-specific 95th percentile from the 2000 CDC Growth Charts. SOURCES: CDC/NCHS, National Health and Nutrition Examination Surveys (NHANES) III 1988–1994 and NHANES 2007–2008.

energy balance. The body's state of energy balance is determined by the amount of energy ingested in food in relation to the amount of energy expended in metabolism and physical activity.[39,40] To maintain a stable body weight, energy intake must, over time, exactly equal energy expenditure. Negative energy balance (in which energy expenditure exceeds energy intake) results in weight loss, whereas positive energy balance (in which energy intake exceeds energy expenditure) results in weight gain.

The body appears to have some ability to actively regulate or adjust energy balance, as altering one component of energy balance can affect other components. For example, chronic changes in the amount of food consumed lead to changes in metabolism that serve to oppose a change in body weight.[41] Similarly, chronic changes in physical activity can affect food intake.[42,43] However, these compensatory physiologic changes are not sufficient to completely prevent changes in body weight in the face of strong, persistent positive or negative energy balance.[42,43] The human physiologic system seems to protect more against body weight loss than against body weight gain. This makes sense in that for most of humankind's history, starvation was a much more serious problem than obesity.[44]

Each component of energy balance can be influenced by genetic, epigenetic, and environmental factors. For example, genes can affect each component of energy balance[45] and can explain some of the differences between individuals in body mass and body composition. Although one can conclude that genes are permissive for weight gain, the gradual weight gain of the population does not seem to be primarily due to genetic factors.

The extent to which the body's physiologic regulatory mechanisms serve to maintain a healthy weight depends on the environment. In an environment in which high levels of physical activity are necessary for securing food and shelter and for transportation, and in which food is inconsistently available, the body's physiologic regulatory mechanisms appear to work best and serve to facilitate sufficient food intake to avoid loss of body mass. However, as the environment has gradually changed to one in which high levels of physical activity are not required in daily life and in which food is abundant, inexpensive, and served in large portions, the physiologic regulation of body weight appears to be insufficient to oppose positive energy balance, weight gain, and obesity. In these situations, becoming obese is an adaptation to the environmental conditions and appears to represent a new "settling point."

Obesity researchers are increasingly recognizing the importance of the physical and social environment in facilitating weight gain and obesity. Our current environment is one in which food is often inexpensive, abundant, and served in very large portions.[40] Similarly, we have created a physical activity environment with only a rare need for significant energy expenditure for food, shelter, and transportation.[40] These environmental influences make it easy for us to overeat and underexercise. The body's physiologic system for adjusting energy balance is not sufficiently strong in most people to completely oppose the positive energy balance that results.

Similarly, evidence suggests that obesity is being facilitated by our social environment. Christakis and Fowler demonstrated that social networks influence whether or not a person develops obesity.[46] With both the physical and social environment facilitating weight gain, it is not surprising that more and more people are gaining weight and becoming obese.

The current environment arose as an unintended consequence of societal progress. In fact, the environment was likely shaped in large part because of people's biological preferences for high-energy foods and lack of biological preference to be physically active. The environment we have created is one to which our ancestors

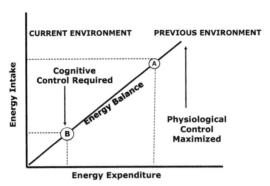

Fig. 7. Both the environment and behavior must be addressed in assessing energy balance.

aspired, and includes a consistent supply of good-tasting, inexpensive, available food and the ability to not have to work hard to secure food, shelter, and transportation.

The realization that the environment is facilitating obesity has increased interest in modifying the environment to help address the obesity epidemic. Although research in this area is only beginning, it represents an exciting new approach to obesity. There are, however, some cautions. First, it is unlikely that modifying the environment alone will solve the obesity problem. The problem is that so many factors that have contributed to obesity also enrich our lives in other ways. For example, we have instant access to information throughout the world through televisions, computers, and personal digital assistants. The fact that these tools contribute to reduced physical activity and thus promote weight gain has only recently been realized. Similarly, the increase in families in which both parents work has increased and contributed to the rise of "fast food restaurants" because few people have the time or energy after work to prepare home-cooked meals. New York City mandated that restaurants place calorie counts on menu items to help people control their intake. However, one study found no change in the number of calories purchased at fast food restaurants before and after menu labeling.[47] It is unlikely that we can ever "go back in time" by giving up these things. It is more likely that we will learn how to modify the environment to support and sustain specific behavioral changes in the population to help people maintain healthy weights.

The need to deal with both the environment and behavior is illustrated in **Fig. 7**. Human biology developed to work best in a different environment—one in which food was inconsistent and high levels of physical activity were required to secure food and shelter and for transportation. In previous environments, physical activity was the "driver" for achieving energy balance, and food intake was "pulled" along.[39] We developed multiple physiologic systems to facilitate eating with no need for physiologic systems for food restriction, and no need to develop a biological preference to be physically active when physical activity was not required. Essentially, our biology tells us to eat whenever food is available and to rest whenever physical activity is not required. In previous environments, this biology was adequate to allow most people to maintain a healthy weight without conscious effort. Body weight regulation was achieved for most with simple physiologic control.

The situation is different in today's environment, which requires very little physical activity. Securing food and shelter and moving around our environment do not require the high levels of physical activity needed in the past.[48] Technology has made it possible to be productive while being largely sedentary. Under such conditions, weight gain can be prevented only with conscious efforts to eat less or to be physically active without the need to be physically active. The minority of Americans who are maintaining a healthy weight are likely exercising cognitive control of eating and physical activity patterns to eat less than they would otherwise and to be physically active without the necessity of doing so. In today's environment, maintaining a healthy body weight cannot be left to physiologic processes but requires cognitive effort. This does not mean that we should not look for ways to modify the environment to make it easy for people to avoid overeating and a sedentary lifestyle. It does mean that we have to focus not exclusively on changing individual behavior or on changing the environment, but on the combination. We must change the environment to facilitate and sustain the behavioral changes required to avoid obesity.

HOW MUCH AND WHAT TYPE OF BEHAVIORAL CHANGE IS REQUIRED?

Hill and colleagues have argued that the obesity epidemic arose from gradual yearly weight gain in the population produced from a slight, consistent degree of positive energy balance (ie, energy intake exceeding energy expenditure).[48] Using longitudinal and cross-sectional data sets, they found that the average US adult has gained an average of 1 to 2 pounds per year for the last 2 to 3 decades. Hill and coworkers[48] concluded that that weight gain in 90% of the adult population is due to a positive energy balance of 100 kcal/day or less. They further suggested that small behavioral changes that impact daily energy balance by as little as 100 kcal/day could help prevent further excessive weight gain in the population.

There is debate in the public health community on whether to focus on changing eating and the food environment or physical activity and the physical activity environment. From an energy balance point of view, it makes no sense to focus on only one side of the equation. While there is a need to modify factors that promote overeating, it may be impossible to manage body weight by food alone in a very sedentary population. In fact, most of the US population may be so physically inactive that it will be virtually impossible for them to eat sufficiently little over the long term to match their low energy expenditure.

DEALING WITH THE COMPLEXITY OF OBESITY

The more that is understood about the etiology of obesity, the more complex it appears. For example, we have learned that the maternal environment may have lasting consequences on body weight regulation and the development of chronic disease in the offspring.[49] Understanding and addressing obesity requires understanding and appreciating our biology, behavior, environment, and culture. Major efforts are underway in the scientific community to focus on each of these areas, but few efforts to integrate among areas. Focusing on only one of these major areas is likely to be incomplete. We need to understand the biology of obesity, but only in rare cases is obesity the result of a biological "defect." Similarly, we need to understand better how to change behavior, but to do this we have to appreciate our biology and the environment in which we live. Figuring out how to change the environment to make a difference in obesity will also require appreciation of biology and behavior. Finally, obesity even involves the ways we have constructed our society, our shared collective worldview, and the material base of this worldview. We need to understand better the complex economic factors that are supporting our current diet and physical activity patterns, and we need to think about how these could be changed to support a healthier lifestyle.[11,50,51] We must begin to examine ways that we can replace those

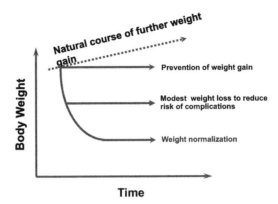

Fig. 8. Strategies to reverse the obesity epidemic. (*Adapted from* Rossner S. Factors determining the long-term outcome of obesity treatment. In: Bjorntorp P, Brodoff BN, editors. Obesity. Philadelphia: J.B. Lippincott; 1992. p. 712–9; with permission.)

aspects of society that support obesity with those that support healthier lifestyles. We need to begin to construct a vision of what our society would look like if it supported maintenance of a healthy body weight and supported obesity prevalence rates that were acceptable.

STRATEGIES FOR GETTING OUT OF THE OBESITY EPIDEMIC

What strategies could we use to reverse the obesity epidemic? **Fig. 8**, adapted from the work of Dr Stephan Rossner,[52] illustrates some possibilities. If we do nothing, the weight of the population will continue to increase until all of those who are not genetically protected will be overweight or obese. How might we reduce obesity prevalence rates to acceptable levels over time?

One possibility is to reduce weight in many of the people who are already overweight or obese. The problem is that our ability to produce and maintain substantial weight loss is not good.[53–55] Most people who lose large amounts of weight regain this weight completely within a few years.[53–55] Rarely does anyone transition permanently from the obese category to the healthy weight category. One meta-analysis showed that obese people were 3.2% below their baseline weight at 5 years, which reflected the maintenance of 23% of their initial weight loss.[56] Another study of NHANES data concluded that only 17% of overweight or obese adults maintained a weight loss of at least 10% for 1 year.[57] Health care professionals now recommend that weight loss goals of 5% to 10% of initial weight can be achieved and maintained in many people.[58] The bottom line is that currently we do not have a good ability to produce and maintain significant weight loss in large numbers of overweight and obese individuals. Although we will certainly improve our obesity treatment strategies over time, we cannot at present rely on this treatment to reverse the obesity epidemic.

It is possible to reverse the obesity epidemic through prevention. This could begin with stopping the gradual weight gain in the adult population and identifying and stopping excessive weight gain in children. It was previously demonstrated that weight gain in most adults can be prevented with small changes in energy balance of 100 kcal/day or less.[39] Preventing further weight gain in the population could have significant positive impacts on health and health care costs of the population because increasing BMI is associated with increasing risk of chronic disease and with increasing health care costs.[59]

Wang and colleagues[60] have estimated that children and adolescents need to shift the energy balance by 150 kcal/day or less to prevent weight gain. This amount is likely significantly less than that required for substantial weight loss.

We and others have found some success with the small changes approach to preventing excessive weight gain. Rodearmel and colleagues demonstrated in two prospective studies that small changes in diet and physical activity could reduce excessive weight gain in overweight and obese children when delivered as part of a family intervention.[61,62] The ASPIRE trial showed that overweight and obese sedentary adults randomized to a 16-week intervention that used small changes in diet and physical activity lost significantly more weight than both the standard didactic group or control group.[63] Although weight loss for the small changes group was small (average of 4.62 kg), it was clinically significant (5% of body weight). Importantly, the small changes group also maintained weight loss, decreased waist circumference, and abdominal fat loss at 3 months after treatment. In addition, a 12-week small changes telephonic intervention was evaluated in sedentary obese veterans.[64] Although not a randomized trial, results were similar to those of the ASPIRE trial in that participants showed significant weight loss.

The cause of preventing and treating childhood obesity was given a boost when the First Lady, Michelle Obama, decided to concentrate on childhood obesity. The White House Task Force on Childhood Obesity was formed, and in May 2010 it released its report, which recommends a multipronged approach to end childhood obesity in one generation. The recommendations include preconceptual and prenatal care, suggestions for early childhood, helping parents and caregivers to make better choices, improving food choices in school cafeterias, increasing access to healthy foods, and increasing physical activity.[65]

By using a strategy of stopping excessive weight gain, the prevalence of obesity would decrease with each successive generation. Although it may take decades to reverse the obesity epidemic using this strategy, the positive view is that we may actually be able to produce and maintain the behavioral changes that would be required to stop excessive weight gain. This can be done through a combination of focusing on specific behavioral change and modifying the environment in ways to support and sustain the desired behavioral changes.

SUMMARY

The obesity epidemic in the United States has proven difficult to reverse. We have not been successful in helping people sustain the eating and physical activity patterns that are needed to maintain a healthy body weight. There is growing recognition that we will not be able to sustain healthy lifestyles until we are able to address the environment and culture that currently support unhealthy lifestyles.

Addressing obesity requires an understanding of energy balance. From an energy balance approach it should be easier to prevent obesity than to reverse it. Further, from an energy balance point of view, it may not be possible to solve the problem by focusing on food alone. Currently, energy requirements of much of the population may be below the level of energy intake than can reasonably be maintained over time.

Many initiatives are underway to revise how we build our communities, the ways we produce and market our foods, and the ways we inadvertently promote sedentary behavior. Efforts are underway to prevent obesity in schools, worksites, and communities. It is probably too early to evaluate these efforts, but there have been no large-scale successes in preventing obesity to date.

There is reason to be optimistic about dealing with obesity. We have successfully addressed many previous threats to public health. It was probably inconceivable in the 1950s to think that major public health initiatives could have such a dramatic effect on reducing the prevalence of smoking in the United States. Yet, this serious problem was addressed via a combination of strategies involving public health, economics, political advocacy, behavioral change, and environmental change. Similarly, Americans have been persuaded to use seat belts and recycle, addressing two other challenges to public health.[66]

But, there is also reason to be pessimistic. Certainly, we can learn from our previous efforts for social change, but we must realize that our challenge with obesity may be greater. In the other examples cited, we had clear goals in mind. Our goals were to stop smoking, increase the use of seatbelts, and increase recycling. The difficulty of achieving these goals should not be minimized, but they were clear and simple goals. In the case of obesity, there is no clear agreement about goals. Moreover, experts do not agree on which strategies should be implemented on a widespread basis to achieve the behavioral changes in the population needed to reverse the high prevalence rates of obesity. We need a successful model that will help us understand what to do to address obesity. A good example is the recent HEALTHY study.[67] This comprehensive intervention was implemented in several schools and aimed to reduce obesity by concentrating on behavior and environment. This intervention delivered most of the strategies we believe to be effective in schools. Although the program produced a reduction in obesity, this reduction was not greater than the reduction seen in the control schools that did not receive the intervention. This does not mean we should not be intervening in schools, but rather that it may require concerted efforts across behavioral settings to reduce obesity.

Although we need successful models, there is a great deal of urgency in responding to the obesity epidemic. An excellent example is the effort to get menu labeling in restaurants, which is moving rapidly toward being national policy. The evaluation of this strategy is still ongoing, and it is not clear what impact it will have on obesity rates. We should be encouraging efforts like this, but we must evaluate them rigorously.

Once we become serious about addressing obesity, it will likely take decades to reverse obesity rates to levels seen 30 years ago. Meanwhile, the prevalence of overweight and obesity remains high and quite likely will continue to increase.

REFERENCES

1. Flegal KM, Carroll MD, Ogden CL, et al. Prevalence and trends in obesity among US adults, 1999–2008. JAMA 2010;303:235–41.
2. Ogden CL, Carroll MD, Curtin LR, et al. Prevalence of high body mass index in US children and adolescents, 2007–2008. JAMA 2010;303:242–9.
3. James WP. WHO recognition of the global obesity epidemic. Int J Obes (Lond) 2008;32(Suppl 7):S120–6.
4. Finucane MM, Stevens GA, Cowan MJ, et al. National, regional, and global trends in body-mass index since 1980: systematic analysis of health examination surveys and epidemiological studies with 960 country-years and 9.1 million participants. Lancet 2011;377:557–67.
5. Expert Panel on the Identification, Evaluation, and Treatment of Overweight in Adults. Clinical guidelines on the identification, evaluation, and treatment of overweight and obesity in adults: executive summary. Am J Clin Nutr 1998;68:899–917.
6. Zhang Q, Wang Y. Trends in the association between obesity and socioeconomic status in U.S. adults: 1971 to 2000. Obes Res 2004;12:1622–32.

7. Molarius A, Seidell JC, Sans S, et al. Educational level, relative body weight, and changes in their association over 10 years: an international perspective from the WHO MONICA Project. Am J Public Health 2000;90:1260–8.
8. Sobal J, Stunkard AJ. Socioeconomic status and obesity: a review of the literature. Psychol Bull 1989;105:260–75.
9. Truong K, Sturm R. Does the obesity epidemic widen sociodemographic health disparities in the US? Santa Monica: Rand Institute; 2004.
10. Drewnowski A, Specter SE. Poverty and obesity: the role of energy density and energy costs. Am J Clin Nutr 2004;79:6–16.
11. Cawley J. An economic framework for understanding physical activity and eating behaviors. Am J Prev Med 2004;27:117–25.
12. Harper S, Lynch J. Trends in socioeconomic inequalities in adult health behaviors among U.S. states, 1990–2004. Public Health Rep 2007;122:177–89.
13. Gordon-Larsen P, Nelson MC, Page P, et al. Inequality in the built environment underlies key health disparities in physical activity and obesity. Pediatrics 2006;117:417–24.
14. Barlow SE, Committee E. Expert committee recommendations regarding the prevention, assessment, and treatment of child and adolescent overweight and obesity: summary report. Pediatrics 2007;120(Suppl 4):S164–92.
15. Allison DB, Saunders SE. Obesity in North America. An overview. Med Clin North Am 2000;84:305–32, v.
16. Geiss LS, James C, Gregg EW, et al. Diabetes risk reduction behaviors among U.S. adults with prediabetes. Am J Prev Med 2010;38:403–9.
17. Terry RB, Wood PD, Haskell WL, et al. Regional adiposity patterns in relation to lipids, lipoprotein cholesterol, and lipoprotein subfraction mass in men. J Clin Endocrinol Metab 1989;68:191–9.
18. Eckel RH, Krauss RM. American Heart Association call to action: obesity as a major risk factor for coronary heart disease. AHA Nutrition Committee. Circulation 1998;97:2099–100.
19. Boeka AG, Lokken KL. Neuropsychological performance of a clinical sample of extremely obese individuals. Arch Clin Neuropsychol 2008;23:467–74.
20. Fergenbaum JH, Bruce S, Lou W, et al. Obesity and lowered cognitive performance in a Canadian First Nations population. Obesity (Silver Spring) 2009;17:1957–63.
21. Gunstad J, Paul RH, Cohen RA, et al. Elevated body mass index is associated with executive dysfunction in otherwise healthy adults. Compr Psychiatry 2007;48:57–61.
22. Gunstad J, Paul RH, Cohen RA, et al. Obesity is associated with memory deficits in young and middle-aged adults. Eat Weight Disord 2006;11:e15–9.
23. Raji CA, Ho AJ, Parikshak NN, et al. Brain structure and obesity. Hum Brain Mapp 2010;31:353–64.
24. Taki Y, Kinomura S, Sato K, et al. Relationship between body mass index and gray matter volume in 1,428 healthy individuals. Obesity (Silver Spring) 2008;16:119–24.
25. Pannacciulli N, Del Parigi A, Chen K, et al. Brain abnormalities in human obesity: a voxel-based morphometric study. Neuroimage 2006;31:1419–25.
26. Stanek KM, Grieve SM, Brickman AM, et al. Obesity is associated with reduced white matter integrity in otherwise healthy adults. Obesity (Silver Spring) 2011;19:500–4.
27. Ho AJ, Raji CA, Becker JT, et al. Obesity is linked with lower brain volume in 700 AD and MCI patients. Neurobiol Aging 2010;31:1326–39.
28. Fitzpatrick AL, Kuller LH, Lopez OL, et al. Midlife and late-life obesity and the risk of dementia: cardiovascular health study. Arch Neurol 2009;66:336–42.

29. Doruk H, Naharci MI, Bozoglu E, et al. The relationship between body mass index and incidental mild cognitive impairment, Alzheimer's disease and vascular dementia in elderly. J Nutr Health Aging 2010;14:834–8.
30. Anstey KJ, Cherbuin N, Budge M, et al. Body mass index in midlife and late-life as a risk factor for dementia: a meta-analysis of prospective studies. Obes Rev 2011;12: e426–37.
31. Gorospe EC, Dave JK. The risk of dementia with increased body mass index. Age Ageing 2007;36:23–9.
32. Matteoni CA, Younossi ZM, Gramlich T, et al. Nonalcoholic fatty liver disease: a spectrum of clinical and pathological severity. Gastroenterology 1999;116:1413–9.
33. Adler M, Schaffner F. Fatty liver hepatitis and cirrhosis in obese patients. Am J Med 1979;67:811–6.
34. Reeves GK, Pirie K, Beral V, et al. Cancer incidence and mortality in relation to body mass index in the Million Women Study: cohort study. BMJ 2007;335:1134.
35. Renehan AG, Tyson M, Egger M, et al. Body-mass index and incidence of cancer: a systematic review and meta-analysis of prospective observational studies. Lancet 2008;371:569–78.
36. Freedman DS, Mei Z, Srinivasan SR, et al. Cardiovascular risk factors and excess adiposity among overweight children and adolescents: the Bogalusa Heart Study. J Pediatr 2007;150:12–7.e2.
37. Fagot-Campagna A, Pettitt DJ, Engelgau MM, et al. Type 2 diabetes among North American children and adolescents: an epidemiologic review and a public health perspective. J Pediatr 2000;136:664–72.
38. Freedman DS, Dietz WH, Srinivasan SR, et al. The relation of overweight to cardio-vascular risk factors among children and adolescents: the Bogalusa Heart Study. Pediatrics 1999;103:1175–82.
39. Peters JC, Wyatt HR, Donahoo WT, et al. From instinct to intellect: the challenge of maintaining healthy weight in the modern world. Obes Rev 2002;3:69–74.
40. Hill JO, Wyatt HR, Melanson EL. Genetic and environmental contributions to obesity. Med Clin North Am 2000;84:333–46.
41. Horton TJ, Drougas H, Brachey A, et al. Fat and carbohydrate overfeeding in humans: different effects on energy storage. Am J Clin Nutr 1995;62:19–29.
42. Blundell JE, Stubbs RJ, Hughes DA, et al. Cross talk between physical activity and appetite control: does physical activity stimulate appetite? Proc Nutr Soc 2003;62: 651–61.
43. Epstein LH, Paluch RA, Consalvi A, et al. Effects of manipulating sedentary behavior on physical activity and food intake. J Pediatr 2002;140:334–9.
44. Prentice AM. Fires of life: the struggles of an ancient metabolism in a modern world. Nutr Bull 2001;26:13–27.
45. Bouchard C, Perusse L, Rice T, et al. Genetics of human obesity. In: Bray G, Bouchard C, editors. Handbook of obesity. New York: Marcel Dekker; 2004. p. 157–200.
46. Christakis NA, Fowler JH. The spread of obesity in a large social network over 32 years. N Engl J Med 2007;357:370–9.
47. Elbel B, Kersh R, Brescoll VL, et al. Calorie labeling and food choices: a first look at the effects on low-income people in New York City. Health Aff (Millwood) 2009;28: w1110–21.
48. Hill JO, Wyatt HR, Reed GW, et al. Obesity and the environment: where do we go from here? Science 2003;299:853–5.
49. Barker DJ, Gluckman PD, Godfrey KM, et al. Fetal nutrition and cardiovascular disease in adult life. Lancet 1993;341:938–41.

50. Sturm R. The economics of physical activity: societal trends and rationales for interventions. Am J Prev Med 2004;27:126–35.
51. Hill JO, Sallis JF, Peters JC. Economic analysis of eating and physical activity: a next step for research and policy change. Am J Prev Med 2004;27:111–6.
52. Rossner S. Factors determining the long-term outcome of obesity treatment. In: Bjorntorp P, Brodoff BN, editors. Obesity. Philadelphia: J.B. Lippincott; 1992. p. 712–9.
53. Wing RR, Hill JO. Successful weight loss maintenance. Annu Rev Nutr 2001;21: 323–41.
54. Brownell KD. Diet, exercise and behavioural intervention: the nonpharmacological approach. Eur J Clin Invest 1998;28(Suppl 2):19–21 [discussion 2].
55. Wadden TA, Foster GD, Letizia KA. One-year behavioral treatment of obesity: comparison of moderate and severe caloric restriction and the effects of weight maintenance therapy. J Consult Clin Psychol 1994;62:165–71.
56. Anderson JW, Konz EC, Frederich RC, et al. Long-term weight-loss maintenance: a meta-analysis of US studies. Am J Clin Nutr 2001;74:579–84.
57. Kraschnewski JL, Boan J, Esposito J, et al. Long-term weight loss maintenance in the United States. Int J Obes (Lond) 2010;34:1644–54.
58. The Surgeon General's call to action to prevent and decrease overweight and obesity. Washington, DC: US Department of Health and Human Services; 2000.
59. Sturm R, Ringel JS, Andreyeva T. Increasing obesity rates and disability trends. Health Aff (Millwood) 2004;23:199–205.
60. Wang YC, Gortmaker SL, Sobol AM, et al. Estimating the energy gap among US children: a counterfactual approach. Pediatrics 2006;118:e1721–33.
61. Rodearmel SJ, Wyatt HR, Barry MJ, et al. A family-based approach to preventing excessive weight gain. Obesity (Silver Spring) 2006;14:1392–401.
62. Rodearmel SJ, Wyatt HR, Stroebele N, et al. Small changes in dietary sugar and physical activity as an approach to preventing excessive weight gain: the America on the Move family study. Pediatrics 2007;120:e869–79.
63. Lutes LD, Winett RA, Barger SD, et al. Small changes in nutrition and physical activity promote weight loss and maintenance: 3-month evidence from the ASPIRE random-ized trial. Ann Behav Med 2008;35:351–7.
64. Damschroder LJ, Lutes LD, Goodrich DE, et al. A small-change approach delivered via telephone promotes weight loss in veterans: results from the ASPIRE-VA pilot study. Patient Educ Couns 2010;79:262–6.
65. White House Task Force on Childhood Obesity Report to the President. Solving the problem of childhood obesity within a generation. May 2010.
66. Economos CD, Brownson RC, DeAngelis MA, et al. What lessons have been learned from other attempts to guide social change? Nutr Rev 2001;59:S40–56 [discussion: S7–65].
67. Foster GD, Linder B, Baranowski T, et al. A school-based intervention for diabetes risk reduction. N Engl J Med 2010;363:443–53.

Regulation of Energy Balance and Body Weight by the Brain: A Distributed System Prone to Disruption

Lucy F. Faulconbridge, PhD[a],*, Matthew R. Hayes, PhD[b]

KEYWORDS

- Energy balance • Cholecystokinin • Glucagon-like-peptide-1
- Leptin • Ghrelin • Reward

Energy balance refers to the physiologic mechanisms that are reciprocally linked to ensure that adequate energy is available for cellular processes required for survival and reproduction. As the term implies, there are two arms of this balance, each equally important in maintaining energy homeostasis: energy intake (ie, food intake) and energy expenditure (eg, physical activity, metabolism, and core body temperature regulation). Any internal or external perturbations to the physiologic mechanisms governing either energy intake or expenditure will almost undoubtedly affect the other arm of the system and result in disruption to the energy balance system as a whole. The coordinated regulation of energy balance is therefore ultimately controlled by the central nervous system (CNS). Given the reciprocal link between energy intake and expenditure, and the fundamental requirement to maintain adequate energy for survival and reproduction, the CNS control of energy balance is one that is multidetermined. Multiple internal signals, neural receptors, and regions of the brain operate with a degree of redundancy to ensure that enough energy exists to sustain life. This article discusses some of the classic internal signals, physiologic mechanisms, the distinct nuclei within the brain, as well as the brain's response to environmental stimuli, that together play an essential role in energy balance regulation.

This work was supported in part by NIH grant K23HL109235 to Lucy F. Faulconbridge and DK085435 to Matthew R. Hayes.

[a] Center for Weight and Eating Disorders, Department of Psychiatry, Perelman School of Medicine, University of Pennsylvania, 3535 Market Street, Philadelphia, PA 19104, USA
[b] Translational Neuroscience Program, Department of Psychiatry, Perelman School of Medicine, University of Pennsylvania, TRL Building, 125 South 31st Street, Philadelphia, PA 19104, USA
* Corresponding author.
E-mail address: lucyhf@mail.med.upenn.edu

Psychiatr Clin N Am 34 (2011) 733–745
doi:10.1016/j.psc.2011.08.008
0193-953X/11/$ – see front matter © 2011 Elsevier Inc. All rights reserved.

CNS CONTROL OF FOOD INTAKE

When discussing how the brain regulates energy intake, we must consider "the meal" as the fundamental unit of energy intake.[1] Thus, physiologic systems exist to negatively or positively influence food intake either during a meal (within-meal) or between a meal, controlling the time between meals and the frequency of meal taking (intermeal interval).[1–4] Once a meal has begun, and the ingested food enters the oral cavity, the brain perceives various components of the meal including the taste and texture of the food, potentially communicating the presence of preferred energy-rich nutrients (eg, fats and sugars) that promote for further feeding.[5–7] As food is swallowed and enters the gastrointestinal (GI) tract, information about the volume of the ingested food through the mechanical distension of the stomach is relayed to the brain. In turn, these gastric-inhibitory signals begin to counteract the positive meal-promoting signals from the oral cavity. In addition, the various chemical and nutritive properties of the food also give rise to the release of a number of gut peptides (hormones) and neurotransmitters from the GI tract that communicate to the brain about the ongoing status of the meal. The majority of these signals are referred to as *satiation signals*, or within-meal intake inhibitory signals.[1] As these satiation signals accumulate, feeding rate slows and eventually *satiety*, or meal termination, is achieved. Satiety then persists from the end of one meal to the start of the next meal.

To date, an extensive number of GI-derived satiation signals have been identified (some are discussed in more detail later), each with a rich literature base unto themselves. A short, noncomprehensive list of some of the classic satiation signals includes: cholecystokinin (CCK), serotonin (5-hydroxytryptamine [5-HT]), peptide-YY (PYY), glutamate, enterostatin, glucagon-like-peptide-1 (GLP-1), and gastric distension. Although specific receptor populations exist within the CNS for many of these GI-derived satiation signals, under normal physiologic conditions, the available circulating levels of these gut peptides and neurotransmitters are not elevated in sufficient quantity to have direct action within the brain.[4,8] Instead, the majority of GI-derived satiation signaling is communicated to the brain via afferent fibers of the vagus nerve (cranial nerve X), which innervates all of the organs within the peritoneal and thoracic cavity.[4,8,9] Thus, the presence of food within the lumen of the GI tract results in the release of the aforementioned gut peptides, which in turn activate specific receptors expressed on the dendritic terminals of vagal afferents that innervate the GI tract. This vagal afferent activation is then relayed to the brainstem, where processing of the inhibitory signals begins. The vagal communication and CNS processing of these signals are discussed in greater detail later.

The physiologic control of meal taking is governed not only by GI-derived vagally mediated satiation signals. The brain also detects a number of circulating hormones and nutrients (eg, glucose, free fatty acids) that communicate the availability of circulating and stored energy. These circulating hormones have been previously termed "long-term energy status signals" or "adiposity signals"[2,10] and include neuropeptides released from the pancreas (eg, insulin, glucagon, amylin), adipose tissue (eg, leptin, adiponectin), as well as the GI tract (eg, ghrelin). Although receptors for many of these signals exist on the vagus nerve, the principal pathway of communication for these long-term energy status signals is one of an endocrine-pathway with direct brain activation. In other words, they circulate in the blood, cross the blood–brain barrier, and act directly on receptors in the brain.

CNS PROCESSING OF GUT-PEPTIDE SATIATION AND ENERGY-STATUS HORMONAL SIGNALS

Historically, much of the field's attention has focused on the role of hypothalamic nuclei in regulating energy balance. Although this hypothalamic-centric work greatly added to our knowledge of the neural control circuitry and intracellular signaling pathways mediating food intake and energy expenditure control,[10–13] it neglected the role of other important brain structures involved in energy balance regulation. Only within the last decade has the field at large started to embrace the perspective that the CNS regulation of energy balance involves a multitude of distributed nuclei that each has a critical role in energy balance regulation.[2,14–19] Reciprocal ascending and descending projections exist between many brain structures to control food intake, as well as energy expenditure. Many of the previously described vagally mediated satiation signals, as well as the circulating energy-status signals, engage processing of the same brain structures, and subsequently influence not only ingestive behavior but also energy expenditure autonomic responses (eg, heart rate, core body temperature, nutrient metabolism and storage).[2,9,16,20]

Among the CNS nuclei controlling energy balance, the more evolutionarily conserved nuclei of the caudal brainstem and hypothalamus are often considered regulatory centers of energy balance from a *homeostatic* (energy need-based) perspective. However, metabolic need (ie, when the body is in a state of negative energy balance) is not the only motivation to consume food. Other factors influencing food intake include the rewarding features of the food, temporal factors (time of day, season), emotion, and cognition (learning, memory, social cues). Collectively, these factors influence the *nonhomeostatic/hedonic* control of food intake and have been discussed in numerous reviews. The hedonic control centers of energy intake are often classified as higher-order nuclei and include, but are not limited to, the hippocampus, amygdala, ventral tegmental area (VTA), nucleus accumbens (NAc), and prefrontal cortex. **Fig. 1** attempts to illustrate (1) the distributed CNS nuclei controlling energy intake and (2) the perspective that circulating energy-status signals, as well as vagally mediated satiation signals, can act either directly or indirectly on both homeostatic nuclei (hypothalamus and nucleus tractus solitarius [NTS] in the brainstem) and hedonic/nonhomeostatic nuclei. Signals considered relevant to homeostatic control of feeding may also affect neural circuitries associated with hedonic feeding, suggesting that the functional descriptors to brain regions as "homeostatic" versus "hedonic" may be too restrictive, as individual brain regions contribute to both homeostatic and nonhomeostatic control functions.[16,21]

SATIATION AND LONG-TERM ENERGY STATUS SIGNALS

The rewarding properties of food, together with the hedonic processes listed previously, and described in more detail later, contribute to the cognitive decision to procure food and initiate feeding. However, it is very clear that the determinants that initiate a meal are not purely appetitive in nature, but also involve internal hunger cues. Although orexigenic (ie, hunger/meal-initiating) hormonal signals do exist (eg, ghrelin) and contribute to overall food intake regulation, the vast majority of evidence suggests that the sensation of hunger occurs in response to (1) the accumulation of these orexigenic signals, (2) the decrease in anorectic satiation signals from the last meal,[1,4] and (3) the decrease in specific energy-status signals (eg, leptin).[2] After digestion, the decrease or absence of nutrient content within the GI tract results in a decrease or cessation of hormonal gut-peptide release from the GI tract. Thus, the satiation gut peptides not only negatively communicate to the brain during a meal,

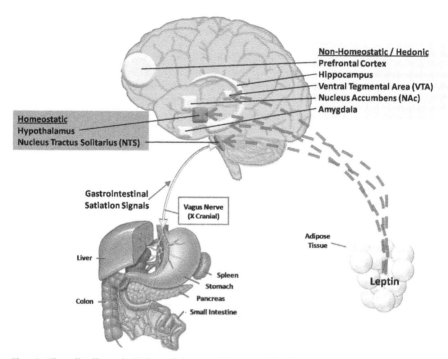

Fig. 1. The distributed CNS nuclei control energy intake. The circulating energy-status signals, as well as vagally mediated satiation signals, can act either directly or indirectly on both homeostatic and hedonic/nonhomeostatic nuclei.

eventually leading to satiety, but the lack of signaling by these hormones can also actually promote meal initiation (as a result of an absence in the vagally mediated inhibitory signal). Among the plethora of GI-derived satiation signals that could be discussed, two hormones have received the most attention over the last four decades for their intake-inhibitory role: CCK and GLP-1. Each is discussed in very brief detail in this article and in much greater detail by others.[3,4,17, 22–24] Likewise, among a wide variety of circulating energy-status signals that contribute to energy balance control, leptin and ghrelin have perhaps been investigated more than others[2,15,25–27] and are also briefly discussed.

CCK

Gibbs and colleagues first reported in 1973 that exogenous administration of CCK produces a dose-dependent decrease in meal size.[28] A number of studies have since revealed that CCK (released from intestinal "I" cells in response to ingestion of nutrients[29,30]) is one of the most biologically potent satiety peptides. Systemic CCK acts via CCK-1 receptors, found densely distributed in the periphery on the vagus nerve and in select regions of the CNS.[31,32] CCK-induced suppression of intake is enhanced when combined with other GI-derived satiation signals, such as serotonin[33–37] or gastric distension.[38,39] Recent evidence also suggests that in addition to the traditional role of CCK as a within-meal inhibitory signal, CCK may interact with specific long-term energy status signals, such as insulin or leptin,[2,18,40–42] demonstrating a role for CCK not only in the control of meal size, but also in long-term body weight regulation and overall energy homeostasis.

GLP-1

GLP-1 is a neuropeptide that is endogenously released, principally from two distinct sources within the body: (1) "L" cells in the GI tract after ingestion of food[43-45] and (2) neurons of the nucleus NTS in the caudal brainstem that project to GLP-1 receptors (GLP-1R), both locally and throughout the brain.[46-48] Exogenous stimulation of either peripheral or central GLP-1Rs results in reduced food intake,[49-53] inhibition of gastric emptying,[49,54] and increased glucose-stimulated insulin secretion.[55-57] Within the periphery, GLP-1 activates GLP-1R on vagal afferent neurons in the small intestine, portal vein, liver, and upper GI tract. GLP-1 afferent signals are processed by CNS neurons that then drive neuroendocrine, behavioral, and physiologic responses that result in improved glycemic control and reduced feeding. One such neuroendocrine response to vagal afferent activation by GLP-1 is the subsequent vagal efferent neural transmission to the pancreatic β-cell, resulting in insulin secretion.[22,58,59]

The effects of GLP-1 in inhibiting food intake and regulating blood glucose/insulin levels have led to two separate emerging pharmacologic approaches in an effort to take advantage of the peripheral GLP-1 system to treat type 2 diabetes mellitus (T2DM) and potentially obesity: (1) development of long-lasting GLP-1R analogues (eg, exendin-4 [Byetta], liraglutide [Victoza]), and (2) dipeptidyl peptidase IV (DPP-IV, an enzyme that degrades GLP-1) inhibitors (eg, sitagliptin [Januvia]), which elevate endogenous GLP-1 levels. Both of these clinical strategies are FDA-approved for the treatment of T2DM for improving blood glucose regulation. Preliminary evidence also suggests that long-acting GLP-1R agonists (liraglutide and exendin-4) may also produce weight loss as a consequence of reduced food intake.[60-63]

Leptin

Discovery of the adipose tissue–derived hormone leptin[64] has transformed our understanding of the function of white adipose tissue from one of a simple energy storage depot to the view that adipose tissue is an active endocrine organ. Thus, the greater the stores of energy in the adipose tissue (ie, the greater the fat mass of an individual), the larger the available circulating levels of leptin. We now appreciate that leptin acting on its receptors (LepRb, or ObRb) in the brain contributes significantly to the control of feeding and energy expenditure.[2,10,15,18,25] Under normal physiologic conditions in a lean human or animal, both the total amount of adiposity, and fluctuation in adiposity levels, is minimal. Under these conditions slight variations in circulating leptin levels, communicating energy storage within the adipose tissue, are sensed by the brain, and appropriate CNS signaling pathways are engaged to either increase or decrease food intake and energy expenditure to normalize energy need. Unfortunately, however, in the case of energy surplus (ie, obesity), leptin levels are chronically elevated, and the brain fails to correctly perceive and respond to the overaccumulation of the leptin signal. Such a response is known as "leptin resistance,"[25,65] discussed in more detail later.

Ghrelin

Ghrelin is a peptide hormone released in the stomach and small intestines,[66,67] and is the only known peripheral peptide to increase food intake. (All other peripheral feeding–related signals act to terminate meals.) Ghrelin binds to the growth hormone secretatogue receptor (GHS-R) located in both homeostatic regions (such as the hypothalamus and caudal brainstem[68,69]) and hedonic brain regions (such as the VTA[70]). Exogenous ghrelin administration to rodents or humans results in potent increases in hunger, food intake, and body weight.[71,72] Studies in rodents suggest that ghrelin augments food intake by increasing primarily the frequency of meals, with smaller effects on meal size.[73] The notion of ghrelin as a physiologic hunger signal is supported by the dramatic increase in plasma ghrelin levels observed before meals, and their rapid decline following food consumption.[71,74] Work to develop ghrelin antagonists and mimetics to interfere with the perception of hunger by the elevation in this hormone is underway as a potential therapeutic tool for obesity, although this work has been largely unsuccessful thus far.

A MODERN ENVIRONMENT DISRUPTS BIOLOGY

The neural control of energy balance is tightly regulated, utilizing an array of internal signals to defend body weight, such that small perturbations in the energy status of the body are detected rapidly and remedied. Yet despite such tight regulation, the system is vulnerable to disruption by environmental manipulations. The areas of the brain controlling the regulation of food intake evolved at a time when food sources were scarce and large amounts of physical activity were required to obtain enough calories for survival. The resulting "thrifty genotype,"[75] which allowed for easy storage of fat, conferred an obvious advantage on the survival of humans and their young. Now, however, this genotype operates in a modern world that is exposed to a "toxic environment,"[76] characterized by the increased availability of cheap, energy-dense foods and a decreased need for physical activity. As such, the neurochemical signals that have evolved to initiate or terminate feeding are no match for the ever-present array of highly palatable, calorie-rich foods that are readily available in the environment. As Egger and Swinburn suggest, obesity is "a normal response to an abnormal environment".[77(p477)]

Leptin and Insulin Resistance

Under conditions in which the body is challenged by a constant oversupply of nutrients, the normal functioning of the physiologic mechanisms maintaining energy balance is disrupted. A state of chronic nutrient excess (caused by overconsumption of calorie-dense foods) leads eventually to a blunting of signaling in the insulin and leptin pathways, a concept referred to as "resistance." As described earlier, under normal conditions, elevated leptin levels act centrally to decrease feeding and prevent obesity. Likewise, insulin, in the nonobese state, acts on peripheral cells (eg, skeletal muscle) to enhance utilization of blood glucose. Under conditions of excess (ie, obesity), even though large amounts of leptin and insulin circulate in the blood, there are disruptions in the receptor and intracellular signaling responses for these hormones. In short, the oversaturation of the hormone at the receptor decreases the receptor response to the hormone, such that leptin fails to suppress food intake and increase energy expenditure. Thus, weight gain continues, further exacerbating the obesity phenotype. Likewise, insulin signaling is blunted in the obese state, such that cells do not effectively utilize the excessive circulating levels of glucose. A vicious cycle develops, such that a person already consuming too many calories now has less sensitivity to the normal neurochemical signals that should be leading to meal termination. Over time this resistance to leptin and insulin signaling further predisposes the individual toward T2DM and obesity.

Our Love of Highly Palatable Foods

Our understanding of humans' preference for highly palatable foods (those typically high in fat and sugar), even in the absence of hunger, has improved over the last decade. It is now clear that two complementary neural systems regulate food intake: homeostatic and hedonic circuits.[78,79] As discussed previously, homeostatic circuits refer to pathways that alter the motivation to eat based on the energy status of the body. Key homeostatic brain areas that integrate neural and peripheral signals are the hypothalamus and caudal brainstem.[5,80–82] In contrast, hedonic neural circuits control the rewarding properties of food. Neural areas implicated include the mesolimbic dopamine system (including the striatum and VTA), the orbitofrontal cortex (OFC), and the amygdala.[83–87] These circuits, which also mediate the rewarding response to drugs of abuse, make highly palatable foods attractive even in the absence of caloric/nutritional deficiency.[79,88]

Substances that are hedonically pleasing, such as food, sex, and drugs of abuse, stimulate dopamine release from neurons in the VTA that project to the NAc (also known as the ventral striatum).[6,89,90] This increased release of dopamine may help to coordinate an organism's attempts to obtain food through increased arousal, psychomotor activation, and increased memory for food-related stimuli.[91] The mechanism by which food intake increases dopamine signaling is not yet clear, although there are bidirectional neuronal projections between the VTA/NAc and several of the hypothalamic nuclei involved in homeostatic regulation.[92–94] Thus, although hedonic and homeostatic pathways frequently work in synergy to control food intake, the hedonic circuit may override homeostatic pathways in the fed state by increasing the desire to ingest foods that are highly palatable.[95]

NEURAL MEDIATION OF FOOD IN THE HUMAN BRAIN

Several recent imaging studies in humans have examined activity in homeostatic and hedonic areas of the brain to understand better why some people do not stop eating, even when satiated. The studies examine neural activation in response to participants merely seeing pictures of food (ie, food cues), or to actually ingesting various food items.

Response to Food Cues

Typically, these investigations have used either positron emission tomography (PET) or functional magnetic resonance imaging (fMRI) to compare responses to nonfood versus food images, or responses to high- vs. low-calorie (or palatability) food images.[96,97] In lean individuals, food cues (and high-calorie food cues in particular) consistently evoke activation in hedonic pathways, including the VTA, NAc, and OFC cortex.[98,99] Interestingly, obese individuals appear to show a greater response to food cues in these areas compared to their lean counterparts.[100,101] These findings present the possibility that obese individuals anticipate greater hedonic reward from eating, and that appetitive food cues may stimulate greater appetitive drive in heavier individuals.

Response to Feeding

Several studies have investigated the neural response to glucose ingestion[102–104] or to calorie-dense preferred foods such as chocolate,[99] and found correlations between regional cerebral blood flow and satiety. Gautier and colleagues investigated differences in neural activation in response to a mixed nutrient meal between lean and obese men[105] and women[106] using PET and the tracer ^{15}O-labeled water. Increases in regional cerebral blood flow were found in the prefrontal and occipital cortex (hedonic areas); decreases were observed in the insular cortex, limbic and paralimbic regions, and the hypothalamus. This pattern is consistent with previous findings.[107]

Gautier and colleagues hypothesized that the hypothalamus, insula, and limbic/paralimbic regions make up a central orexigenic network (including both homeostatic and hedonic components). This network receives inhibitory projections from the prefrontal cortex that dampen orexigenic activity upon consumption of food. Obese subjects showed greater activation of the prefrontal cortex than lean controls, which may be necessary if the orexigenic network needing inhibition is overactive in these individuals. Obese participants also showed an attenuated deactivation of the hypothalamus, thalamus, and cingulate cortex. These findings suggest that orexigenic areas in heavier individuals may not be inhibited to the same extent as in lean individuals after meal ingestion, thus suggesting an impaired satiation response in the obese state.

Collectively, there is accumulating evidence that eating and food choices are controlled by a complex network of neural circuits that are put to the test by the modern environment. We are just beginning to understand why humans may continue to eat energy-dense foods even after they are fully satiated. The decision to continue consuming obesogenic foods in the absence of hunger is likely to be a result of complex integration of neural signals comprising pleasurable feelings of reward, learning, and impaired satiety.

SUMMARY

Maintaining adequate energy supply via regulation of food intake and energy expenditure is crucial for survival and reproduction. The neural control of energy balance is highly complex, occurs across distributed central and peripheral areas, and incorporates multiple domains of control (including homeostatic and hedonic processes). The sheer number of active compounds (such as leptin and GLP-1) involved in the regulation of food intake speaks to the redundancy and complexity of the system. The balance between energy intake and expenditure is under CNS control. Constant bidirectional communication between the brain and the GI tract, as well as between the brain and other relevant tissues (ie, adipose tissue, pancreas, and liver), ensures that the brain constantly perceives and responds accordingly to the energy status/needs of the body. This elegant biological system is subject to disruption by a toxic obesogenic environment, leading to syndromes such as leptin and insulin resistance, and ultimately further exposing obese individuals to further weight gain and T2DM. Recent imaging studies in humans are beginning to examine the influence that higher-order/hedonic brain regions have on homeostatic areas, as well as their responsiveness to homeostatic peripheral signals. With greater understanding of these mechanisms, the field moves closer to understanding and eventually treating the causalities of obesity.

REFERENCES

1. Smith GP. The direct and indirect controls of meal size. Neurosci Biobehav Rev 1996;20:41–6.
2. Grill HJ. Leptin and the systems neuroscience of meal size control. Front Neuroendocrinol 2010;31:61–78.
3. Moran TH. Gut peptide signaling in the controls of food intake. Obesity 2006; 14(Suppl 5):250S–3S.
4. Ritter RC. Gastrointestinal mechanisms of satiation for food. Physiol Behav 2004; 81:249–73.
5. Grill HJ, Kaplan JM. The neuroanatomical axis for control of energy balance. Front Neuroendocrinol 2002;23:2–40.

6. Hajnal A, Smith GP, Norgren R. Oral sucrose stimulation increases accumbens dopamine in the rat. Am J Physiol Regul Integr Comp Physiol 2004;286:R31–7.
7. Nasse J, Terman D, Venugopal S, et al. Local circuit input to the medullary reticular formation from the rostral nucleus of the solitary tract. Am J Physiol Regul Integr Comp Physiol 2008;295:R1391–408.
8. Raybould HE. Gut chemosensing: interactions between gut endocrine cells and visceral afferents. Auton Neurosci 2010;153:41–6.
9. Grill HJ, Hayes MR. The nucleus tractus solitarius: a portal for visceral afferent signal processing, energy status assessment and integration of their combined effects on food intake. Int J Obes 2009;33(Suppl 1):S11–5.
10. Schwartz MW, Woods SC, Porte D Jr, et al. Central nervous system control of food intake. Nature 2000;404:661–71.
11. Morton GJ, Schwartz MW. Leptin and the central nervous system control of glucose metabolism. Physiol Rev 2011;91:389–411.
12. Stefater MA, Seeley RJ. Central nervous system nutrient signaling: the regulation of energy balance and the future of dietary therapies. Annu Rev Nutr 2010;30:219–35.
13. Elmquist JK, Coppari R, Balthasar N, et al. Identifying hypothalamic pathways controlling food intake, body weight, and glucose homeostasis. J Comp Neurol 2005;493:63–71.
14. Grill HJ. Distributed neural control of energy balance: contributions from hindbrain and hypothalamus. Obesity 2006;14(Suppl 5):216S–21S.
15. Myers MG Jr, Munzberg H, Leinninger GM, et al. The geometry of leptin action in the brain: more complicated than a simple ARC. Cell Metab 2009;9:117–23.
16. Narayanan NS, Guarnieri DJ, DiLeone RJ. Metabolic hormones, dopamine circuits, and feeding. Front Neuroendocrinol 2010;31:104–12.
17. Hayes MR, De Jonghe BC, Kanoski SE. Role of the glucagon-like-peptide-1 receptor in the control of energy balance. Physiol Behav 2010;100:503–10.
18. Hayes MR, Skibicka KP, Leichner TM, et al. Endogenous leptin signaling in the caudal nucleus tractus solitarius and area postrema is required for energy balance regulation. Cell Metab 2010;11:77–83.
19. Watts AG. Neuropeptides and the integration of motor responses to dehydration. Annu Rev Neurosci 2001;24:357–84.
20. Bartness TJ, Vaughan CH, Song CK. Sympathetic and sensory innervation of brown adipose tissue. Int J Obes 2010;34(Suppl 1):S36–42.
21. Grill HJ, Skibicka KP, Hayes MR. Imaging obesity: fMRI, food reward, and feeding. Cell Metab 2007;6:423–5.
22. Holst JJ. The physiology of glucagon-like peptide 1. Physiol Rev 2007;87:1409–39.
23. Ritter RC, Covasa M, Matson CA. Cholecystokinin: proofs and prospects for involvement in control of food intake and body weight. Neuropeptides 1999;33:387–99.
24. Raybould HE. Mechanisms of CCK signaling from gut to brain. Curr Opin Pharmacol 2007;7:570–4.
25. Myers MG, Cowley MA, Munzberg H. Mechanisms of leptin action and leptin resistance. Annu Rev Physiol 2008;70:537–56.
26. Dieguez C, da Boit K, Novelle MG, et al. New insights in ghrelin orexigenic effect. Front Horm Res 2010;38:196–205.
27. Castaneda TR, Tong J, Datta R, et al. Ghrelin in the regulation of body weight and metabolism. Front Neuroendocrinol 2010;31:44–60.
28. Gibbs J, Young RC, Smith GP. Cholecystokinin decreases food intake in rats. J Comp Physiol Psychol 1973;84:488–95.

29. Brenner L, Yox DP, Ritter RC. Suppression of sham feeding by intraintestinal nutrients is not correlated with plasma cholecystokinin elevation. Am J Physiol 1993;264:R972–6.

30. Liddle RA, Green GM, Conrad CK, et al. Proteins but not amino acids, carbohydrates, or fats stimulate cholecystokinin secretion in the rat. Am J Physiol 1986;251: G243–8.

31. Moran TH, Norgren R, Crosby RJ, et al. Central and peripheral vagal transport of cholecystokinin binding sites occurs in afferent fibers. Brain Res 1990;526:95–102.

32. Moran TH, Baldessarini AR, Salorio CF, et al. Vagal afferent and efferent contributions to the inhibition of food intake by cholecystokinin. Am J Physiol 1997;272: R1245–51.

33. Helm KA, Rada P, Hoebel BG. Cholecystokinin combined with serotonin in the hypothalamus limits accumbens dopamine release while increasing acetylcholine: a possible satiation mechanism. Brain Res 2003;963:290–7.

34. Esfahani N, Bednar I, Qureshi GA, et al. Inhibition of serotonin synthesis attenuates inhibition of ingestive behavior by CCK-8. Pharmacol Biochem Behav 1995;51:9–12.

35. Hayes MR, Moore RL, Shah SM, et al. 5-HT3 receptors participate in CCK-induced suppression of food intake by delaying gastric emptying. Am J Physiol 2004; 287:R817–83.

36. Hayes MR, Savastano DM, Covasa M. Cholecystokinin-induced satiety is mediated through interdependent cooperation of CCK-A and 5-HT3 receptors. Physiol Behav 2004;82:663–9.

37. Hayes MR, Covasa M. CCK and 5-HT act synergistically to suppress food intake through simultaneous activation of CCK-1 and 5-HT3 receptors. Peptides 2005;26: 2322–30.

38. Kissileff HR, Carretta JC, Geliebter A, et al. Cholecystokinin and stomach distension combine to reduce food intake in humans. Am J Physiol Regul Integr Comp Physiol 2003;285:R992–8.

39. Schwartz GJ, Netterville LA, McHugh PR, et al. Gastric loads potentiate inhibition of food intake produced by a cholecystokinin analogue. Am J Physiol 1991;261: R1141–6.

40. Emond M, Schwartz GJ, Ladenheim EE, et al. Central leptin modulates behavioral and neural responsivity to CCK. Am J Physiol 1999;276:R1545–9.

41. Matson CA, Ritter RC. Long-term CCK-leptin synergy suggests a role for CCK in the regulation of body weight. Am J Physiol Regul Integr Comp Physiol 1999;276: R1038–45.

42. Riedy CA, Chavez M, Figlewicz DP, et al. Central insulin enhances sensitivity to cholecystokinin. Physiol Behav 1995;58:755–60.

43. Creutzfeldt W. The entero-insular axis in type 2 diabetes—incretins as therapeutic agents. Exp Clin Endocrinol Diabetes 2001;109(Suppl 2):S288–303.

44. Mojsov S, Kopczynski MG, Habener JF. Both amidated and nonamidated forms of glucagon-like peptide I are synthesized in the rat intestine and the pancreas. J Biol Chem 1990;265:8001–8.

45. Kokrashvili Z, Mosinger B, Margolskee RF. Taste signaling elements expressed in gut enteroendocrine cells regulate nutrient-responsive secretion of gut hormones. Am J Clin Nutr 2009;90:822S–5S.

46. Larsen PJ, Tang-Christensen M, Holst JJ, et al. Distribution of glucagon-like peptide-1 and other preproglucagon-derived peptides in the rat hypothalamus and brainstem. Neuroscience 1997;77:257–70.

47. Goke R, Larsen PJ, Mikkelsen JD, et al. Distribution of GLP-1 binding sites in the rat brain: evidence that exendin-4 is a ligand of brain GLP-1 binding sites. Eur J Neurosci 1995;7:2294–300.
48. Merchenthaler I, Lane M, Shughrue P. Distribution of pre-pro-glucagon and glucagon-like peptide-1 receptor messenger RNAs in the rat central nervous system. J Comp Neurol 1999;403:261–80.
49. Hayes MR, Skibicka KP, Grill HJ. Caudal brainstem processing is sufficient for behavioral, sympathetic and parasympathetic responses driven by peripheral and hindbrain glucagon-like-peptide-1 receptor stimulation. Endocrinology 2008;149: 4059–68.
50. Kinzig KP, D'Alessio DA, Seeley RJ. The diverse roles of specific GLP-1 receptors in the control of food intake and the response to visceral illness. J Neurosci 2002;22: 10470–6.
51. Schick RR, Zimmermann JP, vorm Walde T, et al. Peptides that regulate food intake: glucagon-like peptide 1-(7–36) amide acts at lateral and medial hypothalamic sites to suppress feeding in rats. Am J Physiol Regul Integr Comp Physiol 2003;284:R1427–35.
52. Abbott CR, Monteiro M, Small CJ, et al. The inhibitory effects of peripheral administration of peptide YY(3–36) and glucagon-like peptide-1 on food intake are attenuated by ablation of the vagal-brainstem-hypothalamic pathway. Brain Res 2005; 1044:127–31.
53. Chelikani PK, Haver AC, Reidelberger RD. Intravenous infusion of glucagon-like peptide-1 potently inhibits food intake, sham feeding, and gastric emptying in rats. Am J Physiol Regul Integr Comp Physiol 2005;288:R1695–706.
54. Imeryuz N, Yegen BC, Bozkurt A. Glucagon-like peptide-1 inhibits gastric emptying via vagal afferent-mediated central mechanisms. Am J Physiol 1997;273:G920–7.
55. Sandoval DA, Bagnol D, Woods SC, et al. Arcuate GLP-1 receptors regulate glucose homeostasis but not food intake. Diabetes 2008;57:2046–54.
56. Knauf C, Cani PD, Perrin C, et al. Brain glucagon-like peptide-1 increases insulin secretion and muscle insulin resistance to favor hepatic glycogen storage. J Clin Invest 2005;115:3554–63.
57. Komatsu R, Matsuyama T, Namba M, et al. Glucagonostatic and insulinotropic action of glucagonlike peptide I-(7–36)-amide. Diabetes 1989;38:902–5.
58. Nakabayashi H, Nishizawa M, Nakagawa A, et al. Vagal hepatopancreatic reflex effect evoked by intraportal appearance of tGLP-1. Am J Physiol 1996;271: E808–13.
59. Balkan B, Li X. Portal GLP-1 administration in rats augments the insulin response to glucose via neuronal mechanisms. Am J Physiol Regul Integr Comp Physiol 2000; 279:R1449–54.
60. Blonde L, Klein EJ, Han J, et al. Interim analysis of the effects of exenatide treatment on A1C, weight and cardiovascular risk factors over 82 weeks in 314 overweight patients with type 2 diabetes. Diabetes Obes Metab 2006;8:436–47.
61. Montanya E, Sesti G. A review of efficacy and safety data regarding the use of liraglutide, a once-daily human glucagon-like peptide 1 analogue, in the treatment of type 2 diabetes mellitus. Clin Ther 2009;31:2472–88.
62. Buse JB, Rosenstock J, Sesti G, et al. Liraglutide once a day versus exenatide twice a day for type 2 diabetes: a 26-week randomised, parallel-group, multinational, open-label trial (LEAD-6). Lancet 2009;374:39–47.
63. Hayes MR, Kanoski SE, Alhadeff AL, et al. Comparative effects of the long-acting GLP-1 receptor ligands, liraglutide and exendin-4, on food intake and body weight suppression in rats. Obesity 2011;19(7):1342–9.

64. Zhang Y, Proenca R, Maffei M, et al. Positional cloning of the mouse obese gene and its human homologue. Nature 1994;372:425–32.
65. Banks WA. Blood-brain barrier as a regulatory interface. Forum Nutr 2010;63: 102–10.
66. Date Y, Kojima M, Hosoda H, et al. Ghrelin, a novel growth hormone-releasing acylated peptide, is synthesized in a distinct endocrine cell type in the gastrointestinal tracts of rats and humans. Endocrinology 2000;141:4255–61.
67. Kojima M, Hosoda H, Date Y, et al. Ghrelin is a growth-hormone-releasing acylated peptide from stomach. Nature 1999;402:656–60.
68. Guan XM, Yu H, Palyha OC, et al. Distribution of mRNA encoding the growth hormone secretagogue receptor in brain and peripheral tissues. Brain Res Mol Brain Res 1997;48:23–9.
69. Lin Y, Matsumura K, Fukuhara M, et al. Ghrelin acts at the nucleus of the solitary tract to decrease arterial pressure in rats. Hypertension 2004;43:977–82.
70. Jerlhag E, Egecioglu E, Dickson SL, et al. Ghrelin administration into tegmental areas stimulates locomotor activity and increases extracellular concentration of dopamine in the nucleus accumbens. Addict Biol 2007;12:6–16.
71. Tschop M, Smiley DL, Heiman ML. Ghrelin induces adiposity in rodents. Nature 2000;407:908–13.
72. Wren AM, Seal LJ, Cohen MA, et al. Ghrelin enhances appetite and increases food intake in humans. J Clin Endocrinol Metab 2001;86:5992.
73. Faulconbridge LF, Cummings DE, Kaplan JM, et al. Hyperphagic effects of brainstem ghrelin administration. Diabetes 2003;52:2260–5.
74. Cummings DE, Purnell JQ, Frayo RS, et al. A preprandial rise in plasma ghrelin levels suggests a role in meal initiation in humans. Diabetes 2001;50:1714–9.
75. Neel JV. Diabetes mellitus: a "thrifty" genotype rendered detrimental by "progress"? Am J Hum Genet 1962;14:353–62.
76. Brownell KD. Get slim with higher taxes. New York Times. Dec 15, 1994; A 29.
77. Egger G, Swinburn B. An "ecological" approach to the obesity pandemic. BMJ 1997;315:477–80.
78. Kringelbach ML. Food for thought: hedonic experience beyond homeostasis in the human brain. Neuroscience 2004;126:807–19.
79. Saper CB, Chou TC, Elmquist JK. The need to feed: homeostatic and hedonic control of eating. Neuron 2002;36:199–211.
80. Berthoud HR. Mind versus metabolism in the control of food intake and energy balance. Physiol Behav 2004;81:781–93.
81. Lenard NR, Berthoud HR. Central and peripheral regulation of food intake and physical activity: pathways and genes. Obesity 2008;16(Suppl 3):S11–22.
82. Woods SC, D'Alessio DA. Central control of body weight and appetite. J Clin Endocrinol Metab 2008;93:S37–50.
83. Killgore WD, Young AD, Femia LA, et al. Cortical and limbic activation during viewing of high- versus low-calorie foods. Neuroimage 2003;19:1381–94.
84. O'Doherty JP, Deichmann R, Critchley HD, et al. Neural responses during anticipation of a primary taste reward. Neuron 2002;33:815–26.
85. Rolls ET. The brain and emotion. New York: Oxford University Press; 1990.
86. Rolls ET. The orbitofrontal cortex and reward. Cereb Cortex 2000;10:284–94.
87. Small DM, Jones-Gotman M, Dagher A. Feeding-induced dopamine release in dorsal striatum correlates with meal pleasantness ratings in healthy human volunteers. Neuroimage 2003;19:1709–15.

88. Batterham RL, ffytche DH, Rosenthal JM, et al. PYY modulation of cortical and hypothalamic brain areas predicts feeding behaviour in humans. Nature 2007;450: 106–9.

89. Berridge KC, Robinson TE. What is the role of dopamine in reward: hedonic impact, reward learning, or incentive salience? Brain Res Brain Res Rev 1998;28:309–69.

90. Nestler EJ. Molecular basis of long-term plasticity underlying addiction. Nat Rev Neurosci 2001;2:119–28.

91. Grigson PS, Twining RC. Cocaine-induced suppression of saccharin intake: a model of drug-induced devaluation of natural rewards. Behav Neurosci 2002;116:321–33.

92. Del-Fava F, Hasue RH, Ferreira JG, Shammah-Lagnado SJ. Efferent connections of the rostral linear nucleus of the ventral tegmental area in the rat. Neuroscience 2007;145:1059–76.

93. Kelley AE. Memory and addiction: shared neural circuitry and molecular mechanisms. Neuron 2004;44:161–79.

94. Usuda I, Tanaka K, Chiba T. Efferent projections of the nucleus accumbens in the rat with special reference to subdivision of the nucleus: biotinylated dextran amine study. Brain Res 1998;797:73–93.

95. Lutter M, Nestler EJ. Homeostatic and hedonic signals interact in the regulation of food intake. J Nutr 2009;139:629–32.

96. Holsen LM, Zarcone JR, Thompson TI, et al. Neural mechanisms underlying food motivation in children and adolescents. NeuroImage 2005;27:669–76.

97. LaBar KS, Gitelman DR, Parrish TB, et al. Hunger selectively modulates corticolimbic activation to food stimuli in humans. Behav Neurosci 2001;115:493–500.

98. Porubska K, Veit R, Preissl H, et al. Subjective feeling of appetite modulates brain activity: an fMRI study. NeuroImage 2006;32:1273–80.

99. Small DM, Zatorre RJ, Dagher A, et al. Changes in brain activity related to eating chocolate: from pleasure to aversion. Brain 2001;124:1720–33.

100. Rosenbaum M, Sy M, Pavlovich K, et al. Leptin reverses weight loss-induced changes in regional neural activity responses to visual food stimuli. J Clin Invest 2008;118:2583–91.

101. Stoeckel LE, Weller RE, Cook EW 3rd, et al. Widespread reward-system activation in obese women in response to pictures of high-calorie foods. NeuroImage 2008; 41:636–47.

102. Matsuda M, Liu Y, Mahankali S, et al. Altered hypothalamic function in response to glucose ingestion in obese humans. Diabetes 1999;48:1801–6.

103. Liu Y, Gao JH, Liu HL, et al. The temporal response of the brain after eating revealed by functional MRI. Nature 2000;405:1058–62.

104. Smeets PA, de Graaf C, Stafleu A, et al. Functional MRI of human hypothalamic responses following glucose ingestion. NeuroImage 2005;24:363–8.

105. Gautier JF, Chen K, Salbe AD, et al. Differential brain responses to satiation in obese and lean men. Diabetes 2000;49:838–46.

106. Gautier JF, Del Parigi A, Chen K, et al. Effect of satiation on brain activity in obese and lean women. Obes Res 2001;9:676–84.

107. Tataranni PA, Gautier JF, Chen K, et al. Neuroanatomical correlates of hunger and satiation in humans using positron emission tomography. Proc Natl Acad Sci USA 1999;96:4569–74.

Obesity, Psychiatric Status, and Psychiatric Medications

Robert I. Berkowitz, MD[a], Anthony N. Fabricatore, PhD[b,c,*]

KEYWORDS

• Obesity • Depression • Psychiatric • Antipsychotic

Obesity is a multidetermined disease with genetic, environmental, and behavioral influences. Hyperphagia and limited physical activity contribute to positive energy balance and, thus, are the most direct behavioral determinants of body weight. These factors, however, are also symptoms of various psychological disorders and can be used as means of coping with psychological distress. In addition, the chronic stress that can be associated with excess adiposity—attributable to stigma, medical comorbidities, quality of life impairments, or other factors—may also predispose obese persons to psychopathology.

The relationship between obesity and psychiatric disorder has long been the subject of both theoretical writings and empirical investigations. The past decade, however, has seen a proliferation of large, methodologically rigorous studies on this topic. This article summarizes the epidemiologic and clinical literature relevant to the intersection of obesity and psychopathology. The early part of the article focuses on four primary areas. The first is the cross-sectional relationship between obesity and psychiatric disorders in community populations. This includes an examination of clinical or demographic variables that might moderate that relationship. The second is the temporal relationship between obesity and psychopathology. We examine evidence that obesity is a risk factor for depression, and that depression is a risk factor for obesity. Third is the presence of psychopathology in obese persons seeking clinical weight loss interventions. Fourth is the question of how weight loss affects, and is affected by, intentional weight loss in obese individuals. The latter portion of the

Dr Fabricatore is an employee of Nutrisystem, Inc. and has received research support from Merck & Co., Inc.
[a] Children's Hospital of Philadelphia, and Center for Weight and Eating Disorders, Department of Psychiatry, Perelman School of Medicine at the University of Pennsylvania, 3535 Market Street, Suite 3029, Philadelphia, PA 19104, USA
[b] Center for Weight and Eating Disorders, University of Pennsylvania School of Medicine, 3535 Market Street, Suite 3108, Philadelphia, PA 19104-3309, USA
[c] Research and Development, Nutrisystem, Inc., 600 Office Center Drive, Fort Washington, PA 19034, USA
* Corresponding author. Center for Weight and Eating Disorders, 3535 Market Street, Suite 3108, Philadelphia, PA 19104-3309.
E-mail address: fabricat@mail.med.upenn.edu

Psychiatr Clin N Am 34 (2011) 747–764
doi:10.1016/j.psc.2011.08.007
0193-953X/11/$ – see front matter © 2011 Elsevier Inc. All rights reserved.

article is dedicated to attending to weight when treating persons with psychiatric disorders.

THE CROSS-SECTIONAL RELATIONSHIP BETWEEN OBESITY AND PSYCHOPATHOLOGY
Depression

The majority of studies that have examined comorbidity between obesity and psychiatric disorders have focused on depression. There has been sufficient research on this topic, in fact, to a support a meta-analysis. De Wit and colleagues identified 17 epidemiologic studies (n = 204,507) of the general adult population that examined the cross-sectional relationship between obesity and depression.[1] Depression was assessed using diagnostic interviews (6 studies) or symptom checklists (11 studies), and obesity was calculated using objective (3 studies) or self-reported (14 studies) measurements. The 17 studies yielded 28 comparisons of obese versus nonobese individuals that were included in the meta-analysis. Significant positive associations between obesity and depression were found in 14 comparisons, negative associations in 2 comparisons, and no significant relationships in the remaining 12. The pooled odds ratio (OR) of 1.18 (95% confidence interval [CI]: 1.01–1.37) indicated that, overall, the odds of being depressed were 18% higher in obese versus nonobese persons.

The researchers then conducted subgroup analyses to determine whether the relationship between obesity and depression was different based on participant or study characteristics.[1] Participant age, study publication date, and methods of assessing obesity (objective vs self-report) and depression (symptom checklist vs diagnostic interview) did not significantly influence the relationship between obesity and depression across studies. Participant gender, however, was a significant moderator. Whereas obese men (11 comparisons) had the same risk of depression as nonobese men (OR = 1.00, 95% CI: 0.76–1.31), obese women (11 comparisons) had a 32% increased risk of depression compared with their nonobese counterparts (OR = 1.32, 95% CI: 1.23–1.40).

The moderating effect of gender clearly shows that the relationship between obesity and psychiatric status can vary between obese subpopulations. The severity of obesity is another variable that has repeatedly been shown to influence the strength of the relationship. For example, Onyike and colleagues found that neither class I (body mass index [BMI] 30–34.9) nor class II (BMI 35–39.9) obesity was significantly related to past-month, past-year, or lifetime depression, but that class III (BMI ≥40, extreme obesity) was associated with significantly greater odds of depression in each time frame (past-month OR = 4.98, 95% CI: 2.07–11.99; past-year OR = 2.92, 95% CI: 1.28–6.67; lifetime OR = 2.60, 95% CI: 1.38–4.91).[2] A similar pattern of results (albeit less pronounced) was reported by Petry and colleagues, who found that the odds of depression were approximately 50% greater among all obese individuals versus nonobese individuals (OR = 1.53, 95% CI: 1.41–1.67), but more than 100% greater among those with extreme obesity (OR = 2.02, 95% CI: 1.74–2.35).[3]

Other Psychiatric Disorders

The use of diagnostic psychiatric interviews in large epidemiologic studies has benefitted not only the quality of the research on obesity and psychopathology, but also the breadth of the investigations. A growing body of evidence (**Tables 1 and 2**) suggests that obese persons are more likely to have an anxiety disorder or bipolar disorder than nonobese individuals.[3–7] As with depression, the relationships are more consistent and are stronger in obese women versus men, and for extremely obese persons, as compared with obese persons in general.

Table 1
ORs of lifetime and current psychiatric disorders in obese persons (both sexes), obese women, and obese men, compared with average weight individuals, found in large epidemiologic studies

Disorder or Category	Simon et al[4]			Mather et al[5]			Barry et al[6]	
	Obese	Obese Men	Obese Women	Obese	Obese Men	Obese Women	Obese Men	Obese Women
Lifetime								
Any mood disorder	1.27 (1.15–1.41)	1.21 (.99–1.46)	1.29 (1.11–1.50)	1.29 (1.12–1.49)	1.17 (.91–1.50)	1.38 (1.16–1.64)	1.39 (1.21–1.60)	1.79 (1.63–1.28)
Major depressive disorder	1.21 (1.09–1.35)			1.41 (1.22–1.64)	1.38 (1.05–1.81)	1.43 (1.21–1.68)	1.35 (1.14–1.59)	1.58 (1.43–1.75)
Bipolar disorder/mania	1.47[a] (1.12–1.93)			1.53 (1.17–2.00)	1.39 (0.88–2.18)	1.67 (1.23–2.28)	1.20 (0.93–1.55)	2.24 (1.80–2.78)
Any anxiety disorder	1.28 (1.05–1.57)	1.17 (0.82–1.67)	1.34 (1.09–1.64)	1.22 (1.10–1.36)	1.25 (1.06–1.46)	1.20 (1.05–1.38)	1.35 (1.18–1.53)	1.76 (1.58–1.96)
Any substance use disorder	0.78 (.65–.93)	0.75 (.60–.93)	0.88 (.65–1.18)					
Alcohol use disorder								
Drug use disorder								
Past year								
Any mood disorder	1.19 (1.00–1.42)			1.20 (0.98–1.46)	1.05 (0.73–1.52)	1.30 (1.04–1.63)	1.33 (1.20–1.59)	1.75 (1.52–2.01)

(continued on next page)

Table 1
(continued)

Disorder or Category	Simon et al[4]	Mather et al[5]			Barry et al[6]	
	Obese	Obese	Obese Men	Obese Women	Obese Men	Obese Women
Major depressive disorder	1.09 (0.89–1.34)	1.24 (1.02–1.52)	1.21 (0.82–1.80)	1.27 (1.02–1.58)	1.31 (1.03–1.67)	1.49 (1.25–1.76)
Bipolar disorder/mania	1.61[a] (1.07–2.43)	1.91 (1.33–2.73)	1.45 (0.82–2.56)	2.44 (1.52–3.91)	1.15 (0.80–1.64)	2.41 (1.84–3.17)
Any anxiety disorder	1.34 (1.07–1.66)	1.29 (1.11–1.48)	1.45 (1.14–1.84)	1.19 (1.00–1.42)	1.36 (1.16–1.61)	1.79 (1.58–1.96)
Any substance use disorder	0.65 (0.40–1.06)	0.88 (0.66–1.16)	0.87 (0.62–1.24)	0.88 (0.55–1.41)		
Alcohol use disorder	1.05[b] (0.80–1.39)					
Drug use disorder	0.53[b] (.31–.89)					

[a] Includes bipolar I and bipolar II.
[b] Includes substance dependence only.

Data from Simon GE, von Korff M, Saunders K, et al. Association between obesity and psychiatric disorders in the US adult population. Arch Gen Psychiatry 2006;63:824–30; Mather AA, Cox BJ, Enns MW, et al. Associations of obesity with psychiatric disorders and suicidal behaviors in a nationally representative sample. J Psychosom Res 2009;66:277–85; and Barry D, Pietrzak RH, Petry NM. Gender differences in associations between body mass index and DSM-IV mood and anxiety disorders: results from the National Epidemiologic Survey on Alcohol and Related Conditions. Ann Epidemiol 2008;18:458–66.

Table 2
ORs of lifetime and current psychiatric disorders in obese and extremely obese individuals, compared with average weight persons, found in large epidemiologic studies

Disorder or Category	Petry et al[3]		Scott et al[7]	
	Obese	Extremely Obese	Obese	Class II–III Obese
Lifetime				
Any mood disorder	1.56 (1.44–1.69)	2.00 (1.74–2.31)		
Major depressive disorder	1.53 (1.41–1.67)	2.02 (1.74–2.35)		
Bipolar disorder/mania	1.55 (1.29–1.86)	2.70 (2.00–3.66)		
Any anxiety disorder	1.54 (1.41–1.68)	1.97 (1.67–2.31)		
Any substance use disorder				
Alcohol use disorder	1.21 (1.11–1.33)	1.33 (1.12–1.58)		
Drug use disorder	1.06 (0.94–1.19)	1.41 (1.07–1.85)		
Past year				
Any mood disorder	1.52 (1.35–1.70)	1.91 (1.58–2.31)	1.1 (1.0–1.3)	1.4 (1.2–1.6)
Major depressive disorder	1.45 (1.28–1.63)	1.95 (1.57–2.42)		
Bipolar disorder/mania	1.63 (1.24–2.14)	2.58 (1.74–3.81)		
Any anxiety disorder	1.56 (1.40–1.73)	2.08 (1.73–2.50)	1.2 (1.1–1.3)	1.5 (1.3–1.7)
Any substance use disorder				
Alcohol use disorder	0.87 (0.75–1.01)	0.88 (0.64–1.20)	0.9 (0.7–1.1)	
Drug use disorder	0.82 (0.64–1.05)	1.01 (0.61–1.69)		

Data from Petry NM, Barry D, Pietrzak RH, et al. Overweight and obesity are associated with psychiatric disorders: results from the National Epidemiologic Survey on Alcohol and Related Conditions. Psychosom Med 2008;70:288–97; and Scott KM, McGee MA, Wells JE, et al. Obesity and mental disorders in the adult general population. J Psychosom Res 2008;64:97–105.

Among patients with bipolar disorder, those who are obese have more frequent manic and depressive episodes and are more likely to attempt suicide than those at normal weight.[8,9] Bond and colleagues found a potential neurobiologic mechanism for the greater vulnerability to bipolar disorder in obese persons—reduced brain volumes.[10] Using magnetic resonance imaging, these researchers found that higher BMI was associated with decreased total brain and gray matter volume in healthy subjects. In those with bipolar disorder, however, BMI was associated with decreased white matter and temporal lobe volume, which had been previously found to be vulnerabilities for bipolar disorder.

Obese persons tend to have a lower risk of substance use problems than those of average weight, although the difference in risk is not consistently significant (see **Tables 1 and 2**).[3–7] One study, however, found that obese and extremely obese persons were more likely to have a lifetime history of an alcohol use disorder than those of average weight.[3] In an investigation of nearly 40,000 US adults, the risk of obesity was found to be 49% and 26% higher among women and men, respectively, with a family history of alcoholism or alcohol problems than in their counterparts without this family history.[11] These elevations in risk became somewhat attenuated, yet remained significant (OR = 1.30, 95% CI: 1.19–1.43 in women; OR = 1.11, 95% CI: 1.01–1.23 in men) after adjustment for race, age, education, income, personal alcohol use, smoking status, and major depression. These findings suggest the possibility of a shared vulnerability toward obesity and substance use, a possibility also suggested by functional neuroimaging studies that have found that food-related stimuli produce similar brain responses in obese individuals as do drug-related stimuli in persons with substance use disorders.[12]

Binge Eating Disorder: A Special Case?

Repeatedly consuming excessively large amounts of food, accompanied by subjective loss of control and subsequent distress, are the key features of binge eating disorder (BED).[13] Several studies have shown that BED commonly co-occurs with other psychopathology—including depressive, anxiety, substance use, and personality disorders—in both clinical and community samples.[14] The findings of a large epidemiologic study are illustrative. Using persons who were of normal weight and free of BED as the reference group, Grucza and coworkers[15] examined the risk of several psychiatric disorders among those who: (1) were obese and free of BED and (2) had BED, at any weight. Those with BED, regardless of weight status, had significantly elevated odds of major depression (OR = 5.4, 95% CI: 2.3–12.9), generalized anxiety disorder (OR = 5.3, 95% CI: 2.3–12.7), panic attacks (OR = 4.9, 95% CI: 2.3–10.4), and suicide attempts (OR = 3.7, 95% CI: 1.6–8.5). By contrast, obese persons who did not have BED were not at increased risk of any of these disorders.

THE TEMPORAL RELATIONSHIP BETWEEN OBESITY AND DEPRESSION

Prospective examinations of the relationship between obesity and depression have been conducted in a variety of age groups, in several settings, and over a range of follow-up periods. There has been sufficient research in this area—much of it published in the past 10 years—to support two systematic reviews,[16,17] including one meta-analysis.[16] Both of these investigations summarized the research on obesity as a risk factor for incident depression, as well as on depression as a risk factor for incident obesity. As shown in **Tables 3 and 4**, the included studies overlapped a great deal between the two reviews. The broad conclusion to be drawn from these analyses is that there is evidence to support both potential temporal pathways.

Obesity to Depression

Luppino and colleagues' meta-analysis[16] found that the OR of developing depression among those with obesity at baseline was 1.55 (95% CI: 1.22–1.98) when unadjusted analyses were pooled and 1.57 (95% CI: 1.23–2.01) when adjusted analyses were pooled. Subgroup analyses found no differences in the ORs for pooled analyses of women (OR = 1.67, 95% CI: 1.11–2.51) versus men (OR = 1.31, 95% CI: 1.13–1.51; P = .81 for difference), but that effects were stronger when conducted in the United States (OR = 2.12, 95% CI: 1.48–3.03) versus Europe (OR = 1.33, 95% CI: 0.98–1.81, P = .05 for difference) and when the presence of depressive disorder was the outcome (OR = 2.15, 95% CI: 1.48–3.12), rather than depressive symptoms (OR = 1.36, 95% CI: 1.03–1.80, P = .05 for difference). Mean age at baseline (<20, 20–59, ≥60 years old), follow-up duration (<10, ≥10 years), and study quality (high, low) did not significantly moderate the obesity-to-depression temporal relationship.

Findings from a large observational study published too late to be included in the reviews by Luppino and colleagues[16] and Faith and colleagues[17] stand in contrast to those reviews' findings. Gariepy and colleagues reported on a nationally representative sample of 10,545 Canadian adults who were assessed seven times over 12

Table 3
Summary of studies included in two systematic reviews assessing the temporal relationship from obesity to depression

Study	Luppino et al[16]	Faith et al[17]	OR (95% CI)	Population	Follow-up (years)
Herva et al[18]	X	X	1.63 (1.16–2.29)	Adolescents—Europe	17
Anderson et al[19]	X	X	2.00 (1.00–4.01)	Adolescents—US	20
Goodman & Whitaker[20]		X	1.16 (0.81–1.65)	Adolescents—US	1
Ball et al [21]		X	1.33 (1.08–1.65)	Young Women—Australia	3
Bjerkeset et al [22]	X	X	1.66 (1.23–2.24)	Adults—Europe	11
Koponen et al[23]	X		0.77 (0.38–1.56)	Adults—Europe	7
Van Gool et al[24]	X		1.01 (0.63–1.63)	Adults—Europe	6
Kasen et al[25]	X		3.96 (1.23–12.75)	Adults—US	28
Roberts et al[26]		X	1.43 (0.85–2.43)	Adults—US	1
Roberts et al[27]		X	1.77 (1.03–3.05)	Adults—US	5
Roberts et al[28]	X	X	2.01 (1.25–3.24)	Older adults—US	5
Sachs-Ericsson et al[29]	X	X	1.76 (0.47–6.57)	Older adults—US	3

Only studies in which obesity was defined categorically as BMI $\geq$30 kg/m^2 are included here.
Note: X indicates study was included in the systematic review.
Data from Luppino FS, de Wit LM, Bouvy PF, et al. Overweight, obesity, and depression: A systematic review and meta-analysis of longitudinal studies. Arch Gen Psychiatry 2010;67:220–9; and Faith MS, Butryn M, Wadden TA, et al. Evidence for prospective associations among depression and obesity in population-based studies. Obesity Rev 2011;12:e438–53.

years.[39] Baseline obesity was measured using self-reported height and weight, and past-year major depression was assessed using a structured clinical interview. The unadjusted hazard ratio (HR) for past-year depression in obese women was 1.03 (95% CI: 0.78–1.36). Adjusting for potential confounds did not alter the ratio. In obese men, the unadjusted HR was 0.70 (95% CI: 0.49–0.99), which remained stable after adjustment (0.71, 95% CI: 0.51–0.98). Thus, in this sample, obesity was found to be unrelated to the development of depression in women, and protective against the development of obesity in men. Whether inclusion of this study in the aforementioned systematic reviews and meta-analysis cited[16,17] would have altered their conclusions is not clear. It seems clear, however, that more research on obesity as a risk factor for the onset of depression is needed.

Depression to Obesity

In Luppino and colleagues' investigation, the pooled depression-to-obesity relationship was significant in both unadjusted (OR = 1.58, 95% CI: 1.33–1.87) and adjusted (OR = 1.40, 95% CI: 1.15–1.71) analyses.[16] Although the relationship was significant in women (OR = 2.01, 95% CI: 1.11–3.65) but not in men (OR = 1.43, 95% CI: 0.96–2.13), sex was not a statistically significant modifier of the depression-to-obesity relationship (P = .50 for difference). In fact, none of the potential moderators tested (sex, age, follow-up, method of assessing depression, study quality, or study location) significantly altered the relationship.

Table 4
Summary of studies included in two systematic reviews assessing the temporal relationship from depression to obesity

Study	Luppino et al[16]	Faith et al[17]	OR (95% CI)	Population	Follow-up (years)
Goodwin et al[30]	X		1.4 (0.9–2.3)	Children (girls)—Finland	15
Pine 2001 et al[31]	X	X	1.93 (0.73–5.10)	Children—US	15
Barefoot et al[32]	X	X	1.58 (1.06–2.36)	Adolescents—US	22
Franko et al[33]	X		3.11 (1.13–5.12)	Adolescent girls—US	5
Goodman & Whitaker[20]	X		2.39 (1.05–5.45)	Adolescents—US	1
Hasler et al[34]	X	X	2.73 (1.16–6.44)	Adolescents—Europe	20
Pine et al[35]		X	1.75 (1.23–2.49)	Adolescents—US	10
Richardson et al [36]	X	X	1.77 (1.13–2.78)	Adolescents—NZ	7
Stice et al[37]	X		2.32 (0.62–8.65)	Adolescent girls—US	4
Koponen et al [23]		X	1.47 (0.80–2.71)	Adults—Europe	7
Van Gool et al[24]		X	1.17 (0.75–1.83)	Adults—Europe	6
Roberts et al[28]	X	X	1.32 (0.65–2.69)	Older adults—US	5
Vogelzangs et al[38]	X	X	1.45 (0.83–2.53)	Older adults—US	5

Only studies in which obesity was defined categorically as BMI $\geq$30 kg/m^2 are included here.
Note: X indicates study was included in the systematic review.
Data from Luppino FS, de Wit LM, Bouvy PF, et al. Overweight, obesity, and depression: a systematic review and meta-analysis of longitudinal studies. Arch Gen Psychiatry 2010;67:220–9; and Faith MS, Butryn M, Wadden TA, et al. Evidence for prospective associations among depression and obesity in population-based studies. Obesity Rev 2011;12:e438–53.

PSYCHOPATHOLOGY IN CLINICAL SAMPLES OF OBESE INDIVIDUALS

Studies investigating the prevalence of psychopathology among obese persons seeking weight loss therapy have yielded a pattern of results similar to those found in epidemiologic studies, albeit with a greater magnitude of effect. A case-control study of 293 obese treatment seekers, compared with matched controls from the general population, found ORs of 3.5 (95% CI: 2.5–4.9) for Axis I mental disorders and 4.3 (95% CI: 2.7–6.9) for Axis II disorders.[40] More specifically (and consistent with epidemiologic studies) the prevalence of mood disorders (31.4% vs 12.3%), anxiety disorders (30.0% vs 12.3%), and eating disorders (15.7% vs 1.0%) was significantly higher in treatment seekers versus controls. There were no differences, however, in the prevalence of psychotic (1.0 % vs 0.3%), substance use (2.1% vs 0.7%), or other disorders (1.7% vs 0.6%).

As in the general population, BED appears to be a marker for comorbid psychopathology in clinical samples, as well. Grilo and colleagues found that the lifetime and current prevalence of at least one Axis I disorder was 74% and 43%, respectively, in a sample of 404 patients with BED.[41] Mood disorders were the most common (54%

lifetime, 26% current), followed by anxiety disorders (37% lifetime, 25% current). However, this study lacked a control group of obese treatment seekers without BED for comparisons.

Psychopathology also appears to be more common in obese treatment seekers with higher BMIs than in their less obese counterparts. Wadden and coworkers compared 146 extremely obese women who sought weight loss with bariatric surgery to 90 mildly to moderately obese women seeking weight reduction with lifestyle modification.[42] In addition to scoring significantly higher on the Beck Depression Inventory-II[43] (13.2 vs 8.1), women with extreme obesity were more likely than less obese women to report a history of clinically significant psychological problems (45.9% vs 29.2%), physical abuse (24.3% vs 6.6%), and sexual abuse (19.9% vs 8.9%).[42]

The presence (and significance) of psychopathology in extremely obese persons seeking bariatric surgery has been the focus of considerable research in the past decade. Like studies assessing psychiatric disorder in the general population, the methodology in investigations of bariatric surgery candidates has become more rigorous. In particular, these studies have included consecutive series of patients, used structured clinical interviews to assess psychopathology, and conducted the interviews independently of the process of selecting appropriate candidates for bariatric surgery. The last of these methodological improvements is made necessary by the tendency of some candidates to minimize psychiatric distress to gain "clearance" for bariatric surgery.[44]

Table 5 summarizes the results of two such studies of bariatric surgery candidates. Kalarchian and colleagues[45] reported on 288 bariatric surgery candidates who were evaluated using structured interviews for Axis I and Axis II disorders, independently of the preoperative screening process. These researchers found that 66% of candidates had at least one lifetime Axis I disorder, and 38% met criteria at the time of the evaluation. In a similar study, Mauri and coworkers[46] found that a smaller percentage of patients (21%) had at least one current Axis I disorder, albeit in a less obese sample (mean BMI = 43.5 kg/m^2, compared with 52.2 kg/m^2 in the study of Kalarchian and colleagues). In both studies, the most common current Axis I conditions were BED and major depressive disorder, and the most common diagnoses on Axis II were avoidant and obsessive–compulsive personality disorders. Although these findings suggest high rates of psychopathology in bariatric surgery candidates, the lack of a control group precludes comparisons with nonobese, less obese, or non–treatment-seeking individuals.

PSYCHOPATHOLOGY AND THE OUTCOMES OF CLINICAL WEIGHT LOSS INTERVENTIONS

Given the known relationship between obesity and psychiatric disorder, two primary questions emerge, relative to treating obesity: (1) how does weight loss affect psychological status and (2) how does psychological status affect weight loss?

Effect of Intentional Weight Loss on Psychopathology

In a classic study, Keys found that normal-weight males who intentionally lost 25% of their body weight experienced a variety of severe psychiatric symptoms (including hallucinations).[47] In addition, Stunkard reported a constellation of distressing emotional symptoms in obese women who participated in weight loss therapy, which he dubbed the "dieting depression."[48] These reports, coupled with more recent findings regarding psychiatric side effects of cannabinoid receptor inverse agonists, are

Table 5
Percentage of bariatric surgery candidates meeting criteria for psychiatric disorders: results of two investigations that employed diagnostic interviews

Disorder or Category	Kalarchian et al[45]		Mauri et al[46]	
	Lifetime	Current	Lifetime	Current
Any Axis I disorder	66.3	37.8	37.6	20.9
Any mood disorder	45.5	15.6	22.0	6.4
Major depressive disorder	42.0	10.4	19.1	4.6
Bipolar disorder (I or II)	3.5	1.7	2.2	1.1
Dysthymic disorder	—	3.8	1.1	1.1
Any anxiety disorder	37.5	24.0	18.1	12.4
Panic disorder	19.4	5.9	8.5	4.6
Agoraphobia	3.5	1.0	2.1	
Social phobia	9.4	9.0	3.2	2.8
Specific phobia	8.0	7.3	5.3	5.0
Obsessive–compulsive disorder	3.8	2.1	2.8	2.1
Posttraumatic stress disorder	11.8	2.8	1.8	1.1
Generalized anxiety disorder	—	6.3	1.1	1.1
Any substance use disorder	32.6	1.7	1.1	
Any eating disorder	29.5	16.3	12.8	7.1
Bulimia nervosa	3.5	0.3	1.8	0.4
Binge eating disorder	27.1	16.0	11.0	6.7
Any Axis II disorder	66.3	37.8	37.6	20.9
Paranoid personality disorder		5.6		0.7
Schizoid personality disorder		2.1		—
Schizotypal personality disorder		0.4		—
Antisocial personality disorder		2.8		—
Borderline personality disorder		4.9		1.8
Histrionic personality disorder		0		—
Narcissistic personality disorder		0.7		0.4
Avoidant personality disorder		17.0		6.8
Dependent personality disorder		1.7		0.4
Obsessive–compulsive personality disorder		7.6		13.9

Data from Kalarchian MA, Marcus MD, Levine MD, et al. Psychiatric disorders among bariatric surgery candidates: relationship to obesity and functional health status. Am J Psychiatry 2007;164:328–34; and Mauri M, Rucci P, Calderone A, et al. Axis I and II disorders and quality of life in bariatric surgery candidates. J Clin Psychiatry 2008;69:295–301.

among the sources of concern that weight loss may induce or exacerbate psychopathology.[49]

A recent meta-analysis, however, found that a variety of weight loss interventions had largely positive effects on symptoms of depression. Fabricatore and colleagues[50] included 31 randomized controlled trials (n = 7937) and categorized treatments as lifestyle modification, non-dieting, dietary counseling, diet-alone, exercise-alone, pharmacotherapy, placebo, or control interventions. Between-groups effect sizes (standardized mean differences [SMD]) were computed for common treatment comparisons. Lifestyle modification (ie, a combination of diet, exercise, and behavior therapy) was found to yield significantly more favorable changes in depressive symptoms than control interventions (SMD = 0.28, 95% CI: 0.17–0.40) and non-dieting interventions (SMD = 0.31, 95% CI: 0.08–0.54), and marginally more favorable changes than dietary counseling (SMD = 0.40, 95% CI: –0.01 to 0.81) and exercise alone (SMD = 0.31, 95% CI: –0.01 to 0.62). Exercise alone, in turn, produced more favorable changes than control interventions (SMD = 0.54, 95% CI: 0.04–1.04). Meta-analysis of within-group effects found that treatment with lifestyle modification, non-dieting, diet-alone, exercise-alone, and orlistat/siburamine all produced significant reductions in symptoms of depression. Interestingly, a meta-regression found no relationship between change in weight and change in depressive symptoms among groups treated with lifestyle modification, suggesting that other aspects of treatment (eg, social support) have a beneficial effect on mood.

The meta-analysis described in the preceding text addressed group-level changes in symptomatology but did not capture changes in depression at the level of the individual. It is possible that some individuals would experience a significant exacerbation of symptoms or would develop a diagnosable depressive disorder during the course of treatment. Faulconbridge and colleagues[51] examined this possibility by measuring depressive symptoms at baseline and six additional times during the course of a year of treatment with lifestyle modification, sibutramine, or their combination. Despite a significant mean reduction in depressive symptoms across treatment groups, 14% of participants experienced a potentially discernible increase in symptoms of depression (ie, ≥5 points on the BDI-II), and 3.6% reported incident suicidal ideation at some point during the 1-year treatment.

Patients who undergo bariatric surgery typically achieve larger weight losses than those produced by behavioral and pharmacological treatments.[52–54] In addition, these patients have been found to achieve, on average, significant reductions in symptoms of depression, anxiety, and BED, and significant improvements in quality of life.[55] As with nonsurgical treatments, the psychological outcomes of bariatric surgery, however, are not uniformly positive. A prospective study of bariatric surgery patients evaluated with structured clinical interviews preoperatively and 6–12 and 24–36 months postoperatively found that the incidence of depressive disorders was 11% at 6–12 months and 4% at 24–36 months.[56] Incident anxiety disorders occurred in 7% and 9% of patients at 6–12 and 24–36 months, respectively. A comparison of bariatric surgery patients with similarly obese controls who did not undergo weight loss surgery found a significant reduction in disease related mortality (HR = 0.60, 95% CI: 0.45–0.67), but elevated risk of non–disease-related mortality (HR = 1.58, 95% CI: 1.02–2.45), including accidents and suicide.[57] These results suggest that bariatric surgery candidates should be screened for psychopathology and, if psychiatric disorders are found, treated accordingly. Although weight loss improves mood for some, it is not an evidence-based intervention for depression or any other psychiatric disorder.

Effect of Psychiatric Disorder on the Outcomes of Weight Loss Interventions

Most clinical weight loss trials exclude persons with significant psychopathology at baseline. Thus, the effects of psychiatric disorders on intentional weight loss are not fully understood. The existing literature is mixed, with some studies showing a deleterious effect of depression or BED on weight loss, some showing no effect, and some showing more favorable outcomes among those with baseline psychopathology.[55,58,59] Whether in surgical or nonsurgical interventions, however, and whether or not a statistically significant effect of psychopathology is found, the results do not appear to justify the exclusion of persons with psychopathology from treatment based on the rationale that they will fail treatment. Reliable psychosocial predictors of treatment failure, to our knowledge, have yet to be identified.

OBESITY AND PSYCHIATRIC MEDICATIONS

More information from pharmaceutical companies and independent investigators now exists about the risk of weight gain and, consequently, of metabolic and lipid changes with psychotropic medications. Several of these drugs are now known to be associated with weight gain. These include the atypical antipsychotic medications, antidepressant medications (selective serotonin reuptake inhibitors [SSRIs], tricyclic antidepressants, and mirtazapine), and mood stabilizers (including lithium and some anticonvulsants).[60] A brief review of the side effects of antipsychotic medications follows because this class of medications presents the greatest concerns.

Antipsychotic Medications

The antipsychotic medications used in the treatment of schizophrenia, bipolar disorder, and related conditions are associated with clinically significant weight gain. A 2004 consensus statement alerted health care professionals to assess patients receiving atypical antipsychotic medications for rapid weight gain and for metabolic effects, including the development of diabetes and dyslipidemia.[61] The consensus statement, published simultaneously in the February 2004 issues of *Diabetes Care* and *Journal of Clinical Psychiatry*, was written by a panel representing the American Association of Clinical Endocrinologists, the American Diabetes Association, the American Psychiatric Association, and the North American Association for the Study of Obesity (now known at The Obesity Society).

The consensus statement reported that antipsychotic medications have been an important therapy for psychotic conditions and other serious psychiatric disorders. The first-generation antipsychotics (FGAs) treated the positive symptoms of psychosis (ie, hallucinations and delusions) but were less effective in managing the negative symptoms of psychotic disorders such as withdrawal, apathy, and affective disorder. The FGAs were more likely to be associated with movement disorders, including dystonic reactions, akathisia, drug-induced parkinsonism, and the potentially irreversible serious side effect of tardive dyskinesia.

The atypical antipsychotic medications, also referred to as second-generation antipsychotics (SGA), were developed with the aims of improving efficacy and minimizing adverse effects.[61] The SGAs indeed are associated with fewer extrapyramidal and other movement disorders. In addition to treating the positive symptoms of psychosis, SGAs are significantly more helpful in treating the negative symptoms. The consensus statement reported that, except for clozapine, SGAs have become widely used as the primary treatment modality for psychotic disorders and other severe psychiatric syndromes. In addition to clozapine, these medications include risperidone, olanzapine, ziprasidone, quetiapine, and aripiprazole. Several SGAs, however, have been associated with weight gain and metabolic abnormalities.

Allison and colleagues[62] reported in a meta-analysis that FGAs and SGAs cause varying degrees of weight gain within the first 10 weeks of treatment. Placebo treatment resulted in a mean weight reduction of 0.74 kg. Of the FGAs, a 3.19 kg weight gain was reported with thioridazine. Among the SGAs, mean increases were

4.45 kg for clozapine, 4.15 kg for olanzapine, 2.92 kg for sertindole, 2.10 kg for risperidone, and 0.04 kg for ziprasidone. Few data were available to evaluate quetiapine at 10 weeks,[62] and aripiprazole was not available.

According to the consensus statement, the precise neurobiology concerning how the SGAs are associated with weight gain is not understood, although both hunger and satiety may be affected by these medications. Investigators hypothesized that the SGAs most likely work by affecting receptor sites for dopamine, serotonin, norepinephrine, and histamine-H1, which also are related to mechanisms involved in weight regulation. It may be that the mechanisms involved in the therapeutic value of these medications also are involved directly in the development of increased food intake and excess weight gain.

In the years after the publication of the consensus panel, only modest increases in screening for metabolic changes were observed in patients using SGAs. The consensus statements' authors recommended greater efforts to screen for diabetes and lipid disorders in patients receiving these medications.[63]

In a comprehensive study of the treatment of schizophrenia, Lieberman and colleagues[64] found that olanzapine was the most effective medication, in terms of less discontinuation, compared with risperidone, quetiapine, ziprasidone, and perphenazine. Olanzapine, however, was associated with the greatest weight gain and worsening of levels of glucose and lipids.

However, a note of caution is required. The risks of developing obesity and other complications (such as diabetes and dyslipidemia) must be considered along with the patient's psychiatric diagnosis and response to treatment with a specific medication. For example, it is not clear whether a patient who is treated successfully for a severe psychiatric condition, taking one antipsychotic, will have as favorable of a response when switched to another medication. Clozapine, for example, may be associated with improved therapeutic gains for patients with treatment-resistant schizophrenia or suicidal risk. At the same time, it may be associated with a higher risk of weight gain and metabolic abnormalities. Clinicians must weigh the risks of not controlling psychiatric symptoms adequately against those of precipitating weight gain and metabolic complications.

Type 2 Diabetes Mellitus and Dyslipidemia

The consensus report found that there was evidence[64–68] for increased risk for diabetes with clozapine and olanzapine. Henderson and colleagues[69] evaluated patients taking clozapine for 5 years and reported that 36.6% had a diagnosis of type 2 diabetes mellitus. Increased insulin resistance, secondary to weight gain, has been suggested as one possible mechanism for this association with antipsychotic medication usage.

Lipids disorders also are associated with the weight gain resulting from the SGAs. Greater increases in low-density lipoprotein (LDL) cholesterol and triglycerides as well as greater reductions in high-density lipoprotein (HDL) have been observed with greater weight gain, particularly in patients treated with clozapine and olanzapine. Aripiprazole and ziprasidone appear to be associated with minimal weight gain and dyslipidemia.

Monitoring

The consensus panel advised that physicians monitor health status at baseline and during treatment in patients who take antipsychotic medications. Panel members suggested that history of obesity, diabetes, dyslipidemia, hypertension, and cardiovascular disease (including family history) be obtained, and height, weight, and waist circumference measured. In addition, they suggested that blood pressure, fasting glucose, and a lipid profile be obtained before treatment. When obesity, hypertension, metabolic disorders, or dyslipidemia are diagnosed, therapy should be initiated, including referral to the appropriate health care professionals.

Although it may be clinically challenging when the patient is acutely psychiatrically ill, both nutritional and physical activity counseling should be initiated when psychiatric treatment is begun, to limit potential weight gain with SGAs. In studies in which patients were switched from olanzapine, for example, to ziprasidone, there was a reduction in body weight of about 2 kg and improvements in metabolic and lipid parameters.[70]

The consensus panel also recommended that health care professionals, patients, and family members be educated to the signs and symptoms of diabetes and to the development of diabetic ketoacidosis (DKA), a potentially fatal condition. The recommendations state that DKA may present uncommonly, but rapidly, and include the following symptoms: polyuria, polydipsia, weight loss, nausea, vomiting, dehydration, rapid respiration, and delirium or coma. In addition, the panel advised that drugs be chosen that minimize the risk of weight gain for patients at higher risk for diabetes who require antipsychotic (or mood-stabilizing) drugs.

The panel recommended that once SGA treatment is started, the patient's weight be measured at 4, 8, and 12 weeks. If the patient has gained more than 5% of initial weight, consideration of switching to another SGA should be made; such a switch should be made in a gradual manner. It is important to assess the psychiatric status of the patient and the potential benefit, however, of the SGA, before discontinuing it. Fasting lipid and glucose values, along with blood pressure readings, should be obtained at 12 weeks. These assessments should continue quarterly, with appropriate referral to other health care providers for management of hypertension, dyslipidemia, hyperglycemia, or symptoms of diabetes or DKA as clinically indicated. The choice of SGA may reduce the frequency of the onset of diabetes or cardiovascular disease. Initial short-term evidence suggests that adding dietary and physical activity intervention may minimize weight gain with the SGAs. More research is needed to evaluate the effectiveness of this strategy.[71]

SUMMARY

This article has shown that obesity is related to several psychiatric disorders, the most thoroughly researched of which is depression. In both community and clinical populations, the observed relationship is more consistent in women than in men, and is stronger in more severely obese individuals. The presence of BED also is associated with elevated risk of additional psychopathology. Longitudinal research provides evidence to support a pathway from obesity to depression, as well as one from depression to obesity. Weight loss, particularly with nonpharmacologic methods, appears to have favorable group-level effects on mood, but may be associated with adverse outcomes for some individuals. Persons who require antipsychotic medications are at risk for weight gain and metabolic abnormalities, and their management should be informed by consensus guidelines.

REFERENCES

1. de Wit L, Luppino F, van Straten A, et al. Depression and obesity: a meta-analysis of community-based studies. Psychiatry Res 2010;178:230–5.
2. Onyike CU, Crum RM, Lee HB, et al. Is obesity associated with major depression? Results from the third National Health and Nutrition Examination Survey. Am J Epidemiol 2003;58: 1136–47.

3. Petry NM, Barry D, Pietrzak RH, et al. Overweight and obesity are associated with psychiatric disorders: results from the National Epidemiologic Survey on Alcohol and Related Conditions. Psychosom Med 2008;70:288–97.
4. Simon GE, von Korff M, Saunders K, et al. Association between obesity and psychiatric disorders in the US adult population. Arch Gen Psychiatry 2006;63:824–30.
5. Mather AA, Cox BJ, Enns MW, et al. Associations of obesity with psychiatric disorders and suicidal behaviors in a nationally representative sample. J Psychosom Res 2009;66:277–85.
6. Barry D, Pietrzak RH, Petry NM. Gender differences in associations between body mass index and DSM-IV mood and anxiety disorders: results from the National Epidemiologic Survey on Alcohol and Related Conditions. Ann Epidemiol 2008;18: 458–66.
7. Scott KM, McGee MA, Wells JE, et al. Obesity and mental disorders in the adult general population. J Psychosom Res 2008;64:97–105.
8. Wang PW, Sachs GS, Zarate CA, et al. Overweight and obesity in bipolar disorders. J Psychiatr Res 2006;40:762–4.
9. Fagiolini A, Kupfer DJ, Rucci P, et al. Suicide attempts and ideation in patients with bipolar I disorder. J Clin Psychiatry 2004;65:509–14.
10. Bond DJ, Lang DJ, Noronha MM, et al. The association of elevated body mass index with reduced brain volumes in first-episode mania. Biol Psychiatry 2011;70:381–7.
11. Grucza RA, Krueger RF, Racette SB, et al. The emerging link between alcoholism risk and obesity in the United States. Arch Gen Psychiatry 2010;67:1301–8.
12. Wang GJ, Volkow ND, Thanos PK, et al. Imaging of brain dopamine pathways: implications for understanding obesity. J Addict Med 2009;3:8–18.
13. American Psychiatric Association. Diagnostic and Statistical Manual of Mental Disorder. 4th edition, text revision. Washington, DC: American Psychiatric Association. 2000.
14. Wonderlich SA, Gordon KH, Mitchell JE, et al. The validity and clinical utility of binge eating disorder. Int J Eat Disord 2009;42:687–705.
15. Grucza RA, Przybeck TR, Cloninger CR. Prevalence and correlates of binge eating disorder in a community sample. Compr Psychiatry 2007;48:124–31.
16. Luppino FS, de Wit LM, Bouvy PF, et al. Overweight, obesity, and depression: a systematic review and meta-analysis of longitudinal studies. Arch Gen Psychiatry 2010;67:220–9.
17. Faith MS, Butryn M, Wadden TA, et al. Evidence for prospective associations among depression and obesity in population-based studies. Obes Rev 2011;12:e438–e453.
18. Herva A, Laitinen J, Miettunen J, et al. Obesity and depression: results from the longitudinal Northern Finland 1966 Birth Cohort Study. Int J Obes 2006;30:520–7.
19. Anderson SE, Cohen P, Naumova EN, et al. Adolescent obesity and risk for subsequent major depressive disorder and anxiety disorder: prospective evidence. Psychosom Med 2007;69:740–7.
20. Goodman E, Whitaker RC. A prospective study of the role of depression in the development and persistence of adolescent obesity. Pediatrics 2002;110:497–504.
21. Ball K, Burton NW, Brown WJ. A prospective study of overweight, physical activity, and depressive symptoms in young women. Obesity 2009;17:66–71.
22. Bjerkeset O, Romundstad P, Evans J, et al. Association of adult body mass index and height with anxiety, depression, and suicide in the general population: the HUNT study. Am J Epidemiol 2008;167:193–202.
23. Koponen H, Jokelainen J, Keinanen-Kiukaanniemi S, et al. Metabolic syndrome predisposes to depressive symptoms: a population-based 7-year follow-up study. J Clin Psychiatry 2008;69:178–82.

24. van Gool CH, Kempen GI, Bosma H, et al. Associations between lifestyle and depressed mood: longitudinal results from the Maastricht Aging Study. Am J Public Health 2007;97:887–94.

25. Kasen S, Cohen P, Chen H, et al. Obesity and psychopathology in women: a three decade prospective study. Int J Obes 2008;32:558–66.

26. Roberts RE, Kaplan GA, Shema SJ, et al. Are the obese at greater risk for depression? Am J Epidemiol 2000;152:163–70.

27. Roberts RE, Strawbridge WJ, Deleger S, et al. Are the fat more jolly? Ann Behav Med 2002;24:169–80.

28. Roberts RE, Deleger S, Strawbridge WJ, et al. Prospective association between obesity and depression: evidence from the Alameda County Study. Int J Obes Relat Metab Disord 2003;27:514–21.

29. Sachs-Ericsson N, Burns AB, Gordon KH, et al. Body mass index and depressive symptoms in older adults: the moderating roles of race, sex, and socioeconomic status. Am J Geriatr Psychiatry 2007;15:815–25.

30. Goodwin RD, Sourander A, Duarte CS, et al. Do mental health problems in childhood predict chronic physical conditions among males in early adulthood? Evidence from a community-based prospective study. Psychol Med 2009;39:301–11.

31. Pine DS, Goldstein RB, Wolk S, et al. The association between childhood depression and adulthood body mass index. Pediatrics 2001;107:1049–56.

32. Barefoot JC, Heitmann BL, Helms MJ, et al. Symptoms of depression and changes in body weight from adolescence to mid-life. Int J Obes Relat Metab Disord 1998;22: 688–94.

33. Franko DL, Striegel-Moore RH, Thompson D, et al. Does adolescent depression predict obesity in black and white young adult women? Psychol Med 2005;35: 1505–13.

34. Hasler G, Pine DS, Kleinbaum DG, et al. Depressive symptoms during childhood and adult obesity: the Zurich Cohort Study. Mol Psychiatry 2005;10:842–50.

35. Pine DS, Cohen P, Brook J, et al. Psychiatric symptoms in adolescence as predictors of obesity in early adulthood: a longitudinal study. Am J Public Health 1997;87:1303–10.

36. Richardson LP, Davis R, Poulton R, et al. A longitudinal evaluation of adolescent depression and adult obesity. Arch Pediatr Adolesc Med 2003;157:739–45.

37. Stice E, Presnell K, Shaw H, et al. Psychological and behavioral risk factors for obesity onset in adolescent girls: a prospective study. J Consult Clin Psychol 2005;73:195–202.

38. Vogelzangs N, Kritchevsky SB, Beekman AT, et al. Depressive symptoms and change in abdominal obesity in older persons. Arch Gen Psychiatry 2008;65:1386–93.

39. Gariepy G, Wang JL, Lesage AD, et al. The longitudinal association from obesity to depression: results from the 12-year National Population Health Survey. Obesity 2010;18:1033–8.

40. Carpiniello B, Pinna F, Pillai G, et al. Psychiatric comorbidity and quality of life in obese patients: results from a case-control study. Int J Psychiatry Med 2009;39:63–78.

41. Grilo CM, White MA, Masheb RM. DSM-IV psychiatric disorder comorbidity and its correlates in binge eating disorder. Int J Eat Disord 2009;42:228–34.

42. Wadden TA, Butryn ML, Sarwer DB, et al. Comparison of psychosocial status in treatment-seeking women with class III vs. class I-II obesity. Surg Obes Relat Dis 2006;2:138–45.

43. Beck AT, Steer RA, Brown GK. Beck Depression Inventory-II (BDI-II). San Antonio (TX): Psychological Corporation; 1996.

44. Fabricatore AN, Sarwer DB, Wadden TA, et al. Impression management or real change? Reports of depressive symptoms before and after the preoperative psychological evaluation for bariatric surgery. Obes Surg 2007;17:1213–9.
45. Kalarchian MA, Marcus MD, Levine MD, et al. Psychiatric disorders among bariatric surgery candidates: relationship to obesity and functional health status. Am J Psychiatry 2007;164:328–34.
46. Mauri M, Rucci P, Calderone A, et al. Axis I and II disorders and quality of life in bariatric surgery candidates. J Clin Psychiatry 2008;69:295–301.
47. Keys A. Biology of human starvation. Minneapolis (MN): University of Minnesota Press; 1950.
48. Stunkard AJ. The dieting depression: incidence and clinical characteristics of untoward responses to weight reduction regimens. Am J Med 1957;23:77–86.
49. Christensen R, Kristensen PK, Bartels EM, et al. Efficacy and safety of the weight loss drug rimonabant: a meta-analysis of randomized trials. Lancet 2007;370:1706–13.
50. Fabricatore AN, Wadden TA, Higginbotham AJ, et al. Intentional weight loss and changes in symptoms of depression: a systematic review and meta-analysis. Int J Obes (Lond) 2011. [Epub ahead of print]. DOI:10.1038/ijo.2011.2.
51. Faulconbridge LF, Wadden TA, Berkowitz RI, et al. Changes in symptoms of depression with weight loss: results of a randomized trial. Obesity 2009;15:1009–16.
52. Dansinger ML, Tatsioni A, Wong JB, et al. Meta-analysis: the effect of dietary counseling for weight loss. Ann Intern Med 2007;147:41–50.
53. Li Z, Maglione M, Tu W, et al. Meta-analysis: pharmacologic treatment of obesity. Ann Intern Med 2005;142:532–46.
54. Padwal R, Klarenbach S, Wiebe N, et al. Bariatric surgery: a systematic review of the clinical and economic evidence. J Gen Intern Med 2011. [Epub ahead of print]. DOI: 10.1007/s11606-011-1721-x.
55. Wadden TA, Sarwer DB, Fabricatore AN. Psychosocial and behavioral status of patients undergoing bariatric surgery: what to expect before and after surgery. Med Clin North Am 2007;91:451–69.
56. de Zwaan M, Enderle J, Wagner S, et al. Anxiety and depression in bariatric surgery patients: a prospective, follow-up study using structured clinical interviews. J Affect Disord 2011;133:61–8.
57. Adams TD, Gress RE, Smith SC, et al. Long-term mortality after gastric bypass surgery. N Engl J Med 2007;357:753–61.
58. Anton SD, Martin CK, Redman L, et al. Psychosocial and behavioral pre-treatment predictors of weight loss outcomes. Eat Weight Disord 2008;13:30–7.
59. Teixeira PJ, Going SB, Sardinha LB, et al. A review of psychosocial pre-treatment predictors of weight control. Obes Rev 2005;6:43–65.
60. Aronne LJ, Bray GA, Pi-Sunyer FX, et al, editors. Management of drug-induced weight gain: a continuing education monograph for physicians. Madison (WI): The University of Wisconsin School of Medicine and Boron LePore Group Companies; 2002.
61. Consensus Development Conference on Antipsychotic Drugs and Obesity and Diabetes. Diabetes Care 2004;27:596–601.
62. Allison DB, Mentore JL, Heo M, et al. Antipsychotic-induced weight gain: a comprehensive research synthesis. Am J Psychiatry 1999;156:1686–96.
63. Marrato EH, Newcomer JW, Kamat S, et al. Metabolic Screening after the American Diabetes Association's Consensus Statement on Diabetes and Antipsychotic Drugs. Diabetes Care 2009;32:1037–42.
64. Lieberman JA, Stroup TS, McEvoy JP, et al. Effectiveness of antipsychotic drugs in patients with chronic schizophrenia. N Engl J Med 2005;353:1209–23.

65. Gianfrancesco FD, Grogg AL, Mahmoud RA, et al. Differential effects of risperidone, olanzapine, clozapine, and conventional antipsychotics on type 2 diabetes: findings from a large health plan database. J Clin Psychopharmacol 2003;23:328–35.

66. Genuth S, Alberti KG, Bennett P, et al. Expert committee on the diagnosis and classification of diabetes mellitus: follow-up report on the diagnosis of diabetes mellitus. Diabetes Care 2003;26:3160–7.

67. Koller EA, Doraiswamy PM. Olanzapine-associated diabetes mellitus. Pharmacotherapy 2002;22:841–52.

68. Newcomer JW, Haupt DW, Fucetola R, et al. Abnormalities in glucose regulation during antipsychotic treatment of schizophrenia. Arch Gen Psychiatry 2002;59: 337–45.

69. Henderson DC, Cagliero E, Gray C, et al. Clozapine, diabetes mellitus, weight gain, and lipid abnormalities: a five-year naturalistic study. Am J Psychiatry 2000;157: 975–81.

70. Alptekin K, Hafez J, Brook S, et al. Efficacy and tolerability of switching to ziprasidone from olanzapine, risperidone, or haloperidol: an international multicenter study. Int Clin Psychopharmacol 2009;24:229–38.

71. Allison DB, Newcomer JW, Dunn AL, et al. Obesity among those with mental disorders: a National Institute of Mental Health meeting report. Am J Prev Med 2009;36:341–50.

Eating Disorders and Obesity

Albert J. Stunkard, MD

KEYWORDS

- Obesity • Night eating syndrome • Binge eating disorder
- Comorbidity

An understanding of the relationship between obesity and eating disorders has grown in recent years. Obesity is characterized by an excessive amount of fat in tissues of the body. Body fat typically is estimated by the body mass index, calculated as weight in kilograms divided by height in meters squared. Persons with a body mass index of 30 kg/m^2 or greater are considered obese.[1] In 2007 and 2008, the prevalence of obesity among US adult men was 32.2% and among adult women was 35.5%, although the rate of increase in prevalence of adult obesity has slowed over the past 10 years.[2] In the past, obesity had itself been considered to be an eating disorder. We have learned, however, that most overweight and obese persons do not overeat in any distinctive pattern. For a smaller number, however, 2 clear patterns of overeating have been identified: Binge eating disorder (BED) and night eating syndrome (NES). Both disorders are more prevalent among overweight and obese persons than among persons of normal weight, and they contribute to the overweight of such persons.

BINGE EATING DISORDER

Binge eating was first described by Hippocrates, who viewed it as a "sick form of hunger."[3] The first proposal of binge eating as a syndrome occurred in 1959 when it was proposed as "BED."[4] Since then, formal diagnostic criteria have been proposed and appear with a provisional diagnosis in the *Diagnostic and Statistical Manual of Mental Disorders, Fourth Edition, Text Revision* (DSM-IV-TR, 2000). These criteria were based on 2 large studies (of 1984 and 1785 persons, respectively) conducted at 12 eating disorder programs.[4,5] Two core features and several associated features have been identified.

Diagnostic Features

The first of 2 "core features" of the diagnosis of BED are "eating within a discreet period of time . . . an amount that is definitely larger than most individuals would eat under similar circumstances."[6] The second "core feature" of BED is experiencing a

Center for Weight and Eating Disorders, Department of Psychiatry, Perelman School of Medicine at the University of Pennsylvania, 3535 Market Street, Suite 3029, Philadelphia, PA 19104, USA
E-mail address: Stunkard@mail.med.upenn.edu

Psychiatr Clin N Am 34 (2011) 765–771
doi:10.1016/j.psc.2011.08.010
0193-953X/11/$ – see front matter © 2011 Elsevier Inc. All rights reserved.

loss of control over eating during this period of time, as if one cannot stop eating or limit the quantity eaten. BED is to be distinguished from bulimia nervosa by the absence of compensatory behaviors such as vomiting, laxative abuse, or compulsive exercising. A sense of shame and disgust with oneself is associated with episodes of BED that cause significant distress. Compared with control (non-BED) obese persons, those with BED suffer from more severe obesity; earlier onset of overweight; earlier onset of, and more frequent, dieting; and greater psychopathology.[4,5]

Prevalence

Estimates of the prevalence of BED vary widely, depending on the method of assessment (eg, survey vs interview) and the definition of a binge. In 2 community surveys, the prevalence was as low as 1.8%[7] and 2.0%.[3] Interview-based studies of treatment-seeking obese persons found higher rates (8.9%[8] and 18.8%[9]). The prevalence of BED is greater the more severe the obesity; thus, rates of BED among severely obese persons undergoing bariatric surgery were 27%,[10] 38%,[11] and 47%.[12] Equal numbers of white men and women are afflicted with BED, whereas black men report the disorder less often than black women.[13–15]

Psychiatric Comorbidity

Two risk factors for BED have been documented: Psychiatric disorders and obesity. Psychopathology, especially depression, has been consistently reported among people with BED.[16–25] Axis II disorders, particularly clusters B (dramatic–emotional) and C (anxious–fearful),[17,19,21] also occur frequently in binge eaters (**Table 1**). In a community study, binge eaters showed several more vulnerabilities than the healthy control subjects, including frequent parental depression; greater susceptibility to obesity; more exposure to negative comments about shape, weight, and eating; morbid perfectionism; and negative self-evaluation.[26] Compared with subjects with other psychiatric disorders, binge eaters were distinctive only by more frequent reports of childhood obesity and awareness of negative comments about shape, weight, and eating.[27] Persons with BED reported less exposure to risk factors for general psychopathology than did those persons with bulimia nervosa.[26]

Table 1					
Percentage of BED patents with lifetime comorbidity of DSM diagnoses, as assessed by SCID					
Study	Major Depression	Any Substance Abuse or Dependence	Any Anxiety Disorder	Any Axis I Disorder	Personality Disorder
Yanovski et al, 1993	51	12		60	35
Specker et al, 1994	47	72	11.6	72.1	33
Mussel et al, 1996	47	23	18.8	70	
Telch & Stice, 1998	49	9		59	20

Data from Stunkard AJ, Allison KC. Binge eating disorder: disorder or marker? Int J Eat Disord 2003;34:S107–16.

Risk Factors

The influence of genetics on BED is unclear. A latent analysis of a large number of twins[28] revealed that one of the generated classes approximated the features of BED, and that monozygotic twin pairs more often fell into the same class than did dizygotic pairs. On the other hand, Lee and co-workers[29] did not find any familial tendency for BED.

A once-popular theory for the cause of BED has been put to rest in recent years; the theory is that dieting causes BED. Spitzer and colleagues[4,5] reported that dieting occurred after the onset of binge eating, a finding that has been confirmed by 5 subsequent studies.[30–35] The National Task Force on the Prevention and Treatment of Obesity concluded that empirical studies do not support the belief that dieting induces binge eating in obese adults.[36,37]

NIGHT EATING SYNDROME

NES is an eating disorder characterized by a phase delay in the circadian pattern of food intake. It is manifested by (1) evening hyperphagia, or (2) awakenings accompanied by nocturnal ingestions, or (3) both.[38] NES was originally described in 1955, based on a single patient and on the subsequent treatment of 25 obese persons referred to a special study clinic because of difficulty in the management of their obesity.[39] The criteria noted in this original study were the consumption of 25% of caloric intake after the evening meal, initial insomnia at least half of the time, and morning anorexia. A revision of the required criteria was proposed in a study by Birketvedt and associates.[40] It reported nighttime awakenings, which were very often the occasion for the consumption of food. At present, provisional criteria for NES include morning anorexia, evening hyperphagia, and awakening accompanied by frequent nocturnal ingestion.[40]

More recently, an item response theory analysis, using data from 1479 Night Eating Questionnaires, examined the symptoms of NES described.[41] Item response theory revealed that evening hyperphagia, defined as eating 25% or more of the daily caloric intake after the evening meal, and/or the presence of nocturnal ingestions, more than half of the time upon awakening, were almost predictive of a diagnosis of NES. Morning anorexia and delayed ingestion of the first meal did not add enough information to be considered essential in diagnosing NES.

Prevalence

NES is uncommon in the general population (1.5%).[42] As in the case of BED, prevalence of NES increases with increasing weight, from 8.9%[43] to 15%[44] in obesity clinics and from 10%[43] to 27%[42] and 42%[12] among obese persons undergoing assessment for bariatric surgery.

A recent discovery has been the occurrence of NES in persons of normal weight. This fact came to light through responses to the NES Web site, which provided the Night Eating Questionnaire.[41] The results showed one major difference between the responses of 40 obese night eaters and 40 nonobese night eaters: The normal weight night eaters were 7 years younger (33.1 ± 10.7 years vs 40.0 ± 14.3 years for the obese night eaters). The younger age of the nonobese subjects suggests that NES may contribute to the later development of obesity. This suggestion is supported by the fact that more than half of obese night eaters reported that their night eating began before their obesity.

Features

Four studies have confirmed aspects of the NES. Gluck and co-workers[43] reported that NES subjects consumed more of their food intake than did controls during the latter part of the day, and that a test meal at this time was larger in night eaters than in control subjects. This study also found elevated levels of depression in NES subjects. Aronoff and colleagues[44] reported that 70% of the 24-hour food intake of night eaters was consumed after 7 pm. Allison and associates[45] found that NES subjects awakened 1.7 times per night, and 73% of these awakenings were associated with snacking. Manni and co-workers[46] found NES (confirmed by polysomnography) in 10 patients who ate during half of these occasions.

Stress plays a strong role in the development and maintenance of NES. In the author's experience, approximately 75% of NES sufferers linked the onset of their disorder to a specific stress-related event. Those who reported a stress-related onset were nearly 15 years older at the age of onset than the 25% of respondents who did not experience such an event (34.2 vs 19.6 years; $P = .001$), suggesting a particular vulnerability to NES among persons with younger age of onset (Allison KC, Sunkard AJ, unpublished data, 2004).

Psychiatric Comorbidity

As in the case of BED, psychiatric comorbidity is common among people with NES.[27,38] More than 75% of NES participants in one study had a lifetime history of an axis I disorder.[38] Specifically, night eaters met *DSM-IV* criteria significantly more often than control subjects for a history of major depressive disorder (47%), any anxiety disorder (37%), and any substance abuse and dependence (24%). Beck Depression Inventory scores were moderately elevated among people with NES.[47] Napolitano and colleagues[47] also reported even higher levels of state and trait anxiety and disinhibition of food intake among obesity clinic patients with NES than among those with BED or with no eating disorder.

Risk Factors

There is a strong familial link in NES. Lundgren and co-workers[48] found that 36% of NES participants reported at least 1 first degree relative with night eating behaviors compared with significantly fewer (16%) matched controls ($P = .03$). This comparison is biased in favor of a higher prevalence among family members of night eaters, because they are far more aware of night eating than are persons without a relative with NES.

Eating Versus Sleep Disorder

The disturbed sleep with frequent ingestions has led to the view that NES is a combined sleeping and eating disorder. The 2004 study by O'Reardon and colleagues,[49] however, revealed no significant differences between night eaters and controls for sleep onset (23:31 ± 1:40 vs 23:32 ± 1:06) and sleep offset (07:24 ± 1:07 vs 6:59 ± 1:12). This finding suggests that, among night eaters, it is the eating pattern that is disturbed and that the sleeping pattern remains undisturbed. NES thus seems to be a disorder of biological rhythm, characterized by a delayed onset of eating (**Fig. 1**). This view encompasses the continuation of overeating into the night and the delay in onset of appetite in the morning.

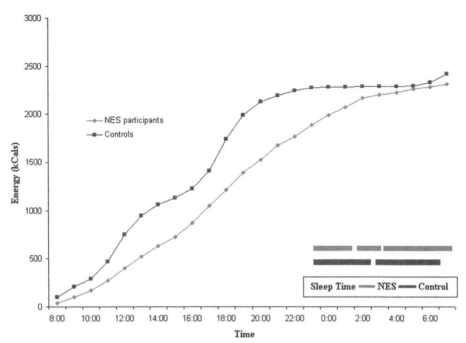

Fig. 1. Cumulative caloric intake for persons with NES. Note that persons with NES have more frequent awakenings than the control group. Note also a delayed circadian shift relative to matched control participants. (*From* O'Reardon JO, Ringel BL, Dinges DF, et al. Circadian eating and sleeping patterns in the night eating syndrome. Obes Res 2004;12:1789–96.)

SUMMARY

In conclusion, 2 types of disordered eating behaviors affect some overweight and obese persons. BED and NES present an excellent opportunity to recognize, treat, and prevent these disorders that, at the least, maintain, and at worst, promote, overweight and obesity. Articles in this volume by Wilson and co-workers and Allison and colleagues discuss current treatment options for BED and NES, respectively. Clinicians are encouraged to evaluate the presence of BED and NES in all patients who seek treatment for their obesity. Although the prevalence of these 2 eating disorders is relatively low, both are associated with significant distress and dysfunction that can be ameliorated with effective treatment.

REFERENCES

1. National Institutes of Health/National Heart, Lung, and Blood Institute. Clinicalguidelines on the identification, evaluation, and treatment of overweight andobesity in adults. Obes Res 1998;6:51S–209S.
2. Katherine FM, Carroll MD, Ogden CL. Prevalence and trends in obesity amongUS adults, 1999–2008. JAMA 2010;303:235–41.
3. Stunkard AJ. A history of binge eating. In: Fairburn CG, Wilson GT, editors.Binge eating: nature, assessment, and treatment. New York: Guilford; 1993. p.15–34.
4. Spitzer RL, Devlin M, Walsh BT, et al. Binge eating disorder: a multisite fieldtrial of the diagnostic criteria. Int J Eat Disord 1992;11:191–203.

5. Spitzer RL, Yanovski S, Wadden TA, et al. Binge-eating disorder; its furthervalidation in a multi-site study. Int J Eat Disord 1993;13:137–50.
6. American Psychiatric Association. Diagnostic and statistical manual of mentaldisorders. 4th edition. Text revision. Washington (DC): American PsychiatricAssociation; 2000. p. 178.
7. Bruce B, Agras WS. Binge eating in females: a population-based investigation.Int J Eat Disord 1992;12:365–73.
8. Stunkard AJ, Berkowitz R, Wadden T, et al. Binge eating disorder and the nighteating syndrome. Int J Obes Metab Disord 1996;20:1–6.
9. Brody ML, Walsh BT, Devlin MJ. Binge eating disorder: reliability and validityof a new diagnostic category. J Consult Clin Psychol 1994;62:381–6.
10. Wadden TA, Sarwer DB, Womble LG, et al. Psychosocial aspects of obesity andobesity surgery. Surg Clin North Am 2001;81:1001–24.
11. Hsu LKG, Betancourt S, Sullivan SP. Eating disorders before and after verticalbanded gastroplasty; a pilot study. Int J Eat Disord 1996;19:23–34.
12. Adami GF, Bandolfo P, Bauer B, et al. Binge eating in massively obese patientsundergoing bariatric surgery. Int J Disord 1995;17:45–50.
13. Grange D, Telch CF, Agras WS. Eating and general psychopathology in a sampleof Caucasian and ethnic minority subjects. Int J Eating Disord 1997;21:285–93.
14. Pike KM, Dohm FA, Striegel-Moore RH, et al. A comparison of black and whitewomen with binge eating disorder. Am J Psychiatry 2001;158:1455–60.
15. Smith DE, Marcus MD, Lewis CE, et al. Prevalence of binge eating disorder,obesity and depression in a biracial cohort of young adults. Ann Behav Med 1998;20:227–32.
16. Marcus MD, Wing RR, Hopkin J. Obese binge eaters: affect, cognitions andresponse to behavioral weight control. J Consult Clin Psychol 1988;56:433–9.
17. Marcus MD, Wing RR, Ewing L, et al. Psychiatric disorders among obese bingeeaters. Int J Eat Disord 1996;9:69–77.
18. Yankovski SZ, Nelson JE, Dubbert BK, et al. Association of binge eatingdisorder and psychiatric comorbidity on obese subjects. Am J Psychiatry 1993;150:1472–9.
19. Mitchell JE, Mussell MP. Comorbidity and binge eating disorder. Addict Behav 1995;20:725–32.
20. Antony MM, Johnson WG, Carr-Nangle RE, et al. Psychopathology correlates ofbinge eating and binge eating disorder. Compr Psychiatry 1994;35:386–92.
21. Specker S, De Zwann M, Raymond N, et al. Psychopathology in subgroups ofobese women with and without binge eating disorder. Compr Psychiatry 1994;35:185–90.
22. Telch C, Stice E. Psychiatric comorbidity in a nonclinical sample of women withbinge eating disorder. J Consult Clin Psychol 1998;66:768–76.
23. Wadden TA, Foster GD, Letiza KA. One-year behavioral treatment of obesity:comparison of moderate and severe caloric restriction and the effects of weightmaintenance therapy. J Consult Clin Psychol 1994;62:165–71.
24. Keunel RH, Wadden TA. Binge eating disorder, weight cycling, andpsychopathology. Int J Eat Disord 1994;15:321–9.
25. Mussel MP, Mitchell JE, de Zwaan M, et al. Clinical characteristics associatedwith binge eating in obese families: a descriptive study. Int J Obes Relat MetabDisord 1996;20:324–31.
26. Fairburn CG, Doll HA, Welch SL, et al. Risk Factors for binge eating disorder: acommunity based, case-control study. Arch Gen Psychiatry 1998;55:425–32.
27. Stunkard AJ, Allison KC. Binge eating disorder: disorder or marker? Int J EatDisord 2003;34:S107–16.
28. Bulick CM, Sullivan PF, Kendler KS. An empirical study of the classification ofeating disorders. Am J Psychiatry 2000;157:851–3.

29. Lee YH, Abbot DW, Seim H, et al. Eating disorders and psychiatric disorders inthe first-degree relatives of obese probands with binge eating disorder and obesenon-binge eating disorder controls. Int J Eat Disord 1999;26:322–32.
30. Wilson GT, Nonas CA, Rosenblum GD. Assessment of binge eating in obesepatients. Int J Eat Disord 1993;150:1427–9.
31. Berkowitz R, Stunkard AJ, Stallings VA. Binge eating disorder in obeseadolescent girls. Annual New York Academy of Medicine 1993;699:200–96.
32. Spurrell EM, Wilfrey DE, Tanofsky MB, et al. Age of onset of binge eatingdisorder: are there different pathways to eating? Int J Eat Disord 1997;21:55–65.
33. Grilo CM, Masheb RM. Onset of dieting vs. binge eating in outpatients withbinge eating disorder. Int J Obes Relat Metab Disord 2000;24:404–9.
34. Abbot DW, de Zwaan M, Mussel MP, et al. Onset of binge eating and dieting inoverweight women: implications for etiology, associated features and treatment. JPsychosom Res 1998;44:367–74.
35. Mussell MP, Mitchell JE, Fenna CJ, et al. A comparison of onset binge eatingversus dieting in the development of bulimia nervosa. Int J Disord 1997;12:353–60.
36. National Task Force on the Prevention and Treatment of Obesity. Dieting anddevelopment of eating disorders in overweight and obese adults. Arch Intern Med 2000; 160:2581–9.
37. Wadden TA, Foster GD, Sarwer DB, et al. Dieting and development of eatingdisorders in obese women: results of a randomized controlled trial. Am J ClinNutr 2004;80: 560–8.
38. Stunkard AJ, Allison KC. Two forms of disordered eating in obesity: binge eatingand night eating. Int J Obes Relat Metab Disord 2003;27:1–12.
39. Stunkard AJ, Grace WJ, Wolff HG. The night eating syndrome: a pattern of foodintake among certain obese patients. Am J Med 1955;19:78–86.
40. Birketvedt G, Florholmen J, Sundsfjord J, et al. Behavioral and neuroendocrinecharacteristics of the night eating syndrome. JAMA 1999;282:657–63.
41. Rand CSW, Macgregor MD, Stunkard AJ. The night eating syndrome in thegeneral population and among post-operative obesity surgery patients. Int J EatDisord 1997;22:65-9.
42. Stunkard AJ. Eating patterns and obesity. Psychiatr Q 1959;33:284–94.
43. Gluck ME, Geliebter A, Satov T. Night eating syndrome is associated withdepression, low self esteem, reduced daytime hunger, and less weight loss inobese outpatients. Obes Res 2001;9:264–7.
44. Aronoff NJ, Geliebter A, Zammit G. Gender and body mass index as related tOthe night eating syndrome in obese outpatients. J Am Diet Assoc 2001;101:102–4.
45. Allison KC, O'Reardon J, Stunkard AJ, et al. Characterizing the night eatingsyndrome. Obes Res 2001;9:93S.
46. Manni R, Ratti MT, Tartara A. Nocturnal eating: prevalence and features in 120insomniac referrals. Sleep 1997;20:734–8.
47. Napolitano MA, Head S, Babyak MA, et al. Binge eating disorder and nighteating syndrome: psychological and behavioral characteristics. Int J Eat Disord 2001;30: 193-30.
48. Lundgren JD, Allison KC, Stunkard AJ. Familial aggregation in the night eatingsyndrome. Int J Eat Disord 2006;39:516–518.
49. O'Reardon JO, Ringel BL, Dinges DF, et al. Circadian eating and sleepingpatterns in the night eating syndrome. Obes Res 2004;12:1789–96.

Treatment of Binge Eating Disorder

G. Terence Wilson, PhD

KEYWORDS

- Binge eating disorder • Cognitive behavior therapy
- Guided self-help • Behavioral weight loss treatment
- Pharmacotherapy

Binge eating disorder (BED) was originally included in the *Diagnostic and Statistical Manual of Mental Disorders, 4th edition* (DSM-IV) as a provisional eating disorder diagnosis within the category of Eating Disorder Not Otherwise Specified.[1] It is now listed as a free-standing diagnosis among the proposed *Draft Revisions to DSM Disorders and Criteria for DSM-5*.[2] BED is defined by recurrent binge eating (once a week, on average, over the previous 3 months) without the regular use of inappropriate compensatory weight control methods. Binge eating itself is characterized by (a) eating, in a discrete period of time, an amount of food that is unambiguously greater than most people would eat in a similar period of time under similar conditions, and (b) a sense of lack of control over eating during the episode. The criteria also include marked distress over binge eating and 3 or more of the following indicators of loss of control (LOC), namely "eating much more rapidly than normal, eating until feeling uncomfortably full, eating large amounts of food when not feeling physically hungry, eating alone because of feeling embarrassed by how much one is eating, and feeling disgusted with oneself, depressed, or very guilty afterwards."[2]

BED can be reliably differentiated from other eating disorders,[3] although accumulating evidence reveals that patients with BED often have levels of overvaluation of body shape and weight that are comparable to those diagnosed with bulimia nervosa. The presence of high overvaluation in BED has been shown to indicate greater disturbance.[4,5] BED is reliably associated with overweight and obesity in treatment-seeking individuals. Nevertheless, BED is different from obesity. For example, compared with obese individuals without BED, those with BED consume more calories in laboratory studies of eating behavior, report greater functional impairment and lower quality of life, and show significantly greater levels of psychiatric comorbidity.[3]

Rutgers–The State University of New Jersey, Graduate School of Applied and Professional Psychology, 152 Frelinghuysen Road, Piscataway, NJ 08854, USA
E-mail address: tewilson@rci.rutgers.edu

Psychiatr Clin N Am 34 (2011) 773–783
doi:10.1016/j.psc.2011.08.011
0193-953X/11/$ – see front matter © 2011 Elsevier Inc. All rights reserved.

TREATMENT

A variety of different psychological and pharmacologic interventions have been used to treat BED. The collective evidence establishes that BED is not simply a nonspecific disorder that responds equally well to virtually any treatment. Rather, the research shows that a diagnosis of BED has distinctive clinical utility in yielding differential outcomes across alternative therapies.[3,6]

Specialized Psychological Treatment

Cognitive-behavioral therapy

Several existing reviews document that manual-based cognitive-behavioral therapy (CBT) is arguably the current treatment of choice for BED given its extensive evaluation and strong empirical support.[7,8] CBT generally achieves total remission from binge eating in more than 50% of patients, along with broad improvement in specific eating disorder psychopathology (eg, overvaluation of body shape and weight), associated depression, and psychosocial functioning. The present article selectively illustrates the evidence with a focus on the more recent and methodologically superior studies.

CBT versus behavioral weight loss treatment

A long-standing question regarding the treatment of BED has been whether a specialty psychological treatment beyond the standard behavioral weight loss treatment (BWL) approach is needed. Two recent studies have addressed this issue with manual-based CBT.

In the first, a comparison of 16 weekly sessions of CBT with BWL for obese patients with BED showed that CBT was significantly more effective than BWL in producing remission from binge eating at posttreatment but not at the 12-month follow-up.[9] In the second, Grilo and colleagues[10] randomly assigned 125 obese patients with BED to 16 sessions of either group CBT, BWL, or a sequential condition in which CBT was administered first, followed by BWL (CBT + BWL). Attrition rates were relatively high (24% for CBT; 31% for BWL; 40% for CBT + BWL), especially in the combined condition. No significant differences in remission rates emerged, although CBT produced significantly greater reductions in frequency of binge eating at the 6- and 12-month follow-ups. BWL resulted in a statistically greater but modest percent body mass index loss. As in other studies,[11,12] remission from binge eating was associated with greater weight loss.

A secondary analysis of the findings of the Grilo and co-workers study[10] showed that rapid response to treatment, defined as 70% or greater reduction in binge eating by week 4, was evident in 57% of patients (67% of CBT; 47% of BWL).[13] Those treated with CBT did equally well regardless of rapid response in terms of reduced binge eating, but did not show weight loss. In patients treated with BWL, however, rapid responders were significantly more likely to achieve binge eating remission (62% vs 13%) and greater reductions in binge eating frequency, eating disorder psychopathology, and weight loss.

Two other studies evaluated the effects of differing combinations of CBT and BWL. Agras and co-workers[11] previously reported that, after BWL, CBT did little to reduce frequency of binge eating. These results do not support the utility of the longer and more costly combined treatment. Devlin and associates,[14] however, did find that adding CBT to BWL resulted in improved binge eating reduction. The reason for the discrepancy between the two sets of findings is unclear.

CBT versus pharmacologic treatment

Despite some inconsistent findings, treatment with antidepressant medication has been shown to be superior to pill placebo. Hence, comparisons with CBT provide a stringent test of the specific effectiveness of CBT. In a randomized, double-blind, placebo-controlled trial, Grilo and colleagues[15] found that CBT was significantly more effective than either fluoxetine or placebo in producing remission from binge eating. An earlier study of the open-label administration of fluoxetine showed the same outcome.[16] Agras and co-workers[11] found that sequentially adding desipramine to CBT did not improve reduction of binge eating frequency. In like fashion, Devlin and associates[14] showed that combining BWL with fluoxetine was significantly less effective than combining BWL and CBT.

Guided self-help

A growing body of research has focused on the implementation of self-help interventions based on the principles of CBT. Guided self-help (CBTgsh) combines the use of a self-help manual with a limited number of brief treatment sessions administered by health care providers of varying degrees of experience and expertise in CBT. Two early, relatively small studies compared CBTgsh to pure self-help in which BED participants were provided with a copy of the Fairburn[17] self-help volume *Overcoming Binge Eating* and instructed to follow its guidance. The Carter and Fairburn[18] study found that the interventions did not differ but were superior to a wait-list control in reducing binge eating and associated psychopathology. The study by Loeb and associates,[19] however, indicated that CBTgsh was significantly more effective than pure self-help in eliminating binge eating and reducing associated psychopathology.

Subsequent research has provided strong empirical support for the effectiveness of CBTgsh in the treatment of BED. Grilo and Masheb[20] found that CBTgsh was significantly more effective in producing remission from binge eating than both a manual-based BWL guided self-help intervention and a third comparison treatment designed to control for nonspecific therapeutic influences. A second study from this group of investigators showed that combining CBTgsh with orlistat (a non-centrally acting lipase inhibitor) resulted in significantly greater remission from binge eating than a combination of CBTgsh and pill placebo at posttreatment, but not at the 3-month follow-up (52% remission rate in both treatments).[21]

In the largest controlled treatment study of BED to date, Wilson and co-workers[22] compared CBTgsh (using the Fairburn[17] manual) with BWL and interpersonal psychotherapy (IPT) in a sample of 205 overweight and obese patients. BWL and IPT consisted of 20 sessions of individual treatment administered over a 6-month period, whereas CBTgsh comprised 10 sessions over this period, 9 of which had a maximum duration of 25 minutes. CBTgsh was provided by beginning graduate students in clinical psychology with little therapeutic experience, whereas IPT was provided by intensively trained and supervised doctoral-level clinical psychologists. Posttreatment analyses revealed no differences among the three treatments on remission from binge eating, whereas at the 2-year follow-up both CBTgsh and IPT not only successfully maintained their improvement, but were also significantly superior to BWL in producing remission from binge eating. BWL produced greater weight loss than either IPT or CBTgsh at posttreatment, but not at follow-up. The results provide further evidence that specialty psychological treatments are more effective than BWL in eliminating binge eating in obese patients.

An exploratory moderator analysis showed that, at the 2-year follow-up, low self-esteem undermined the effects of BWL in eliminating binge eating.[22] CBTgsh was unaffected by low self-esteem in patients with low levels of specific eating disorder psychopathology, but was substantially less effective in interaction with high levels. IPT was equally effective in patients with high or low levels of eating disorder psychopathology. Evidence on predictors of outcome is limited. Both rapid response[23] and high negative affect[24] have been shown to be nonspecific predictors of binge eating reduction in CBTgsh.

In the studies by Wilson and colleagues[22] and Grilo and co-workers,[15] CBTgsh was administered within a specialty eating disorders clinic setting. In contrast, Striegel-Moore and associates[25] compared 8 sessions of CBTgsh with treatment-as-usual over a 12-week period in a large health maintenance organization in the United States. Of the full sample of 123 patients diagnosed with recurrent binge eating (once a week on average for the previous 3 months), 48% met criteria for BED. Based on the Eating Disorder Examination, widely accepted as the gold standard means of assessing eating disorder psychopathology, the remission rates from binge eating at the 12-month follow-up were 64.0% and 44.6% for CBTgsh and treatment-as-usual, respectively. The diagnosis of BED did not moderate outcome. Significant CBTgsh-induced improvement was also evident on measures of eating-related psychopathology as well as depression and functional impairment. CBTgsh proved highly acceptable in this setting, with 74% of the sample attending at least 7 sessions. Only 12% attended 2 or fewer treatment sessions. The cost effectiveness of CBTgsh was also documented.[26]

IPT

Originally developed as a short-term, manual-based psychotherapy for depression, IPT has been adapted for the treatment of both bulimia nervosa and BED.[27] The primary emphasis is on helping patients to identify and change current interpersonal problems that are hypothesized to be maintaining the eating disorder. The treatment is both nondirective and noninterpretive. Two initial studies compared group manual-based CBT with group IPT.[12,28] In the study from Wilfley and colleagues,[12] there were impressive remission rates of 79% and 73% for CBT and IPT, respectively, at posttreatment, and 59% and 62% at the 1-year follow-up. Both treatments also produced clinically significant reductions in specific eating disorder psychopathology and general psychopathology. Patients who do not respond with first-line CBT treatment similarly failed to show much improvement with subsequent IPT.[29,30]

As noted, Wilson and colleagues[8] compared IPT with both BWL and CBTgsh. The advantage of IPT in that study was its effectiveness with a full range of BED patients, including those with high levels of specific eating disorder psychopathology. Another noteworthy finding was the low attrition rate in IPT (7%) compared with 28% and 30% for BWL and CBTgsh, respectively. IPT is readily acceptable to patients with BED.

As with other psychiatric disorders, BED is a heterogeneous category. A latent transition analysis identified 4 different classes.[31] Class 1 was characterized by a lower mean body mass index and increased physical activity. Class 2 patients reported the most binge eating, shape and weight concerns, compensatory behaviors, and negative affect. Class 3 patients reported similar binge eating frequencies to class 2 with lower levels of specific eating disorder psychopathology and compensatory activities, and class 4 was characterized by the highest average body mass index, the most overeating episodes, fewest binge eating episodes, and an absence of compensatory behaviors. A subsequent latent transition analysis found a greater probability of total remission from binge eating among patients who received IPT in class 2 and CBTgsh in class 3. The superiority of IPT for class 2 patients is consistent with the finding from Wilson and co-workers[22] that IPT was more effective than CBTgsh in patients with a high global Eating Disorder Examination score. These two analyses hold the promise of matching specific treatments to particular patient subgroups with BED.

Pharmacologic Therapy

Three classes of drugs have been used to treat BED, namely, antidepressant, antiobesity, and antiepileptic medications. Two recent, rigorous reviews of this literature are available.[32,33] In their comprehensive meta-analysis, Reas and Grilo[33] concluded that drugs are more effective than pill placebo in producing remission from binge eating in the short term (48.7% vs 28.5%). The least effective of the 3 classes of drugs were the selective serotonin reuptake inhibitors, which also produced minimal weight loss effects.

A limitation of this analysis is that it comprised only 14 randomized controlled trials of mainly short-term studies with small sample sizes. Moreover, despite the overall meta-analysis finding, inconsistencies among individual studies are apparent with some showing no differences between drug and placebo.[15] Reas and Grilo[33] concluded that their findings "highlight the potential utility of antiobesity (sibutramine) and antiepileptic (topiramate) medications" (p. 2036). It should be noted that sibutramine was subsequently withdrawn from use in the United States in 2010 because of negative side effects and that topiramate, long associated with serious neurocognitive side effects, has not received approval from the US Food and Drug Administration as a weight loss agent.

Orlistat (a lipase inhibitor) is approved by the US Food and Drug Administration as an antiobesity medication. As noted, combining orlistat with CBTgsh resulted in significantly higher remission from binge eating at posttreatment compared with placebo plus CBTgsh, but not at a 3-month follow-up during which both medication and CBTgsh were discontinued.[34] The combined CBTgsh and orlistat treatment produced significantly greater weight reduction at follow-up than CBTgsh plus placebo, although the absolute amount of weight lost was modest.

Reviews by Bodell and Devlin[32] and Reas and Grilo[33] underscored the reality that both the longer term effects of pharmacotherapy and the impact of discontinuation of medication are generally unknown. The absence of such information regarding the safety and effectiveness of pharmacotherapy for BED is striking. The American Psychiatric Association Practice Guideline for the Treatment of Eating Disorders[35] has cautioned that long-term use of selective serotonin reuptake inhibitors has been associated with weight gain.

Finally, studies to date have shown that pharmacotherapy for BED is significantly less effective than CBT and that combining medication with CBT fails to enhance the latter's success. In one study, however, patients who showed a rapid response to fluoxetine continued to improve, and the absence of an early response predicted treatment failure.[36] Early response to fluoxetine has also been shown to be a clinically important predictor of outcome in patients with bulimia nervosa.[37] The practical implications of this finding are that, should BED patients be treated with an SSRI, the absence of a rapid response should lead to switching to an alternative treatment such as CBT or IPT.

Bariatric Surgery

BED is a common comorbid disorder in obese patients seeking surgery, with rates ranging from 5% to 25% as determined by structured clinical interviews.[38] Research has consistently shown that BED is radically reduced if not eliminated after surgery.[38]

Niego and associates,[39] however, have suggested that if the requirement of a "large amount of food" is dropped from the definition of binge eating then patterns of disturbed eating and LOC occur more frequently postoperatively. Moreover, the latter has been linked with poorer outcomes as summarized below.

Is BED a negative prognostic indicator for weight loss outcomes in obesity treatment?

Early studies of the influence of binge eating on BWL treatment of obese individuals produced conflicting findings, with some showing a negative effect on weight loss, whereas others indicated no effect. Collectively, these studies were limited by relatively small sample sizes, self-report measures of binge eating, and a focus on binge eating per se rather than BED.[40] More recent studies of BWL for BED in overweight and obese patients have shown that whereas BWL is more effective than either CBT or IPT in producing short-term weight loss, the absolute amount of weight loss was much less than what is typically achieved in studies of obese patients in general.[10,9,22] In contrast, in their study of selected BED participants, Wadden and colleageus[38] reported a 1-year weight loss rate of 10.3%. Whether the inconsistencies in weight loss outcomes in these studies are attributable to the negative impact of BED itself, co-occurring psychopathology, or the quality of the BWL treatments cannot be answered at this point. Other research provides evidence that obese individuals with BED lose less weight than comparably obese patients without BED in response to BWL.[41,42] In a rare study of obese adolescents, Bishop-Gilyard and associates[43] found that the presence of binge eating had no significant impact on weight loss at a 12-month follow-up. A limitation of this study is its small sample size, with only 13 of the 82 patients meeting diagnostic criteria for BED.

Several studies have addressed the question of whether binge eating or BED influences weight loss after surgery. Some have found no differences in weight loss between patients with and without BED before surgery. Others have shown that binge eating might predict poorer outcome. The mixed findings could be due to several methodologic differences. One is the manner of assessment of binge eating and BED; self-report questionnaires are inferior to structured clinical interviews. Another is that it is the postoperative presence of LOC over eating, whether or not it was present preoperatively, that results in poorer outcome. For example, in a large study of 361 gastric bypass patients, White and co-workers[44] found that patient reports of LOC postoperatively—but not preoperatively—were associated with less weight loss and more psychosocial disturbance than the absence of LOC at the 1- and 2-year follow-up assessments. A well-controlled study used the Eating Disorder Examination to identify BED in a prospective study of the outcome of bariatric surgery after 1 year.[38] No differences in weight loss were found between patients with (22.1% weight loss) or without BED (24.2%) before surgery. Both groups of patients experienced significant reductions in several cardiovascular disease risk factors. In contrast with previous research, rates of subjective bulimic episodes (defined by LOC) were minimal at the 1-year follow-up and unrelated to weight loss.

In their comprehensive review of the literature, Wonderlich and colleagues[3] concluded that the hypothesis that BED influences the outcome of different weight loss treatments "is inconsistently supported in the empirical literature and the overall effect appears small. This is significant because these studies do not indicate that BWL experts or bariatric surgeons should modify their treatments for individuals with BED"[(p695)].

SUMMARY

The two specialty psychological therapies of CBT and IPT remain the treatments of choice for the full range of BED patients, particularly those with high levels of specific eating disorder psychopathology such as overvaluation of body shape and weight. They produce the greatest degree of remission from binge eating as well as improvement in specific eating disorder psychopathology and associated general psychopathology such as depression.

The CBT protocol evaluated in the research summarized above was the original manual from Fairburn and colleagues.[45] Fairburn[46] has subsequently developed a more elaborate and sophisticated form of treatment, namely, enhanced CBT (CBT-E) for eating disorders. Initial research suggests that CBT-E may be more effective than the earlier version with bulimia nervosa and Eating Disorder Not Otherwise Specified patients.[47] CBT-E has yet to be evaluated for the treatment of BED, although it would currently be the recommended form of CBT. Of relevance in this regard is that the so-called broad form of the new protocol includes 3 optional treatment modules that could be used to address more complex psychopathology in BED patients. One of the modules targeted at interpersonal difficulties is IPT, as described earlier in this chapter. Thus, the broader protocol could represent a combination of the two currently most effective therapies for BED. Whether this combined treatment proves more effective than either of the components alone, particularly for a subset of BED patients with more complex psychopathology, remains to be tested.

CBT-E also includes a module designed to address what Fairburn[46] terms "mood intolerance" (problems in coping with negative affect) that can trigger binge eating and purging. The content and strategies of this mood intolerance module overlap with the emotional regulation and distress tolerance skills training of Linehan's[48] dialectical behavior therapy (DBT). Two randomized controlled trials have tested the efficacy of an adaptation of DBT for the treatment of BED (DBT-BED) featuring mindfulness, emotion regulation, and distress tolerance training. A small study by Telch and colleagues[49] found that modified DBT-BED was more effective than a wait list control in eliminating binge eating. A second study showed that DBT-BED resulted in a significantly greater remission rate from binge eating at posttreatment than a group comparison treatment designed to control for nonspecific therapeutic factors such as treatment alliance and expectations.[50] This difference between the two treatments disappeared over a 12-month follow-up, indicating the absence of DBT-BED-specific influences on long-term outcomes.

Both CBT and IPT have been shown to be more effective in eliminating binge eating than BWL in controlled, comparative clinical trials. Nonetheless, BWL has been effective in reducing binge eating and associated eating problems in BED patients in some studies and might be suitable for treatment of BED patients without high levels of specific eating disorder psychopathology.[31,22] A finding worthy of future research is the apparent predictive value of early treatment response to BWL, indicating when BWL is likely to prove effective or not.[13] No evidence supports the concern that BWL's emphasis on moderate caloric restriction either triggers or exacerbates binge eating in individuals with BED.[43,51]

Initially, CBTgsh was recommended as a feasible first-line treatment that might be sufficient treatment for a limited subset of patients in a stepped care approach.[7] More recent research, however, has shown that CBTgsh seems to be as effective as a specialty therapy, such as IPT, with a majority of BED patients.[31,22] The subset of patients that did not respond well to CBTgsh in this research were those with a high level of specific eating disorder psychopathology, as noted. A plausible explanation for this moderator effect is that the original Fairburn[17] CBTgsh manual does not include an explicit emphasis on body shape and weight concerns. Subsequent implementation of this treatment has incorporated a module that directly addresses overvaluation of body shape and weight.[25] Future research should determine whether an expanded form of CBTgsh is suitable for the full range of patients with BED.

CBTgsh is recommended as a treatment for BED on two other counts. First, its brief and focused nature makes it cost effective.[26] Second, its structured format makes it more readily disseminable than other longer, multicomponent psychological therapies. It can be implemented by a wider range of treatment providers than more technically complex, time-consuming, and clinical expertise-demanding specialty therapies such as CBT-E and IPT. The latter evidence-based therapies are rarely available to patients with BED in routine clinical care settings.[6,52] Nevertheless, it must be noted that much of the research on CBTgsh to date has been conducted in an eating disorder specialty clinic setting. The degree to which the treatment can be adapted to a range of clinical service settings remains to be determined. In addition, little is known about the specific provider qualifications and level of expertise required to implement CBTgsh successfully. Despite its brief and focal nature, specific provider skills regarding what and what not to address in treatment are required.

Currently available pharmacologic treatments cannot be recommended for treatment of BED. Aside from the inconsistent results of existing studies, the striking absence of controlled long-term evaluation of such treatment argues against its use.

As summarized, the evidence-based treatments of CBT, IPT, and CBTgsh result in significant improvement and large treatment effects on multiple outcome measures aside from binge eating in overweight and obese patients. These include specific eating disorder psychopathology (eg, overvaluation of body shape and weight), general psychopathology (eg, depression), and psychosocial functioning. Moreover, these changes are typically well-maintained over 1 to 2 years of follow-up. The exception to this profile of improvement remains weight loss and its maintenance over time. These specialty psychological treatments do not produce weight loss, although successfully eliminating binge eating might protect against future weight gain. BWL consistently produces short-term weight loss, the extent of which has varied across different studies. Long-term weight loss has yet to be demonstrated, however. In this regard, the findings with obese patients with BED are not different than those on the treatment of obesity in general, in which there is little robust evidence of enduring weight loss effects of BWL.[53,54]

ACKNOWLEDGMENTS

The author thanks Laurie Zandberg, PsyM, and Rebecca Greif, PsyM, for the helpful comments in the preparation of this chapter.

REFERENCES

1. American Psychiatric Association. Diagnostic and statistical manual of mental disorders. 4th ed. Washington (DC): American Psychiatric Press; 1994.
2. American Psychiatric Association. Available at: www.DSM-5.org. Accessed May 2011.
3. Wonderlich SA, Gordon KH, Mitchell JE, et al. The validity and clinical utility of binge eating disorder. Int J Eat Disord 2009;42:687–705.
4. Goldschmidt AB, Hilbert A, Manwaring JL, et al. The significance of overvaluation of shape and weight in binge eating disorder. Behav Res Ther 2010;48:187–93.

5. Grilo CM, Hrabosky JI, White MA, et al. Overvaluation of shape and weight in binge eating disorder and overweight controls: refinement of BED as a diagnostic construct. J Abnorm Psychol 2008;117:414–9.
6. Wilson GT, Grilo C, Vitousek K. Psychological treatment of eating disorders. Am Psychol 2007;62:199–216.
7. National Institute for Clinical Excellence. Eating disorders— core interventions in the treatment and management of anorexia nervosa, bulimia nervosa and related eating disorders. NICE Clin. Guideline No. 9. London: NICE; 2004.
8. Wilson GT. Cognitive behavior therapy for eating disorders. In: Agras WS, editor. Handbook of eating disorders. New York: Oxford University Press; 2010. p. 331–47.
9. Munsch S, Biedert E, Meyer A, et al. A randomized comparison of cognitive behavioral therapy and behavioral weight loss treatment for overweight individuals with binge eating disorder. Int J Eat Disord 2007;40:102–13.
10. Grilo CM, Masheb RM, Wilson GT, et al. Cognitive-behavioral therapy, behavioral weight loss, and sequential treatment for obese patients with binge eating disorder: a randomized controlled trial. J Consult Clin Psychol 2011. [Epub ahead of print].
11. Agras WS, Telch CF, Arnow B, et al. Weight loss, cognitive-behavioral, and desipramine treatments in binge eating disorder: an additive design. Behav Ther 1994;25: 225–38.
12. Wilfley DE, Welch RR, Stein RI, et al. A randomized comparison of group cognitive-behavioral therapy and group interpersonal psychotherapy for the treatment of overweight individuals with binge eating disorder. Arch Gen Psychiatry 2002;59: 713–21.
13. Grilo CM, White MA, Wilson GT, et al. Rapid response predicts 12-month post-treatment outcomes in binge eating disorder: theoretical and clinical implications. Psychol Med 2011. [Epub ahead of print].
14. Devlin MJ, Goldfein JA, Petkova E, et al. Cognitive behavioral therapy and fluoxetine for binge eating disorder: two-year follow-up. Obes Res 2007;15:1702–9.
15. Grilo CM, Masheb RM, Wilson GT. Efficacy of cognitive behavioral therapy and fluoxetine for the treatment of binge eating disorder: a randomized double-blind placebo-controlled comparison. Biol Psychiatry 2005;57:301–9.
16. Ricca V, Mannucci E, Mezzani B, et al. Fluoxetine and fluvoxamine combined with individual cognitive-behavioral therapy in binge eating disorder: a one-year follow-up study. Psychother Psychosom 2001;70:298–306.
17. Fairburn CG. Overcoming binge eating. New York: Guilford Press; 1995.
18. Carter JC, Fairburn CG. Cognitive-behavioral self-help for binge eating disorder: a controlled effectiveness study. J Consult Clin Psychol 1998;66:616–23.
19. Loeb KL, Wilson GT, Gilbert JS, et al. Guided and unguided self-help for binge eating. Behav Res Ther 2000;38:259–72.
20. Grilo CM, Masheb RM. A randomized controlled comparison of guided self-help cognitive behavioral therapy and behavioral weight loss for binge eating disorder. Behav Res Ther 2005;43:1509–25.
21. Grilo CM, Masheb RM. Rapid response predicts binge eating and weight loss in binge eating disorder: findings from a controlled trial of orlistat with guided self-help cognitive behavioral therapy. Behav Res Ther 2007;45:2537–50.
22. Wilson GT, Wilfley DE, Agras WS, et al. Psychological treatments for Binge Eating Disorder. Arch Gen Psychiatry 2010;67:94–101.
23. Masheb RM, Grilo CM. Rapid response predicts treatment outcomes in binge eating disorder: implications for stepped care. J Consult Clin Psychol 2007;75:639–44.

24. Masheb RM, Grilo CM. Prognostic significance of two sub-categorization methods for the treatment of binge eating disorder: negative affect and overvaluation predict, but do not moderate, specific outcomes. Behav Res Ther 2008;46:428–37.
25. Striegel-Moore R, Wilson GT, DeBar L, et al. Guided self-help for the treatment of recurrent binge eating. J Consult Clin Psychol 2010;78:312–21.
26. Lynch FL, Dickerson J, Perrin N, et al. Cost-effectiveness of treatment for recurrent binge eating. J Consult Clin Psychol 2010;78:322–33.
27. Tanosky-Kraft M, Wilfley DE. Interpersonal psychotherapy for Bulimia Nervosa and Binge-Eating Disorder. In: Grilo C, Mitchell J, editors. The treatment of eating disorders: a clinical handbook. New York: Guilford Press; 2010. p. 271–93.
28. Wilfley DE, Agras WS, Telch CF, et al. Group cognitive-behavioral therapy and group interpersonal psychotherapy for the nonpurging bulimic individual: a controlled comparison. J Consult Clin Psychol 1993;61:296–305.
29. Agras WS, Telch CF, Arnow B, et al. Does interpersonal therapy help patients with binge eating disorder who fail to respond to cognitive-behavioral therapy? J Consult Clin Psychol 1995;63:356–60.
30. Mitchell JE, Halmi K, Wilson GT, et al. A randomized secondary treatment study of women with bulimia nervosa who fail to respond to CBT. Int J Eat Disord 2002;32: 271–81.
31. Sysko R, Hildebrandt T, Wilson GT, et al. Heterogeneity moderates treatment response among patients with Binge Eating Disorder. J Consult Clin Psychol 2010;78: 681–90.
32. Bodell P, Devlin MJ. Pharmacotherapy for Binge-Eating Disorder. In: Grilo C, Mitchell J, editors. The treatment of eating disorders: a clinical handbook. New York: Guilford Press; 2010. p. 402–14.
33. Reas DL, Grilo CM. Review and meta-analysis of pharmacotherapy for binge-eating disorder. Obesity 2008;16:2024–38.
34. Grilo CM, Masheb RM, Salant SL. Cognitive behavioral therapy guided self-help and orlistat for the treatment of binge eating disorder: a randomized, double-blind, placebo-controlled trial. Biol Psychiatry 2005;57:1193–201.
35. American Psychiatric Association. Practice guideline for treatment of patients with eating disorders. 3rd edition. Washington (DC): American Psychiatric Press; 2006.
36. Grilo CM, Masheb RM, Wilson GT. Rapid response to treatment for binge eating disorder. J Consult Clin Psychol 2006;74:602–12.
37. Walsh BT, Sysko R, Parides MK. Early response to desipramine among women with bulimia nervosa. Int J Eat Disord 2006;39:72–5.
38. Wadden T, Faulconbridge L, Jones-Corneille L, et al. Binge eating disorder and the outcome of bariatric surgery at one year: a prospective, observational study. Obesity 2011;19:1220–8.
39. Niego SH, Kofman MD, Weiss JJ, et al. Binge eating in the bariatric surgery population: a review of the literature. Int J Eat Disord 2007;40:349–59.
40. Wilfley DE, Wilson GT, Agras WS. The clinical significance of binge eating disorder. Int J Eat Disord 2003;34:S96–S106.
41. Blaine B, Rodman J. Responses to weight loss treatment among obese individuals with and without BED: a matched-study meta-analysis. Eat Weight Disord 2007;12: 54–60.
42. Pagoto S, Bodenlos J, Kantor L, et al. Association of major depression and binge eating disorder with weight loss in a clinical setting. Obesity (Silver Spring) 2007;15: 2557–9.
43. Bishop-Gilyard CT, Berkowitz RI, Wadden TA, et al. Weight reduction in obese adolescents with and without binge eating. Obesity 2011;19:982–7.

44. White MA, Kalarchian MA, Masheb RM, et al. Loss of control over eating predicts outcomes in bariatric surgery patients: a prospective, 24-month follow-up study. J Clin Psychiatry 2010;71:175–84.
45. Fairburn CG, Marcus MD, Wilson GT. Cognitive-behavioral therapy for binge eating and bulimia nervosa: A comprehensive treatment manual. In: Fairburn CG, Wilson GT, editors. Binge eating: nature, assessment and treatment. New York: Guilford Press; 1993. p. 361–414.
46. Fairburn CG. Cognitive behavior therapy and eating disorders. New York: Guilford Press; 2008.
47. Fairburn CG, Cooper Z, Doll HA, et al. Transdiagnostic cognitive-behavioral therapy for patients with eating disorders: a two-site trial with 60-week follow up. Am J Psychiatry 2009;166:311–9.
48. Linehan MM. Skills training manual for treating borderline personality disorder. New York: Guilford Press; 1993.
49. Telch CF, Agras WS, Linehan MM. Dialectical behavior therapy for binge eating disorder. J Consult Clin Psychol 2001;69:1061–5.
50. Safer DL, Robinson AH, Jo B. Outcome from a randomized controlled trial of group therapy for binge eating disorder: comparing dialectical behavior therapy adapted for binge eating to an active comparison group therapy. Behav Ther 2010;41:106–20.
51. National Task Force on the Prevention and Treatment of Obesity. Dieting and the development of eating disorders in overweight and obese adults. Arch Intern Med 2000;160:2581–9.
52. Crow SJ, Peterson C, Levine AS, et al. A survey of binge eating and obesity treatment practices among primary care providers. Int J Eat Disord 2004;35:348–53.
53. Brownell K. The humbling experience of treating obesity: should we persist or desist? Behav Res Ther 2010;48:717–9.
54. Cooper Z, Doll H, Hawker D, et al. Testing a new cognitive behavioral treatment for obesity: a randomized controlled trial with three-year follow-up. Behav Res Ther 2010;48:706–13.

Treatment of Night Eating Syndrome

Kelly C. Allison, PhD[a],*, Ellen P. Tarves, MA[b]

KEYWORDS

- Evening hyperphagia • Nocturnal ingestions
- Eating disorder-not otherwise specified
- Cognitive behavior therapy
- Selective serotonin reuptake inhibitors • Light therapy

The night eating syndrome (NES) was first described in 1955 as a disorder defined by morning anorexia, evening hyperphagia (consuming 25% of the daily food intake after the evening meal), and insomnia.[1] NES was originally thought to be a maladaptive response to stress in obese persons who were unsuccessful in weight loss treatment.[1] Attention to NES was neglected until the late 1990s, when the focus of eating-related research shifted in response to the growing prevalence of obesity in the United States.[2] The increased attention to NES within the past decade has prompted several modifications to its core diagnostic criteria, aided in a better understanding of its causes, and promoted interest in developing effective treatments. This article outlines the basic features of the syndrome and summarizes the treatment approaches that have been developed for NES.

CONCEPTUALIZATION AND CLINICAL CHARACTERISTICS

NES has been attributed to a delay in the circadian rhythm of eating, characterized by appetite suppression during morning hours and appetite increase during evening hours.[3] The diagnostic criteria of NES have been varied and disputed in the literature. NES is not listed in the *Diagnostic and Statistical Manual of Mental Disorders, Fourth Edition, Text Revision*,[4] although a consensus regarding its core diagnostic criteria was recently reached by a panel of NES experts (First International Night Eating Symposium, April 28, 2008).[5] According to proposed criteria, an individual must first endorse evening hyperphagia (consumption of at least 25% of daily intake after the evening meal) and/or 2 or more nocturnal ingestions (defined as waking up at night to eat) per week. In addition, an individual must experience at least three of the five following features: morning anorexia (defined as absence of morning appetite), a

[a] Department of Psychiatry, Perelman School of Medicine at the University of Pennsylvania, 3535 Market Street, 3rd Floor, Philadelphia, PA 19104-3309, USA
[b] Department of Psychology, LaSalle University, Philadelphia, PA, USA
* Corresponding author.
E-mail address: kca@mail.med.upenn.edu

Psychiatr Clin N Am 34 (2011) 785–796
doi:10.1016/j.psc.2011.08.002
0193-953X/11/$ – see front matter © 2011 Elsevier Inc. All rights reserved.

strong urge to eat between dinner and sleep onset and/or during nocturnal awakenings, insomnia at least 4 to 5 times per week, a belief that eating is necessary to initiate or return to sleep, and depressed mood that worsens during evening hours. Finally, an awareness and ability to recall evening or nocturnal ingestions must be present; this criterion is necessary to differentiate NES and sleep-related eating disorder (SRED), in which nocturnal ingestions occur without awareness and are unable to be recalled.[6] The host of symptoms associated with NES makes the syndrome best conceptualized as a combination of eating, sleeping, mood, and stress disorder features. Using the proposed criteria can help standardize NES assessment and diagnosis and can create a framework for future research of NES characteristics and treatments.

TREATMENT OF NIGHT EATING SYNDROME

Research on effective treatments specific to NES has been minimal, with just one randomized controlled trial published to date. Case reports and open-label trials have suggested benefit from a variety of strategies including pharmacologic treatment,[7] cognitive behavior therapy (CBT)[8] and several other treatment alternatives such as progressive muscle relaxation,[9] phototherapy,[10] and behavior therapy.[11] The authors present the information currently available, with the recommendation that further research be conducted within each of the treatment modalities to build upon the nascent literature base of effective treatments for NES.

Pharmacologic Interventions

Pharmacotherapy has received the most research attention of any NES treatment. To date, one case series,[12] two open-label trials,[13,14] and one randomized placebo-controlled trial[7] have examined the effectiveness of pharmacotherapy in the reduction of NES symptoms.

In the first pharmacotherapy study of NES, Miyaoka and colleagues[12] followed 4 NES patients throughout a treatment course of either paroxetine or fluvoxamine (selective serotonin reuptake inhibitors; SSRIs) and found that each patient reported a significant decrease in several core night eating symptoms. O'Reardon and colleagues[13] conducted a 12-week open-label trial of sertraline for 17 night eaters and found a significant reduction in the number of awakenings per week, number of nocturnal ingestions per week, and percentage of caloric intake consumed after the evening meal (**Table 1**). Patients whose NES symptoms remitted also averaged a 5-kg weight reduction at the end of active treatment, whereas patients whose symptoms did not remit averaged a 0.6-kg weight gain.

These results were supported by Stunkard and colleagues'[14] long-distance treatment trial of 50 NES patients. Patients who contacted the authors' program through their Web site consented to participate in an innovative trial in which they would receive treatment with sertraline prescribed by their own physician. Over the course of the 8-week study, they participated in phone or e-mail check-ins with study staff and completed questionnaires every 2 weeks to assess treatment effect. Significant improvements were noted on all core aspects of NES, including the Night Eating Symptom Scale (NESS),[13] nocturnal ingestions, percentage of intake after the evening meal, and weight (among overweight and obese participants) (see **Table 1**).

O'Reardon and colleagues[7] conducted the first randomized placebo-controlled trial of sertraline for the treatment of NES. Thirty-four participants diagnosed with NES were randomized to either an 8-week course of sertraline (n = 17) or to a placebo condition (n = 17). Sertraline dosages were administered flexibly and ranged from 50 mg/d to 200 mg/d across participants. The sertraline group reported significantly

Table 1
Treatment response (% reduction) across treatment trials for NES

Study	Treatment Delivered	No. of Participants	Duration (wk)	Mean Dose (mg)	NESS	Percentage of Intake After Dinner	No. of Total Awakenings	No. of Nocturnal Ingestions	Weight (kg)	BDI-II	QLES-Q
Pawlow et al[9]	APMR	10 active, 10 control	1	NA				0.8 vs 2.2 in 1 wk	−0.8 0.3	50% −5%	
O'Reardon et al[13]	Sertraline	17	12	188	24%	50%	60%	67%	−4.8 vs +0.6[a]	33%	−6%
Stunkard et al[14]	Sertraline	50	8	122	42%	66%	64%	70%	−3[b]	58%	19%
O'Reardon et al[7]	Sertraline or placebo	17 active, 17 placebo	8	127	57% 16%	68% 29%	74% 14%	81% 14%	−2.9[b] −0.3	55% 46%	15%
Allison et al[6]	Cognitive behavior therapy	25	12 (10 sessions)	NA	43%	29%	37%	70%	−3.1	28%	5%

Abbreviations: APMR, abbreviated progressive muscle relaxation; BDI-II, Beck Depression Inventory-II; NA, not applicable; NESS, Night Eating Symptom Scale; QLES-Q, Quality of Life, Satisfaction, and Enjoyment Questionnaire.
[a] Mean weight loss for those whose NES remitted on sertraline vs those who did not respond.
[b] Mean weight loss among overweight and obese participants.

greater reductions than the placebo group in the number of nocturnal ingestions, the number of total awakenings, and scores on the NESS. The percentage of calories consumed after the evening meal was reduced by 68% in the sertraline group and 29% in the control group, although this difference was not significant after statistical correction for multiple comparisons. Overweight patients in the sertraline group lost significantly more weight than overweight patients in the control group (2.9 kg vs 0.3 kg). Overall, 71% of patients on sertraline were classified as responders on the Clinical Global Impression of Improvement Scale as compared with 18% in the placebo group.

Improvements on the primary outcome measures were not significantly correlated with improvements on the Beck Depression Inventory-II (BDI),[15] suggesting that the participants did not decrease their night eating symptoms because of an improvement in mood. Instead, it seems that the sertraline had an independent effect on the disordered eating behaviors. The authors suggest that this research demonstrates the use of sertraline as a promising treatment for NES and its associated weight gain.

Sertraline case example

Julie was a high-functioning professional. She was married and the mother of two young adult children. Her daughter had been born prematurely and required 24-hour care for over a year. During this time Julie began eating while she was up caring for her daughter. Even after her daughter required less and less nighttime attention, Julie's nightly nocturnal ingestions continued.

Julie sought treatment 18 years after the onset of her nocturnal ingestions. She recalled that her father had also risen from bed to eat. Julie also described herself as a night owl; she would often stay up late at night and would graze on snacks during this time. Coupled with frequent breakfast skipping, she was consuming at least a quarter of her intake after dinner. Her nocturnal ingestions became more frequent, and at her initial evaluation she was eating 3 times per night. Typically she would have peanut butter and jelly sandwiches, cookies, fruit, other snacks, or leftovers. As she reached menopause, she found it increasingly difficult to lose weight even though she exercised regularly. At the time she sought treatment, her body mass index (BMI) was 31.5 kg/m^2 with her weight loss attempts through various structured programs, never yielding more than a 5-lb loss.

Julie also reported a history of restless legs syndrome and generalized anxiety disorder. She had been prescribed venlafaxine (75 mg) for her anxiety, gabapentin (600 mg) for her restless legs symptoms, and zolpidem (10 mg) for insomnia and restless legs symptoms. Julie stated that she had not thought to mention her night eating symptoms to her sleep doctor when she sought help for her restless legs syndrome and insomnia. After a comprehensive assessment by a psychiatrist with knowledge of NES, it was evident that the venlafaxine was increasing her restless legs symptoms, making it necessary to increase her dose of gabapentin over time, neither of which was helping her nocturnal ingestions. She was tapered from venlafaxine and simultaneously began taking sertraline. Within the first 2 weeks, Julie's nocturnal ingestions decreased to 2 episodes per week. She currently takes 100 mg of sertraline at dinnertime, and her dose of gabapentin has been decreased to 300 mg. She continues taking zolpidem. Most weeks she has reported no nocturnal ingestions, although breakthrough ingestions occur occasionally, typically related to pain due to an injury. She was looking forward to having surgery to alleviate this discomfort so that she could continue to experience nights free of eating. She was amazed that after all of these years she could sleep more soundly and start to lose weight more consistently. She still struggles to some extent with after-dinner snacking, but, overall she perceived a significant improvement in her control over her eating during this time.

Possible future therapeutic medication targets

The trials with sertraline are promising, but more treatment trials with other SSRIs and other agents are warranted. Some successful case reports of NES treatment with topiramate have been published, but no open-label or randomized trials have been conducted. These initial reports have described treatment with topiramate for persons with SRED, as well as those with NES. In these case descriptions, patients experience significant decreases in nocturnal ingestions, weight, and the percentage of calories consumed after dinner.[16,17] Controlled trials of topiramate and/or other similar antiepileptic agents may be warranted. Particular attention should be given to the neurologic side effects that may accompany topiramate such as confusion, memory difficulties, and difficulty concentrating. If these occur, the medication must be discontinued.

Contraindications

O'Reardon and colleagues[13] assessed previous medication trials for each of the participants presenting in their NES study. Not many of these trials had an effect, but of note, none of the participants described success with zolpidem or over-the-counter hypnotics. In fact, the participants reported that these agents promoted SRED. These medications helped them to fall asleep initially, but they still rose from bed during the night seeking food. The participants described little to no recollection of their eating during these occasions, and they found evidence of consuming larger amounts of foods than they typically ate when not taking the hypnotics. Others have since described this phenomenon in case studies.[18,19] Whereas the patient in the case study, Julia, did not experience SRED while taking zolpidem, if night eating is the presenting concern, hypnotics should not be the first line treatment. If patients are already taking a hypnotic, an assessment of the onset of nocturnal eating and level of awareness should be determined.

Cognitive Behavior Therapy

The first study to investigate cognitive behavioral therapy (CBT) for NES was conducted by Allison and colleagues[8] in response to the observed cognitive component of night eating behavior. A central feature of this disorder is, "If I don't eat, I won't be able to fall asleep." Vinai and colleagues[20] have found that this thought distinguishes persons with NES from those with binge eating disorder. Allison and colleagues[8] designed a cognitive behavioral treatment to target NES-specific symptoms by adapting features from CBT protocols for binge eating disorder[21] and behavioral weight loss.[22] The primary goal of CBT for NES is to correct the delay in circadian eating rhythms by shifting food intake to earlier in the day, while simultaneously interrupting the overlearned relationship between nighttime eating, faulty cognitions, and sleep onset.[23] The strategies used to achieve these treatment goals include a combination of behavioral weight management components (monitoring food consumption, regulating meals and snacks, restricting daily caloric intake) and cognitive therapy components (identifying, evaluating, and restructuring maladaptive thoughts).

Allison and colleagues[8] studied 25 participants with NES who were enrolled in a 10-session uncontrolled CBT intervention that lasted 12 weeks; 14 participants completed the treatment. It is difficult to know with certainty why the attrition rate was so high, but clinical observations suggested factors that included (1) feeling overwhelmed with keeping a food and sleep log each day and (2) not losing as much weight as desired in the early weeks. Future studies should stress the importance of daily logging and should set realistic weight management goals to help maximize treatment adherence.

Similar to observations from the sertraline treatment studies, significant reductions in all primary and secondary treatment outcomes were noted following completion of the 10-week CBT program, including reductions in the proportion of calories consumed after dinner, falling from 35% to 25%, and the number of nocturnal ingestions, falling from 8.7 per week to 2.6 per week (see **Table 1**). Mixed modeling regression models were used to account for participant drop-out. Closer examination of nighttime eating showed a significant reduction in the proportion of calories consumed between sleep onset and morning awakening (15% to 5%) but not in the proportion of calories consumed between the evening meal and sleep onset (21.8% to 21.0%). Results from secondary outcome measures indicated significant decreases in daily caloric intake (2365 kcal/d to 1759 kcal/d), total number of awakenings (13.5/wk to 8.5/wk), body weight (−3.1kg), and NESS scores (29 to 16). Finally, BDI-II scores significantly decreased (9 to 6.5) and Quality of Life, Satisfaction, and Enjoyment Questionnaire scores significantly increased (47.2 to 49.6), suggesting improved mood and quality of life, respectively. However, these latter improvements are small in magnitude when examining the clinical relevance of these changes. Study limitations, including the high attrition rate and the absence of a control group, require a tentative interpretation of the findings until these results are replicated under more controlled settings.

The implications from this research are promising and highlight the need for future randomized controlled trials. In particular, the CBT treatment seemed to be more effective in reducing eating during the night than in reducing the proportion of eating before bedtime. This result suggests that more time during sessions may be dedicated to addressing eating during the evening. It may be that more distress is associated with eating during the night, such that more effort is expended trying to eliminate that behavior. Future CBT studies for this population should improve intervention efforts in shifting this evening eating to earlier in the day.

Although food log data are imperfect, Allison and colleagues'[8] study suggested that patients can engage in behavioral weight loss while decreasing their nocturnal ingestions. The data revealed that participants had reduced their total daily intake by about 600 kcal/d, starting after week 3 when calorie counting was introduced. Given this information, the lack of change in the proportion of intake after the evening meal suggests that the circadian delay in energy intake remained present at the end of treatment, although not as pronounced when nocturnal ingestions were more frequent. It therefore seems that these individuals may benefit from maintaining their current level of energy intake but distributing it more evenly across breakfast, lunch, and daytime snacks. A recent study suggests that a positive and independent relationship exists between intake after 8 PM and BMI,[24] although larger studies are needed to confirm this finding.

CBT case example

Carol presented for treatment of her NES, stating that her night eating began in her teen years. She offered that both of her parents had NES and that her husband also now gets up to eat with her. When she married her husband and first lived independently at the age of 20, she did not think her NES was significant, because her parents did it too. Now in her 40s, the behavior had become particularly distressing because she was having trouble controlling her weight, which had risen to a BMI of

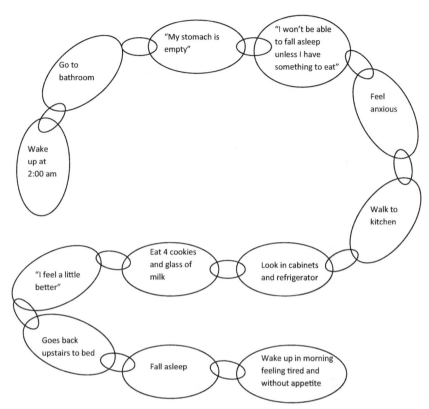

Fig. 1. Behavioral chain for Carol's typical night eating episode.

26 kg/m^2 from 21 kg/m^2 that she had maintained since the birth of her children about 20 years prior.

Carol woke most days before 7 AM. She drank coffee but did not eat until the afternoon, sometime between 12 and 2 PM; a couple days per week she did not eat anything until dinnertime. She prepared a home-cooked meal for dinner at 6 PM. Carol enjoyed coffee afterward but generally did not snack. Her bedtime has varied over the years, but at treatment intake she was going to bed at 9 or 10 PM without any initial insomnia. Then, every night at 2 AM, she awoke and felt compelled to eat. She would occasionally use the bathroom first, but then head to the kitchen where she would eat milk and cookies, pasta, peanut butter and jelly, and/or raisins (**Fig. 1**). She reported that before she goes to bed, she knows she will wake up to eat. She makes it a priority to have food on hand, even when traveling. She stated that she would surely be up all night if she did not have something to eat. She described her experience as feeling the need for her stomach to be full before she could go back to sleep.

At treatment baseline, she was consuming 25.1% of her intake after dinner, and she reported 6 awakenings with 6 nocturnal ingestions in the previous week. Her average daily caloric intake from her food and sleep journal was 2078 kcal, and her baseline NESS score was a 29. She reported no significantly depressed mood, with a BDI score of 5.

Carol successfully started using stimulus control techniques by ridding her kitchen of the foods she most often ate during the night. Living with her husband and son prevented complete control of these foods, but her nocturnal ingestions decreased slowly and consistently across the weeks. She also worked to eat earlier in the day and to monitor her caloric intake while aiming for a goal of 1200 to 1500 kcal/d. She also engaged in cognitive restructuring regarding her beliefs about her need to eat during the night. The authors framed their approach with the idea that she needed to retrain her body not to expect food during the night.

At the end of the 10 sessions, Carol reported her first week without any nocturnal ingestions. Her proportion of calories consumed after dinner had decreased to 16.3%, based on her food journal, and her NESS score decreased to 13. Her BDI score stayed low throughout treatment, ranging between a score of 0 and 3. Carol moved out of the country after treatment. At an 8-month follow-up, her NESS score remained at a 14, and she was consuming 14% of her intake after dinner. However, she reported 4 awakenings and 2 nocturnal ingestions in that previous week, suggesting that she could have benefitted from a longer duration of treatment or occasional booster sessions.

Behavioral and Light Therapies

Behavior therapy

Therapies traditionally used for the treatment of mood and anxiety disorders, such as behavior therapy, may also be adapted to successfully treat NES. To date, two case study reports have examined the effectiveness of behavioral therapy for NES. Coates[25] reported partial success for one NES client through behavioral techniques like leaving notes, restricting access to food, and chaining the refrigerator closed. After several modifications to his behavioral prevention plan, the client's night eating symptoms remitted and his morning anorexia improved. This behavioral plan remained effective in controlling the client's night eating symptoms at an 18-month follow up, but his symptoms reportedly returned if his plan was not in place.

Williamson and colleagues[26] designed a behavior contingency plan to target night eating symptoms in a woman with bulimia nervosa and rumination. This contingency plan was designed to extinguish the client's night eating by rewarding increasingly difficult treatment goals (eg, 1 night/wk without a binge episode, 2 nights/wk without a binge episode). Although the client experienced several lapses in the first phase of treatment, her symptoms remitted completely by treatment end and she remained symptom-free at 3-month and 2-year follow-up assessments. Because the client was also undergoing cognitive behavioral group therapy for her bulimia symptoms, the authors cautioned against drawing firm conclusions about the contingency plan's unique impact on her night eating symptoms.

Because NES has been associated with obesity, behavioral weight management may also represent a possible treatment approach. Gluck and colleagues[27] reported that patients with NES did not lose as much weight in a behavioral weight loss group as patients without NES. More recently, however, Dalle Grave and colleagues[11] compared obese night eaters pursuing weight loss treatment and matched controls following intensive inpatient weight loss treatment. Treatment included psychoeducation, a low-calorie diet, and regular exercise. At program completion, patients with NES and matched controls did not differ in weight loss at program completion or at the 6-month follow-up assessment. However, only 8 of the 32 patients with NES continued to endorse clinically significant night eating symptoms at the 6-month follow up. Although night eating symptoms were not a specific treatment target, the authors posited that the intensity of the dietary and behavioral weight loss strategies effectively treated NES by reducing nighttime hunger and resetting circadian eating rhythms. Dalle Grave and colleagues'[11] results suggest a promising future for behavioral weight management in NES treatment, although future studies should explore the efficacy of less intensive programs.

Progressive muscle relaxation

Progressive muscle relaxation (PMR) is a therapeutic technique designed to achieve muscular relaxation through the tension and release of various muscle groups.[28] Additionally, PMR has been shown to alleviate a variety of cognitive and physical conditions including anxiety[29] and psychological and physiologic stress.[30] Pawlow and colleagues[9] conducted the first controlled treatment trial of PMR for NES. Ten participants who met criteria for NES and received 1 week of abbreviated progressive muscle relaxation (APMR) were compared with a control group of NES participants who did not receive the APMR intervention. The intervention group demonstrated a significant reduction in evening hyperphagia and increase in morning appetite. The treatment group also evidenced reductions in stress, anxiety, fatigue, anger, depression, and cortisol levels. The authors concluded that APMR represents a valid treatment choice for NES patients.

A major limitation of this trial was its brevity. Future studies should follow adherence and outcome over a longer period of time. This criticism applies to all of the trials described thus far. None has demonstrated efficacy longer than 12 weeks, which is a clear weakness of this literature.

Phototherapy

Phototherapy was first introduced as a treatment for seasonal affective disorder in 1984 by Rosenthal and colleagues.[31] After witnessing changes in mood that followed seasonal patterns, Rosenthal and colleagues[31] proposed that melatonin played a role in the onset of seasonal depression and that adjusting the levels of melatonin in the body would lead to symptom improvement. Because NES has been conceptualized as a disorder of circadian rhythm and because melatonin is involved in the regulation of circadian rhythms, phototherapy has been proposed as a logical treatment choice for NES.

Two case studies of phototherapy for NES have been published. In one, a 51-year-old obese woman presented with comorbid depression and night eating; she was already receiving pharmacotherapy (paroxetine) for her symptoms, but it was not effective in significantly reducing them. She was exposed to 30-minute sessions of 10,000-lux white light therapy each morning for a period of 2 weeks.[32] After completing her phototherapy program, the client no longer met clinical criteria for major depression or night eating. Although the woman's night eating symptoms returned at the 1-month follow-up assessment, they fully remitted following 12 additional days of phototherapy.

A second case study involved a 46-year-old nonobese man presenting to treatment with nonseasonal recurrent major depression and NES.[10] This client was prescribed 30 minutes of phototherapy (10,000 lux) every morning for 14 days. Upon completing the 2-week phototherapy program, both depressive and NES symptoms significantly improved, and the client no longer met diagnostic criteria for either disorder. The results of these case studies suggest that phototherapy may have a role in treating comorbid depression and NES. However, future research is needed to confirm the validity of these initial findings, as well as the effect on NES for patients presenting without comorbid depression.

SUMMARY

Although treatment research for NES remains limited, several options are available for patients whose symptoms require clinical attention. Pharmacotherapy has received the most empirical support of the proposed treatments. Controlled trials are needed to confirm the initial results from pilot studies with CBT, behavioral therapy, and phototherapy, and an extended controlled trial of progressive muscle relaxation would be useful.

In their comprehensive review of the field, Striegel-Moore and colleagues[33] have questioned the clinical utility of NES as a diagnostic entity and stress the very limited nature of treatment studies to date. Research in this field has to provide a systematic examination of the approaches described here, as well as others yet to be identified. This pursuit seems warranted given that persons suffering with the cluster of symptoms identified as NES are approaching health care providers for relief and are often frustrated by the lack of recognition of this syndrome.[34]

Future studies should test a wider variety of medications that would target serotonin or the circadian timing of eating. Additionally, trials comparing and combining medication treatments and CBT (or progressive muscle relaxation alone) would also be useful in addressing which treatment should be used as a first line treatment. With NES being considered for inclusion as a Feeding and Eating Condition Not Elsewhere Classified (FEC-NEC) in the *Diagnostic and Statistical Manual of Mental Disorders, Fifth Edition*,[35] it is likely that more clinical attention and studies will address these important issues in the coming years.

REFERENCES

1. Stunkard AJ, Grace WJ, Wolff HG. The night-eating syndrome: a pattern of food intake among certain obese patients. Am J Med 1955;19:78–86.
2. Birketvedt GS, Florholmen J, Sundsfjord J, et al. Behavioral and neuroendocrine characteristics of the night-eating syndrome. JAMA 1999;282:657–63.
3. Stunkard AJ, Allison KC. Two forms of disordered eating in obesity: binge eating and night eating. Int J Obesity Relat Metab Disord 2003;27:1–12.
4. American Psychiatric Association. Diagnostic and Statistical Manual of Mental Disorders. 4th edition. Text Revision. Washington, DC: American Psychiatric Association; 2000.
5. Allison KC, Lundgren JD, O'Reardon, J, et al. Proposed diagnostic criteria for night eating syndrome. Int J Eat Disord 2010;43:241–7.
6. Howell MJ, Schenck CH, Crow SJ. A review of nighttime eating disorders. Sleep Med Rev 2009;13:23–34.
7. O'Reardon JP, Allison KC, Martino NS, et al. A randomized placebo controlled trial of sertraline in the treatment of the night eating syndrome. Am J Psychiatry 2006;163: 893–8.
8. Allison KC, Lundgren J, Moore RH, et al. Cognitive behavior therapy for night eating syndrome: a pilot study. Am J Psychother 2010;64:91–106.
9. Pawlow LA, Jones GE. The impact of abbreviated progressive muscle relaxation on salivary cortisol. Biol Psychol 2002;60:1–16.
10. Friedman S, Even C, Dardennes R, et al. Light therapy, non-seasonal depression, and night eating syndrome. Can J Psychiatry 2004;49:790.
11. Dalle Grave R, Calugi S, Ruocco A, et al. Night eating syndrome and weight loss outcome in obese patients. Int J Eat Disord 2011;44:150–6.

12. Miyaoka T, Yasukawa R, Tsubouchi K, et al. Successful treatment of nocturnal eating/drinking syndrome with selective serotonin reuptake inhibitors. Int Clin Psychopharmacol 2003;18:175-7.

13. O'Reardon JP, Stunkard AJ, Allison KC. A clinical trial of sertraline in the treatment of the night eating syndrome. Int J Eat Disord 2004;35:16-26.

14. Stunkard AJ, Allison KC, Lundgren JD, et al. A paradigm for facilitating pharmacotherapy at a distance: sertraline treatment of the night eating syndrome. J Clin Psychiatry 2006;67:1568-72.

15. Beck AT, Steer RA, Brown GK. BDI-II manual. San Antonio (TX): Harcourt Brace; 1996.

16. Winkelman JW. Treatment of nocturnal eating syndrome and sleep-related eating disorder with topiramate. Sleep Med 2003;4:243-6.

17. Allison KC. Treatment of the night eating syndrome. Symposium talk presented at: Annual meeting of the Eating Disorders Research Society. Toronto (Canada), September 30, 2005.

18. Morgenthaler TI, Silber MH. Amnestic sleep-related eating disorder associated with zolpidem. Sleep Med 2002;3:323-7.

19. Najjar M. Zolpidem and amnestic sleep related eating disorder, J Clin Sleep Med 2007;3:637-8.

20. Vinai P, Allison KC, Cardetti S, et al. Psychopathology and treatment of night eating syndrome: a review. Eat Weight Disord 2008;13:54-63.

21. Fairburn CG, Marcus MD, Wilson GT. Cognitive-behavioral therapy for binge eating and bulimia nervosa: a comprehensive treatment manual. In: Fairburn CG, Wilson GT, editors. Binge eating: nature, assessment, and treatment. New York: Guilford Press; 1993. p. 361-404.

22. Brownell KD. The LEARN program for weight management. 10th edition. Dallas (TX): LEARN—The Lifestyle Company; 2004.

23. Allison KC, Stunkard AJ. Treatment for night eating syndrome. In: Grilo CM, Mitchell JE, editors. The treatment of eating disorders. New York: Guilford Press; 2010. p. 458-70.

24. Baron KG, Reid KJ, Kern AS, et al. Role of sleep timing in caloric intake and BMI. Obesity (Silver Spring) 2011;19:1374-81.

25. Coates TJ. Successive self-management strategies towards coping with night eating. J Behav Ther Exper Psychiatry 1978;9:181-3.

26. Williamson DA, Lawson OD, Bennett SM, et al. Behavioral treatment of night bingeing and rumination in an adult case of bulimia nervosa. J Behav Ther Exper Psychiatry 1989;20:73-7.

27. Gluck ME, Geliebter A, Satov T. Night eating syndrome is associated with depression, low self-esteem, reduced daytime hunger, and less weight loss in obese outpatients. Obes Res 2001;9:264-7.

28. Jacobson E. Progressive relaxation. 2nd edition. Oxford (England): University of Chicago Press; 1938.

29. Conrad A, Roth WT. Muscle relaxation therapy for anxiety disorders: it works but how? J Anxiety Disord 2007;21:243-64.

30. Pawlow LA, O'Neil PM, Malcolm RJ. Night eating syndrome: Effects of brief relaxation training on stress, mood hunger and eating patterns. Int J Obes Relat Metab Disord 2003;27:970-8.

31. Rosenthal NE, Sack DA, Gillin C, et al. Seasonal affect disorder: a description of the syndrome and preliminary findings with light therapy. Arch Gen Psychiatry 984;41:72-80.

32. Friedman S, Even C, Dardennes R, et al. Light therapy, obesity, and night-eating syndrome. Am J Psychiatry 2002;159:875-6.

33. Striegel-Moore RH, Franko D, Garcia J. The validity and utility of night eating syndrome. Int J Eat Disord 2009;42:720–38.

34. Goncalves MD, Moore RH, Stunkard AJ, et al. The treatment of night eating: the patient's perspective. Eur Eat Disord Rev 2009;17:184–90.

35. American Psychiatric Association. DSM-5 development Web site. Available at: http://www.dsm5.org. Accessed August 1, 2011.

Medical and Behavioral Evaluation of Patients with Obesity

Robert F. Kushner, MD[a],*, David B. Sarwer, PhD[b]

KEYWORDS
• Overweight • Obesity • Behavior change • Weight loss

Overweight and obesity are the most common medical problems seen in primary care practice, together affecting over 68% of adults and 31.7% of children and adolescents in the United States.[1,2] Obesity is known to affect at least nine organ systems and is linked to the most prevalent and costly medical problems seen in daily practice. Successful treatment and control of obesity has the potential to have a significant impact on several chronic diseases. Yet despite the importance of screening and evaluating for obesity—and the recommendation to do so from multiple organizations[3–10]—detection and counseling rates among physicians remain low.[11–14] On the other hand, several observational studies have shown that physician acknowledgment of patients' excess weight increases the likelihood of behavior change.[15–17] Reasons for this delayed action include lack of education and training in obesity management, time restraints, lack of reimbursement for obesity as a diagnostic code, and clinician attitudes of futility and lack of perceived benefit and reward. The ill fortune of this "clinical inertia" toward obesity care is that the most successful treatment is likely to be early intervention and prevention, prior to development of more severe obesity and comorbid conditions.

Here, we review the current recommendations for medical evaluation of the obese adult patient as would be done by a physician. We begin with an overview of the identification and evaluation of the patient who could benefit from weight reduction. We detail the central aspects of obtaining a patient's history with obesity, with a particular focus on dietary, behavioral, and psychosocial contributions to the devel-

Portions of this article were previously published in Kushner RF, Roth JL. Medical evaluation of the obese individual. Psychiatr Clin N Am 2005;89–103.
[a] Northwestern Comprehensive Center on Obesity, Northwestern University Feinberg School of Medicine, 750 North Lake Shore Drive, Rubloff 9-976, Chicago, IL 60611, USA
[b] Departments of Psychiatry and Surgery, Center for Weight and Eating Disorders, Perelman School of Medicine at the University of Pennsylvania, 3535 Market Street, Suite 3026, Philadelphia, PA 19104, USA
* Corresponding author.
E-mail address: rkushner@northwestern.edu

opment and maintenance of obesity. We then turn to the physical examination of the obese patient and conclude with a brief discussion of the high-risk patient.

IDENTIFICATION AND EVALUATION OF THE OBESE PATIENT

In 1998, the National Heart, Lung, and Blood Institute (NHLBI) published the Clinical Guidelines on the Identification, Evaluation, and Treatment of Overweight and Obesity in Adults to provide guidance to physicians and associated health professionals and evidence for the effects of obesity treatment.[3] This 228-page document contains over 750 references and is an excellent resource on the research supporting the relationship between obesity and comorbid conditions, and on various treatment approaches. The Practical Guide to the Identification, Evaluation, and Treatment of Overweight and Obesity in Adults was subsequently developed cooperatively by the NHLBI and North American Association for the Study of Obesity (NAASO; now called The Obesity Society) and published in 2000.[18] The expert panel for the update of the Clinical Guidelines on the Identification, Evaluation, and Treatment of Overweight and Obesity in Adults (Obesity II) is currently underway. Guidelines specific to children and adolescents have been published by the American Academy of Pediatrics.[19] The guidelines recommend proactive obesity care beginning with identification, classification, and categorization of risk. Readers are also referred to the American Medical Association's Assessment and Management of Adult Obesity: A Primer for Physicians.[20] The Primer consists of 10 booklets covering: the evaluation process; assessing readiness and making treatment decisions; setting up the office environment; communication and counseling strategies; using dietary, physical activity, pharmacological and surgical management; and suggested resources. Each booklet begins with a case presentation and is subdivided by targeted patient care oriented questions that emphasize practical tips and expected outcomes. Much of the information from the resources is summarized below.

TAKING AN OBESITY-FOCUSED HISTORY

The first step in initiating obesity care is to take a comprehensive history that addresses issues and concerns specific to obesity treatment. This "obesity-focused" history allows the physician to develop tailored treatment recommendations that are more consistent with the needs and goals of the individual patient. Information from the history should address the following six general questions:

1. *What factors contribute to the patient's obesity?*
2. *How is the obesity affecting the patient's health?*
3. *What is the patient's level of risk regarding obesity?*
4. *What are the patient's goals and expectations for weight control?*
5. *Is the patient motivated and engaged to enter a weight management program?*
6. *What kind of help does the patient need?*

The following specific information is pertinent to an obesity-focused history.

CHRONOLOGICAL HISTORY OF WEIGHT GAIN

Age at onset, description of weight gain (and loss), and precipitating events provide clues to potential factors contributing to the patient's obesity and how the patient views his or her weight. Asking the patient to graph her weight pattern over time is a useful reflective and oftentimes therapeutic activity. This material also may be available in an electronic medical record. Common patterns include progressive weight gain, weight cycling, "yo-yo" dieting, and periods of weight stability followed

Table 1
Medications associated with body fat weight gain
Psychiatric/Neurological
Anti-psychotic agents: phenothiazines, olanzapine, clozapine, risperidone
Mood stabilizers: lithium
Anti-depressants: tricyclics, MAOIs, SSRIs (paroxetine), mirtazapine
Antiepileptic Drugs: gabapentin, valproate, carbamazepine
Steroid Hormones
Corticosteriods
Progestational steroids
Anti-diabetes Agents
Insulin, Sulfonylureas, Thiazolidinediones
Anti-hypertensive Agents
Beta- and alpha-1 adrenergic receptor blockers
Antihistamines
Cyproheptadine
HIV Protease inhibitors: lipodystrophy (central obesity)

by weight gain. Rapid cycling of weight often reflects mood instability or "all-or-nothing thinking" with respect to a patient's perceived ability to successfully control her eating behavior and, subsequently, weight. For many patients, weight gain initially occurs or is accelerated coincident to smoking cessation, initiation of a medication, or change in life events, such as a change in marital status, occupation, or illness. At-risk times for women include pregnancy, child rearing years (25–34 years old), and menopause. A familial predisposition should be considered if at least one first-degree relative is also obese and/or if the patient reports an onset of obesity prior to puberty.

Although the vast majority of overweight and obesity can be attributed to behavioral changes in diet and physical activity patterns, the patient's history may suggest several less common secondary causes that may warrant further evaluation. Endocrinologic disorders causing obesity are exceedingly uncommon, with the exception of polycystic ovarian syndrome (PCOS),[21] which should be considered in a woman who has clinical evidence of hyperandrogenism (ie, hirsutism, acne or alopecia), irregular menstrual cycles, and obesity. Although it is not a diagnostic criterion, approximately 50% of women with PCOS are obese, and 50% to 70% have insulin resistance and hyperinsulinemia.[22] Other endocrinologic etiologies include hypothyroidism, Cushing's syndrome, and hypothalamic tumors or damage to this part of the brain as a consequence of irradiation, infection, or trauma.

MEDICATION HISTORY

A thorough medication history should always be taken to uncover possible drug-induced weight gain, as well as for medications interfering with weight loss.[23–26] **Table 1** provides a list of medications that are associated with body fat weight gain. Medications should always be considered when there is a change in the trajectory of body weight coincident with starting a new medication. Other drugs such as nonsteroidal anti-inflammatory drugs and calcium-channel blockers have been associated with peripheral edema rather than body fat weight gain. When possible, an alternative medication that is weight-neutral or weight-losing should be prescribed.

With the recent growth in popularity of bariatric surgery, there is concurrent concern about patients' abilities to appropriately absorb medications postoperatively. This is of particular concern for psychiatric medications.[27] Unfortunately, there is little research to guide clinical practice in this area.

ENVIRONMENTAL FACTORS
Diet

The environmental factors and eating behaviors of the patient are important causes to consider. It is useful to review patients' eating habits—when and where they eat, who shops and cooks in the home, etc. Portion sizes, snacking, and beverage intake are evaluated. This information provides a sense of overall nutritional knowledge and also can be used to target specific problematic behaviors that need to be improved. Although other members of the treatment team, such as a nurse, registered dietitian, or clinical psychologist, may review this information, we believe it is useful to be reviewed by the physician, as well. At a minimum, the repetition underscores to patients the importance of changing these behaviors to optimize weight loss.

A dietary history can be obtained either by having the patient fill out a short questionnaire while in the waiting room or by assessing it as part of the patient interview. A useful and convenient technique is to ask the patient to describe a typical day. *"I want to learn more about your diet. Can you take me through a typical day or an example of a day, starting first thing in the morning and continuing into the evening?"* This open-ended and nonjudgmental approach allows patients to reveal their dietary pattern without guilt, shame, or embarrassment.

The purpose of this question is to obtain a description of the patient's habitual diet regarding meal and snack patterns, selection of types of foods and beverages, frequency of intake of food groups, and portion sizes. Since weekday dietary patterns are often different from weekend patterns, a brief dietary recall of both may be useful. Dietary behaviors such as where food is eaten, what triggers eating, and whether the patient engages in binge eating is also important information. For some patients, their habitual diet may be well managed but episodically uncontrolled due to stress or mood. More detailed information can be obtained by asking the patient to keep a food and activity diary for several days to a week. This can be easily done with the use of one of several electronic tracking programs that are available on the Internet. This exercise serves to increase the patient's awareness of their dietary habits and forms the basis for targeted changes. It also may provide clues about a patient's ability and willingness to follow behavioral recommendations.

The eating behavior and dietary intake of patients often ranges greatly. Many patients are likely consuming more than the 2000 kcal/day recommended by the United States Department of Agriculture and other government agencies.[28] Some patients will report eating 3000 to 4000 kcal/day with many meals consisting of food from fast food or take-out restaurants and including sweetened beverages. In contrast, some patients, often those working diligently to control their type 2 diabetes, will report quite healthy eating habits. Nevertheless, many patients who present for weight loss report difficulties controlling their eating behavior in response to emotional or social cues.

Persons with obesity often consume large amounts of high-caloric beverages, including regular soda, iced tea, fruit juice, and sports drinks. Unfortunately, many individuals are unaware that these calories may be making a significant contribution to their weight problem. Thus, the physician should always ask about beverage intake. If patients will be returning for treatment, they should be instructed to begin recording their food and beverage intake following the assessment.

The presence of disordered eating should be assessed. One disorder that warrants particular attention is binge eating disorder (BED), which is characterized by the consumption of an objectively large amount of food in a brief period of time (eg, 2 hours) with the patient's report of loss of control during the overeating episode.[29,30] (Patients do not engage in a compensatory behavior, such as vomiting, laxative abuse, or excessive exercise, which distinguishes BED from bulimia nervosa.) Binge eating occurs in only about 2% of the general population, but is found in approximately 15% to 20% of obese persons treated in specialty clinics.[31] Obese binge eaters may require psychotherapeutic treatment either before or in addition to weight reduction.

Another condition to be assessed is night eating. Night eating is defined as a circadian delay in the pattern of eating, characterized by evening hyperphagia (ie, the consumption of 25% or greater of total daily caloric intake after the evening meal) and/or three or more nocturnal ingestions (ie, waking during the sleep period to eat).[32,33] The presence of night eating also may contribute to the development and maintenance of obesity.

Physical Activity

The physician also should inquire about the patient's current level of physical activity. Patients should be asked about their participation in traditional forms of exercise, such as jogging or aerobics. In addition, patients should be asked about their daily lifestyle activity, such as stair use and daily walking.[34] Many obese individuals are quite sedentary, frequently due to the physical discomfort associated with activity.

An informative open-ended question to begin the discussion around the issue of physical activity is, *"What is the most physically active thing you do over the course of a week?"* In today's society, walking to or from the car, train, or bus often represents the extent of daily physical activity for many individuals.

Previous Weight Loss History

Patients should be asked about their experience with self-directed diets, commercial weight loss programs, dietary counseling, portion-controlled or meal replacement programs, as well as over-the-counter and prescription weight loss medications. Some patients also choose complementary and alternative medicine approaches to weight control based on their beliefs and attitudes.[35]

Many patients with obesity are "dieting veterans" who have tried numerous weight loss programs, some of which may have been appropriate and others that may have been less appropriate and potentially dangerous. Questions from the physician should focus on why they felt they were (or were not) successful, what elements of the programs were most useful or not helpful, and what led to eventual recidivism of behaviors. Exploration of the reasons for triggering entry into past weight loss attempt as well as what factors caused disengagement of the attempts are often quite revealing. A helpful empathic question is, *"What is hard about managing your weight?"*

PSYCHOSOCIAL ISSUES

The physician should assess psychological, behavioral, and social factors that may contribute to obesity and weight loss. This includes an assessment of patients' psychiatric status and history, as should be done routinely during a history and physical exam. Particular attention should be paid to the presence of mood and anxiety disorders, which are the most common disorders in the general population and also occur with high rates among persons with obesity.

Although obesity has never been categorized as a psychiatric disorder in the Diagnostic and Statistical Manual,[29] many lay persons and professionals erroneously believe that obesity is a direct result of psychopathology. Among obese patients treated in university and hospital-based clinics, approximately 25% to 35% of individuals present with comorbid psychopathology.[36] Many of these conditions can negatively affect behavioral weight control strategies and contraindicate treatment. Bulimia nervosa warrants mental health treatment independent of weight reduction. Persons with an active substance abuse disorder and those with an active psychosis are inappropriate for weight loss treatment.[37]

Several studies have suggested a relationship between excess body weight and depression. Persons with extreme obesity, for example, are almost five times more likely to have experienced an episode of major depression in the past year compared with average weight individuals.[38] This relationship appears to be stronger for women than men, perhaps because of our society's emphasis on female physical appearance. Obese women were more likely to experience a major depressive episode in the past year as compared with average weight women.[39] In contrast, in men, obesity was associated with significantly reduced risks of depression as compared with men of average weight.

The directionality of the relationship between obesity and depression is unclear.[40] For many obese persons, increased symptoms of depression may be a result of their obesity rather than a cause of it. The physical discomfort and challenges of being obese, as well as the associated health problems, may have a quite understandable impact on an individual's mood. Even as experts attempt to educate the public on the multifactoral nature of obesity, many individuals see obesity as a result of depression, an inability to control one's impulses, or even a moral failing. Unfortunately, some physicians and other medical professionals who work with obese individuals also hold these beliefs, which likely compromises their ability to effectively treat these persons. For these reasons, the physician should assess the presence of depressive symptoms.

The mood, affect, and overall presentation of the patient will provide important clues to the presence of a mood disorder. If one is suspected, neurovegetative symptoms should be assessed, including sleep, appetite, and concentration. Patients who endorse these symptoms also should be asked about the frequency of crying, irritability, social isolation, feelings of hopelessness, and the presence of suicidal thoughts. Mild forms of depression, or those related to the patient's current body weight, can frequently be treated simultaneously with weight management. The occurrence of a major depressive episode, however, may contraindicate behavioral weight control efforts until the mood disorder is treated and stabilized.[41]

The physician also should obtain a psychiatric treatment history. This should include directed questions about both outpatient psychopharmacological and psychotherapeutic treatments, as well as psychiatric hospitalizations. Large numbers of persons with obesity are engaged in mental health treatment. For example, up to 40% of patients with extreme obesity who present for bariatric surgery are engaged in some form of mental health treatment, and approximately 50% report a history of mental health treatment.[42] The most common form of treatment appears to be the use of a psychiatric medication (typically relatively low dosages of the serotonin reuptake inhibitors for depression and anxiety), prescribed by a primary care physician.

Beyond screening for psychopathology, it is important to assess other areas of psychosocial functioning. Numerous studies have shown a relationship between excess body weight and decreases in quality of life.[43–45] Individuals with obesity often report significant difficulties with physical functioning (eg, climbing stairs) and occupational functioning. These impairments likely motivate many individuals to seek weight loss.

Body image is an important aspect of quality of life for many individuals. Body image dissatisfaction is common in overweight and obese individuals, as it for women and girls of average weight.[46] The degree of dissatisfaction seems to be directly related to the amount of excess weight a person has, although persons can report dissatisfaction with their entire bodies or with specific features.[47] Body image dissatisfaction is believed to motivate patients to pursue appearance-enhancing behaviors, including health club memberships and cosmetic surgery.[48] It also is believed to play an influential role in the decision to seek weight loss.

Obesity also may affect marital and sexual relationships. The impact of excess body weight on marital relationships is complex. Many patients intuitively believe that weight loss will improve romantic relationships. Others fear that the changes in weight and physical appearance will change these relationships in less positive ways. Similarly, little is known about the relationship between excess body weight and sexual function, although studies have suggested that excess body weight can negatively affect sexual functioning (Sarwer DB, Spitzer JC, Lavery M. A review of the relationships between extreme obesity, quality of life, and sexual function. Submitted for publication.). Given the complexity of these relationships, individuals interested in weight loss are encouraged to discuss with their partners the impact of weight loss on their romantic relationships.

Other individuals, particularly those with extreme obesity, may report experiences of discrimination. Persons with obesity are less likely to complete high school, are less likely to marry, and earn less money compared with average weight persons.[49,50] They often report overt discrimination in a number of settings, including educational, employment, and even health care settings.

Timing of Weight Loss

Another important part of the assessment is the timing of the weight loss effort. Ideally, patients are motivated to engage in weight loss at a time that is relatively free of major life stressors. Thus, the presence of these stressors should be assessed. Increased stress is associated with attrition from weight reduction treatment.[51] Thus, the patient should be relatively free of stressors when undertaking weight loss surgery. Weight maintenance rather than weight loss should be encouraged during periods of high stress. An understanding of patient's motivation and stress level will help both the patient and practitioner determine the patient's readiness to change maladaptive behaviors.

According to the health belief behavior model, individuals are not likely to initiate behavior change unless they feel that their health is threatened and that the threat can be lessened by taking action. In many circumstances, the current or presenting complaint is linked to the burden of excess body weight. Targeted questions, such as *"How does your body weight affect you?"* and *"Is there anything that you cannot do because of your weight?"* are useful in obtaining this information. These triggers also serve as useful motivators that should be monitored during weight management.

Weight Loss Expectations

The assessment of weight loss expectations is another important part of the initial evaluation. Unrealistic expectations may result in disappointment and frustration regardless of the weight loss outcome. Patient goals are often stated as achieving specific body weights, wearing certain clothes sizes, gaining a more attractive physical appearance, or improving their overall health status or an obesity-related medical problem.

One of the greatest challenges for health professionals working with obese patients is helping them adopt more realistic weight loss goals. Unrealistic expectations are common regardless of the weight loss approach. Individuals enrolled in behavioral modification programs have been shown to have "goal" weight losses of 33%, comparable to the weight losses seen with bariatric surgery.[52] Although these unrealistic expectations were once thought to put individuals at risk for weight regain, recent studies have suggested that they are unrelated to weight loss.[53]

Studies suggest that a 10% weight loss, even if the patient remains overweight, often improves many of the health complications of obesity.[3] The health benefits of the loss should be emphasized to the patient. Patients also should be educated about improvements in mobility, appearance, body image, and self-esteem that are associated with these losses.[54] Such discussion may be particularly important for patients with a biological predisposition for obesity. These patients may be able to achieve these weight losses; however, it may be unlikely that these individuals will attain an average body weight (BMI ≤25) and maintain that weight for an extended period of time.

PHYSICAL EXAMINATION OF THE OBESE PATIENT

According to the NHLBI guidelines, assessment of risk status due to overweight or obesity is based on the patient's body mass index, waist circumference, and the existence of comorbid conditions. BMI is calculated as weight (kg)/height (m)^2, or as weight (in pounds $\times$ 703)/height (inches)^2. A BMI table is more conveniently used for simple reference (**Fig. 1**). The BMI is recommended because it provides an estimate of body fat and is related to risk of disease. A desirable or healthy BMI is 18.5 to 24.9 kg/m^2, overweight is 25 to 29.9 kg/m^2, and obesity is $\geq$ 30 kg/m^2. Obesity is further subdefined into class I (30.0–34.9 kg/m^2), class II (35.0–39.9 kg/m^2) and class III ($\geq$40 kg/m^2); **Table 2**. Although 'morbid obesity' is still listed in the ICD-9-CM and ICD-10-CM for coding purposes, other descriptive terms include class III obesity, extreme obesity, or clinically severe obesity.

In practice, after obtaining the patient's measured height and weight, the BMI Table (**Fig. 1**) and Classification Table (see **Table 2**) should be used to categorize overweight and obesity and to document this information in the medical record. Actual measurement of weight and height may not be a routine process of care in the psychiatric office. However, this is an important first step in the identification of an at-risk individual and during re-evaluation. Small amounts of weight gain will likely be missed if the patient is not weighed. To protect privacy, consideration should be given to placing the scale in a private area of the office to avoid unnecessary embarrassment.

In addition to BMI, the risk of overweight and obesity is independently associated with excess abdominal fat and fitness level. Population studies have shown that people with large waist circumferences have impaired health and increased cardiovascular risk compared with those with normal waist circumferences[55,56] within the healthy, overweight, and class I obesity BMI categories.[57] The threshold for excessive abdominal fat is clinically defined as a waist circumference greater than or equal to 102 cm ($\geq$40 inches) in men and greater than or equal to 88 cm ($\geq$35 inches) in women. According to the Practical Guide,[18] "To measure waist circumference, locate the upper hip bone and the top of the right iliac crest. Place a measuring tape in a horizontal plane around the abdomen at the level of the iliac crest. Before reading the tape measure, ensure that the tape is snug, but does not compress the skin, and is

BMI	19	20	21	22	23	24	25	26	27	28	29	30	31	32	33	34	35
Height (inches)							Body Weight (pounds)										
58	91	96	100	105	110	115	119	124	129	134	138	143	148	153	158	162	167
59	94	99	104	109	114	119	124	128	133	138	143	148	153	158	163	168	173
60	97	102	107	112	118	123	128	133	138	143	148	153	158	163	168	174	179
61	100	106	111	116	122	127	132	137	143	148	153	158	164	169	174	180	185
62	104	109	115	120	126	131	136	142	147	153	158	164	169	175	180	186	191
63	107	113	118	124	130	135	141	146	152	158	163	169	175	180	186	191	197
64	110	116	122	128	134	140	145	151	157	163	169	174	180	186	192	197	204
65	114	120	126	132	138	144	150	156	162	168	174	180	186	192	198	204	210
66	118	124	130	136	142	148	155	161	167	173	179	186	192	198	204	210	216
67	121	127	134	140	146	153	159	166	172	178	185	191	198	204	211	217	223
68	125	131	138	144	151	158	164	171	177	184	190	197	203	210	216	223	230
69	128	135	142	149	155	162	169	176	182	189	196	203	209	216	223	230	236
70	132	139	146	153	160	167	174	181	188	195	202	209	216	222	229	236	243
71	136	143	150	157	165	172	179	186	193	200	208	215	222	229	236	243	250
72	140	147	154	162	169	177	184	191	199	206	213	221	228	235	242	250	258
73	144	151	159	166	174	182	189	197	204	212	219	227	235	242	250	257	265
74	148	155	163	171	179	186	194	202	210	218	225	233	241	249	256	264	272
75	152	160	168	176	184	192	200	208	216	224	232	240	248	256	264	272	279
76	156	164	172	180	189	197	205	213	221	230	238	246	254	263	271	279	287

BMI	36	37	38	39	40	41	42	43	44	45	46	47	48	49	50	51	52	53	54
58	172	177	181	186	191	196	201	205	210	215	220	224	229	234	239	244	248	253	258
59	178	183	188	193	198	203	208	212	217	222	227	232	237	242	247	252	257	262	267
60	184	189	194	199	204	209	215	220	225	230	235	240	245	250	255	261	266	271	276
61	190	195	201	206	211	217	222	227	232	238	243	248	254	259	264	269	275	280	285
62	196	202	207	213	218	224	229	235	240	246	251	256	262	267	273	278	284	289	295
63	203	208	214	220	225	231	237	242	248	254	259	265	270	278	282	287	293	299	304
64	209	215	221	227	232	238	244	250	256	262	267	273	279	285	291	296	302	308	314
65	216	222	228	234	240	246	252	258	264	270	276	282	288	294	300	306	312	318	324
66	223	229	235	241	247	253	260	266	272	278	284	291	297	303	309	315	322	328	334
67	230	236	242	249	255	261	268	274	280	287	293	299	306	312	319	325	331	338	344
68	236	243	249	256	262	269	276	282	289	295	302	308	315	322	328	335	341	348	354
69	243	250	257	263	270	277	284	291	297	304	311	318	324	331	338	345	351	358	365
70	250	257	264	271	278	285	292	299	306	313	320	327	334	341	348	355	362	369	376
71	257	265	272	279	286	293	301	308	315	322	329	338	343	351	358	365	372	379	386
72	265	272	279	287	294	302	309	316	324	331	338	346	353	361	368	375	383	390	397
73	272	280	288	295	302	310	318	325	333	340	348	355	363	371	378	386	393	401	408
74	280	287	295	303	311	319	326	334	342	350	358	365	373	381	389	396	404	412	420
75	287	295	303	311	319	327	335	343	351	359	367	375	383	391	399	407	415	423	431
76	295	304	312	320	328	336	344	353	361	369	377	385	394	402	410	418	426	435	443

Fig. 1. Body Mass Index (BMI) Table. (*From* National Institutes of Health, National Heart, Lung, and Blood Institute.)

parallel to the floor. The measurement is made at the end of a normal expiration." Measurement of abdominal girth is not a difficult procedure and only takes a few seconds. Overweight persons with waist circumferences exceeding these limits should be urged more strongly to pursue weight reduction because it categorically increases disease risk for each BMI class. The importance of measuring and documenting waist circumference in patients with a BMI less than 35 kg/m^2 is due to the independent contribution of abdominal fat to the development of comorbid diseases, particularly the metabolic syndrome.

Determination of fitness level is another modifier to assessing risk associated with BMI. Ross and Katzmarzyk[58] found that high cardiorespiratory fitness is associated with lower levels of total and abdominal obesity for a given BMI. Longitudinal studies have shown that cardiorespiratory fitness (as measured by a maximal treadmill exercise test) is an important predictor of all-cause mortality independent of BMI and body composition. More specifically, fit obese men had a lower risk of all-cause and CVD mortality that did unfit lean men.[59] Similarly, among women, cardiorespiratory fitness was a more important predictor of all-cause mortality than was baseline BMI.[60]

Table 2
Classification of weight status and risk of disease (If patient is 18 years or older, use the body mass index (BMI) and waist circumference to estimate weight status and relative risk for diabetes, high blood pressure or heart disease.)

		Risk of Disease (relative to having a healthy weight and waist size)	
		Waist circumference:[a]	Waist circumference:[a]
		35" or less (women) 40" or less (men)	More than 35" (women) More than 40" (men)
Underweight	BMI below 18.5		
Healthy weight	BMI 18.5–24.9		
Overweight	BMI 25.0–29.9	Increased	High
Obesity Class I	BMI 30.0–34.9	High	Very High
Obesity Class II	BMI 35.0–39.9	Very High	Very High
Obesity Class III (Extreme Obesity)	BMI 40 or more	Extremely High	Extremely High

[a] Measure waist circumference at the level of the iliac crest. An increased waist circumference may indicate increased disease risk even at a normal weight.

Adapted from National Institutes of Health, National Heart, Lung, and Blood Institute. Clinical Guidelines on the Identification, Evaluation, and Treatment of Overweight and Obesity in Adults.[3]

These observations highlight the importance of taking an exercise history during the assessment as well as emphasizing the incorporation of moderately vigorous physical activity as a treatment approach.

ASSESSING PATIENT'S READINESS TO CHANGE BEHAVIOUR

Determining a patient's readiness for weight loss is the next essential part of the initial evaluation. Initiating change when the patient is not ready often leads to frustration and may hamper future efforts. Patients who are ready and have thought about the benefits and difficulties of weight management are more likely to succeed.

The NHLBI's Practical Guidelines for readiness recommend that physicians assess patient motivation and support, stressful life events, psychiatric status, time availability and constraints, as well as appropriateness of goals and expectations to help establish the likelihood of lifestyle change.[18] It is not enough to simply ask a patient, "Are you ready to lose weight?" Inquiring about readiness necessitates a more in depth assessment of patients and their environment. Readiness can be viewed as the balance of two opposing forces: motivation, or the patient's desire to change, and resistance, or the patient's resistance to change.[61] It is important to remember that most patients are ambivalent about changing long-standing lifestyle behaviors, fearing that it will be difficult, uncomfortable, or depriving. One helpful method to begin a readiness assessment is to 'anchor' the patient's interest and confidence to change on a numerical scale. To measure this, simply ask the patient, "*On a scale from 0 to 10, with 0 being not at important and 10 being very important, how important is it for you to lose weight at this time?*" and "*Also on a scale from 0 to 10, with 0 being not confident and 10 being very confident, how confident are you that you can lose weight at this time?*"[62] This is a very useful exercise to initiate further dialogue such as, *"What would it take to increase your confidence score from a 4 to a 7?"*

The Transtheoretical or Stages of Change Model proposes that at any specific time, patients are in one of six discrete stages of change: precontemplation, contemplation, preparation, action, maintenance, and relapse.[63] Assessing which stage of change the patient is in helps to tailor the advice and intensity of intervention. For example, if the patient is in the precontemplation stage regarding weight control ("I'm not really interested in losing weight at this time"), the appropriate action would be to provide information about health risks and benefits of weight loss and encourage taking action when ready. In contrast, if the patient is in the preparation stage ("I have to lose weight, and I've already talked to my wife about supporting me"), a reasonable action would be to begin dietary and physical activity counseling.

There are known determinants of whether a patient is likely to institute behavioral changes. Whitlock and colleagues[64] define certain change-predisposing attributes that typically lead to behaviors that promote weight loss. Assessing these qualities helps determine a ready candidate for lifestyle modification. Although it is unlikely that every patient will display all seven qualities, they provide a useful benchmark for assessment. These patients:

- strongly want and intend to change for clear, personal reasons
- face a minimum of obstacles to change
- have the requisite skills and self-confidence to make a change
- feel positively about change and believe it will result in meaningful benefit
- perceive the change as congruent with self-image and social group norms
- receive encouragement and support to change from valued persons.

IDENTIFYING THE HIGH-RISK OBESE PATIENT

According to the Practical Guide, patients at very high absolute risk, which triggers the need for intense risk factor modification and management, show the following factors: established coronary heart disease; presence of other atherosclerotic diseases such as peripheral arterial disease, abdominal aortic aneurysm, or symptomatic carotid artery disease; type 2 diabetes; and sleep apnea. Presence of the metabolic syndrome and high likelihood of insulin resistance should also prompt urgent treatment.[65] The Third Report of the National Cholesterol Education Program Expert Panel on Detection, Evaluation, and Treatment of High Blood Cholesterol in Adults (Adult Treatment Panel III) defines the metabolic syndrome as presence of three or more of the following criteria: (1) abdominal obesity; (2) hypertriglyceridemia ($\geq$150 mg/dL); (3) low HDL cholesterol (<40 mg/dL in men and <50 in women); (4) high blood pressure ($\geq$130/85 mm Hg); and (5) high fasting glucose ($\geq$110 mg/dL).[35] Other symptoms and diseases that are directly or indirectly related to obesity are listed in **Table 3**.[66] Although individuals will vary, the number and severity of organ specific comorbid conditions usually rises with increasing levels of obesity.[67] Even though many of these conditions may not be life threatening, they are often the chief concern and determine the quality of life for the patient and therefore should trigger active obesity treatment. See **Table 3** for a checklist to use during the review of systems section of the history and when developing an obesity-related problem list. If additional examination is warranted, it is important to note the unique aspects of the patient with obesity when performing a physical examination.[68]

There is no single laboratory test or diagnostic evaluation that is indicated for all patients with obesity. The specific evaluation performed should be based on

Table 3	
Obesity-related Organ Systems Review	
Cardiovascular	**Respiratory**
Hypertension	Dyspnea
Congestive heart failure	Obstructive sleep apnea
Cor pulmonale	Hypoventilation syndrome
Pulmonary embolism	Pickwickian syndrome
Coronary artery disease	Asthma
Varicose veins	
Endocrine	**Gastrointestinal**
Metabolic syndrome	Gastroesophageal reflux disease (GERD)
Type 2 diabetes	Non-alcoholic fatty liver disease (NAFLD)
Dyslipidemia	Cholelithiasis
Polycystic ovarian syndrome (PCOS)/hyperandrogenism	Hernias
Amenorrhea/infertility/menstrual disorders	Colon cancer
Musculoskeletal	**Genitourinary**
Hyperuricemia and gout	Urinary stress incontinence
Immobility	Obesity-related glomerulopathy
Osteoarthritis (knees and hips)	Hypogonadism (male)
Low back pain	Breast and uterine cancer
	Complications of pregnancy
Psychological	**Neurologic**
Depression/low self esteem	Stroke
Body image disturbance	Idiopathic intracranial hypertension
Social stigmatization	Meralgia paresthetica
Integument	
Striae distensae (stretch marks)	
Stasis pigmentation of legs	
Lymphedema	
Cellulitis	
Intertrigo, carbuncles	
Acanthosis nigricans/skin tags	

presentation of symptoms, risk factors, and index of suspicion. However, based on several other screening guideline recommendations, most if not all patients should have a fasting lipid panel (total, LDL, and HDL cholesterol and triglyceride levels) and blood glucose measured at presentation along with blood pressure determination. Checking the blood pressure in the obese patient requires special consideration, however. A bladder cuff that is not the appropriate width for the patient's arm circumference will cause a systematic error in blood pressure measurement; if the bladder is too narrow, the pressure will be overestimated and lead to a false diagnosis of hypertension. To avoid errors, the bladder width should be 40% to 50% of upper arm circumference. Therefore, a large adult cuff (15 cm wide) should be chosen for patients with mild to moderate obesity whereas a thigh cuff (18 cm wide) should be used for patients whose arm circumference is greater than 16 inches.[69]

SUMMARY

Obesity may be the most significant medical problem that health care providers will face over the coming decades. Physicians must aggressively address this chronic disease, providing both preventive and therapeutic care. Since this topic has not been traditionally taught in medical school or residency training, physicians and other health providers will need to acquire the knowledge, skills, and attitudes necessary to be effective obesity care providers. Performing a detailed initial assessment, including an obesity focused history, physical examination, and selected laboratory and diagnostic tests is fundamental to the process of care.

REFERENCES

1. Flegal KM, Carroll MD, Ogden CL, et al. Prevalence and trends in obesity among US adults, 1999-2008. JAMA 2010;303:235–41.
2. Ogden CL, Carroll MD, Curtin LR, et al. Prevalence of high body mass index in US children and adolescents, 2007–2008. JAMA 2010;303:242–9.
3. National Institutes of Health. Clinical guidelines on the identification, evaluation, and treatment of overweight and obesity in adults–the evidence report. Obes Res 1998; 6(Suppl 2):51S-210S.
4. U.S. Preventive Services Task Force. Screening for obesity in adults: recommendations and rationale. Ann Intern Med 2003;139:930–2.
5. Mechanick JI, Kushner RF, Sugerman HJ, for the writing group. AACE/TOS/ASMBS Guidelines. The American Association of Clinical Endocrinologists, The Obesity Society, and American Society for Metabolic & Bariatric Surgery medical guidelines for clinical practice for the perioperative nutritional, metabolic, and nonsurgical support of the bariatric surgery patient. Obesity 2009;17(Suppl 1):S1–70.
6. American Academy of Family Physicians. Recommendations for periodic health examination (RPHE) of the American Academy of Family Physicians. Leawood (KS): American Academy of Family Physicians; 1997.
7. Lyznicki JM, Young DC, Riggs JA, et al. Obesity: assessment and management in primary care. Am Fam Physician 2001;63:2185–96.
8. Nawaz H, Katz DL. American College of Preventive Medicine Practice Policy statement. Weight management counseling of overweight adults. Am J Prev Med 2001; 21:73–8.
9. Pearson TA, Blair SN, Daniels SR, et al. AHA Guidelines for Primary Prevention of Cardiovascular Disease and Stroke: 2002 Update: Consensus panel guide to comprehensive risk reduction for adult patients without coronary or other atherosclerotic vascular diseases. American Heart Association Science Advisory and Coordinating Committee. Circulation 2002;106:388–91.
10. The Surgeon General's vision for a healthy and fit nation 2010. Rockville (MD): USDHHS, Public Health Service, Office of the Surgeon General; 2010.
11. Kushner RF. Tackling obesity: is primary care up to the challenge? Arch Intern Med 2010;170:121–3.
12. Haire-Joshu D, Klein S. Is primary care practice equipped to deal with obesity? Arch Intern Med 2011;171:313–5.
13. Jackson JE, Doescher MP, Saver BG, et al. Trends in professional advice to lose weight among obese adults, 1994-2000. J Gen Intern Med 2005;20:814–8.
14. McAlpine DD, Wilson AR. Trends in obesity-related counseling in primary care: 1995–2004. Med Care 2007;45:322–9.
15. Kristeller JL, Hoerr RA. Physician attitudes toward managing obesity: differences among six specialty groups. Prev Med 1997;26:542–9.

16. Loureiro ML, Nayga RM Jr. Obesity, weight loss, and physician's advice. Soc Sci Med 2006;62:2458–68.

17. Post RE, Mainous AG 3rd, Gregorie SH, et al. The influence of physician acknowledgment of patients' weight status on patient perceptions of overweight and obesity in the United States. Arch Intern Med 2011;171:316–21.

18. National Heart, Lung, and Blood Institute and North American Association for the Study of Obesity. The practical guide–Identification, evaluation, and treatment of overweight and obesity in adults. Bethesda (MD): National Institutes of Health; NIH Publ 00-4084; 2000.

19. Krebs NF, Himes JH, Jacobson D, et al. Assessment of child and adolescent overweight and obesity. Pediatrics 2007;120(Suppl 4):S193-228.

20. Kushner RF. Roadmaps for clinical practice series: assessment and management of adult obesity. Chicago: American Medical Association; 2003. Available at: www.ama-assn.org/ama/pub/category/10931.html). Accessed May 7, 2011.

21. Sarwer DB, Allison KC, Gibbons LM, et al. Pregnancy and obesity: a review and agenda for future research. J Womens Health (Larchmt) 2006;15:720–33.

22. Azziz R, Carmina E, Dewailly D, et al. The Androgen Excess and PCOS Society criteria for the polycystic ovary syndrome: the complete task force report. Fertil Steril 2009;91:456–88.

23. Aronne LJ. Drug-induced weight gain: non-CNS medications. In: Aronne LJ, editor. A practical guide to drug-induced weight gain. Minneapolis: McGraw-Hill; 2002. p. 77–91.

24. Zimmermann U, Kraus T, Himmerich H, et al. Epidemiology, implications and mechanisms underlying drug-induced weight gain in psychiatric patients. J Psychiatr Res 2003;37:193–220.

25. American Diabetes Association, American Psychiatric Association, American Association of Clinical Endocrinologists, and North American Association for the Study of Obesity. Consensus development conference on antipsychotic drugs and obesity and diabetes. Obes Res 2004;12:362–8.

26. Fontaine KR, Heo M, Harrigan EP, et al. Estimating the consequences of antipsychotic induced weight gain on health and mortality rate. Psychiatry Res 2001;101:277–88.

27. Sarwer DB, Faulconbridge LF, Steffen KJ, et al. Bariatric procedures: managing patients after surgery. Curr Psychiatr 2010;10:3–9.

28. Wright JD, Wang C-Y. Trends in intake of energy and macronutrients in adults from 1999–2000 through 2007–2008. NCHS Data Brief No. 49: November 2010.

29. American Psychiatric Association. Diagnostic and statistical manual of mental disorders (4th edition, text revision). Author: Washington, DC; 2000.

30. Spitzer RL, Devlin MJ, Walsh BT, et al. Binge eating disorder: a multisite field trial of the diagnostic criteria. Int J Eat Disord 1992;11:191–203.

31. Allison KC, Stunkard AJ. Obesity and eating disorders. Psychiatr Clin North Am 2005;28:55–67.

32. Allison KC, Lundgren JD, O'Reardon JP, et al. Proposed diagnostic criteria for night eating syndrome. Int J Eat Disord 2010; 43:241–7.

33. Allison KC, Stunkard AJ, Their SL. Overcoming night eating syndrome. Oakland (CA): New Harbinger; 2004.

34. Jakicic JM, Otto AD. Physical activity recommendations in the treatment of obesity. Psychiatr Clin North Am 2005;28:141–50.

35. Blanck HM, Khan LK, Serdula MK. Use of nonprescription weight loss products: results from a multistate survey. JAMA 2001;286:930–5.

36. Carpiniello B, Pinna F, Pillai G, et al. Psychiatric comorbidity and quality of life in obese patients. Results from a case-control study. Int J Psychiatry Med 2009;39:63–78.
37. Wadden TA, Sarwer DB. Behavioral assessment of candidates for bariatric surgery: a patient-oriented approach. Surg Obes Relat Dis 2006;2:171–9.
38. Onyike CU, Crum RM, Lee HB, et al. Is obesity associated with major depression? Results from the Third National Health and Nutrition Examination Survey. Am J Epidemiol 2003;158: 1139–47.
39. Carpenter KM, Hasin DS, Allison DB, et al. Relationships between obesity and DSM-IV major depressive disorder, suicide ideation, and suicide attempts: results from a general population study. Am J Publ Health 2000;90:251–7.
40. Faith MS, Butryn M, Wadden TA, et al. Evidence for prospective associations among depression and obesity in population-based studies. Obes Rev 2011;12:e438–53.
41. Fabricatore AN, Wadden TA, Higginbotham AJ, et al. Intentional weight loss and changes in symptoms of depression: a systematic review and meta-analysis. Int J Obes (Lond) 2011. [Epub ahead of print].
42. Sarwer DB, Cohn NI, Gibbons LM, et al. Psychiatric diagnoses and psychiatric treatment among bariatric surgery candidates. Obes Surg 2004;14:1148–56.
43. Søltoft F, Hammer M, Kragh N. The association of body mass index and health-related quality of life in the general population: data from the 2003 Health Survey of England. Qual Life Res 2009;18:1293–9.
44. Mond JM, Baune BT. Overweight, medical comorbidity and health-related quality of life in a community sample of women and men. Obesity (Silver Spring) 2009;17:1627–34.
45. Yancy WS Jr, Olsen MK, Westman EC, et al. Relationship between obesity and health-related quality of life in men. Obes Res 2002;10:1057–64.
46. Sarwer DB, Dilks RJ, Spitzer JC. Weight loss and changes in body image. In: Cash TF, Smolak L, editors. Body image, a handbook of science, practice and prevention. New York: Guilford Press; 2011. p. 369–77.
47. Sarwer DB, Wadden TA, Foster GD. Assessment of body image dissatisfaction in obese women: specificity, severity, and clinical significance. J Consult Clin Psychol 1998;66:651–4.
48. Sarwer DB, Magee L. Body image and plastic surgery. In: Sarwer DB, Pruzinsky T, Cash TF, et al, editors. Psychological aspects of reconstructive and cosmetic plastic surgery: empirical, clinical, and ethical issues. Philadelphia: Lippincott Williams & Wilkins; 2006. p. 23–36.
49. Crosnoe R. Gender, obesity, and education. Sociol Educ 2007;80:241–60.
50. Enzi G. Socioeconomic consequences of obesity: the effect of obesity on the individual. Pharmacoeconomics 1994;5(Suppl 1):54–7.
51. Wadden TA, Letizia KA. Predictors of attrition and weight loss in patients treated by moderate and severe calorie restriction. In: Wadden TA, Van Itallie TB, editors. Treatment of the seriously obese patient. New York: Guilford Press; 1992. p. 383–410.
52. Fabricatore AN, Wadden TA, Womble LG, et al. The role of patients' expectations and goals in the behavioral and pharmacological treatment of obesity. Int J Obes (Lond) 2007;31:1739–45.
53. White MA, Masheb RM, Rothschild BS, et al. Do patients' unrealistic weight goals have a prognostic significance for bariatric surgery? Obes Surg 2007;17:74–81.
54. Foster GD, Wadden TA, Vogt RA. Body image in obese women before, during, and after weight loss treatment. Health Psychol 1997;16:226–9.
55. Lean ME, Han TS, Seidell JC. Impairment of health and quality of life in people with large waist circumference. Lancet 1998;351:853–6.

56. Han TS, van Leer EM, Seidell JC, et al. Waist circumference action levels in the identification of cardiovascular risk factors: prevalence study in a random sample. BMJ 1995;311:1401–5.
57. Janssen I, Katzmarzyk PT, Ross R. Body mass index, waist circumference, and health risk: evidence in support of current National Institutes of Health guidelines. Arch Intern Med 2002;162:2074–9.
58. Ross R, Katzmarzyk PT. Cardiorespiratory fitness is associated with diminished total and abdominal obesity independent of body mass index. Int J Obesity 2003;27:204–10.
59. Lee CD, Blair SN, Jackson AS. Cardiorespiratory fitness, body composition, and all-cause and cardiovascular disease mortality in men. Am J Clin Nutr 1999;69: 373–80.
60. Farrell SW, Braun L, Barlow CE, et al. The relation of body mass index, cardiorespiratory fitness, and all-cause mortality in women. Obes Res 2002;10:417–23.
61. Katz DL. Behavior modification in primary care: the pressure system model. Prev Med 2001;32:66–72.
62. Rollnick S, Mason P, Butler C. Health behavior change: a guide for practitioners. London: Churchill Livingstone; 1999.
63. Prochaska JO, DiClemente CC. Toward a comprehensive model of change. In: Miller WR, editor. Treating addictive behaviors. New York: Plenum; 1986. p. 3–27.
64. Whitlock EP, Orleans CT, Pender N, et al. Evaluating primary care behavioral counseling intervention: an evidence-based approach. Am J Prev Med 2002;22:267–84.
65. Reaven GM. Importance of identifying the overweight patient who will benefit the most by losing weight. Ann Intern Med 2003;138:420–3.
66. Expert panel on detection, evaluation, and treatment of high blood cholesterol in adults. Executive summary of the third reports of the National Cholesterol Education Program (NCEP) expert panel on detection, evaluation, and treatment of high blood cholesterol in adults (Adult Treatment Panel III). JAMA 2001;285:2486–97. Available at: http://www.nhlbi.nih.gov/guidelines/cholesterol/atp3xsum.pdf. Accessed May 7, 2011.
67. Must A, Spadano J, Coakley EH, et al. The disease burden associated with overweight and obesity. JAMA 1999;282:1523–9.
68. Silk AW, McTigue KM. Reexamining the physical examination for obese patients. JAMA 2011;305:193–4.
69. Pickering TG, Hall JE, Appel LJ, et al. Recommendations for blood pressure measurement in humans and experimental animals: part 1: blood pressure measurement in humans: a statement for professionals from the Subcommittee of Professional and Public Education of the American Heart Association Council on High Blood Pressure Research. Circ 2005;111:697–716.

Dietary Approaches to the Treatment of Obesity

Angela Makris, PhD, RD, Gary D. Foster, PhD*

KEYWORDS
- Obesity • Dietary strategy • Low fat • High protein
- Low carbohydrate • Glycemic index

Popular dietary approaches for weight loss have generated widespread interest and considerable debate. While energy balance remains the cornerstone of weight control (ie, calories still count), new diets and books promising weight loss by limiting certain foods or macronutrients rather than energy are constantly emerging and hitting the best seller list. Although their names and approaches may change over time, their basic premise has not. They market "success" as a large weight loss over a short period with little effort. Given the allure of a quick fix, overweight and obese individuals are often in search of the next "best" diet. The public's willingness to try diverse and, in some cases, poorly researched dietary approaches underscores their long-standing struggle to control their weight and the need for more effective strategies to help create an energy deficit. To develop more effective strategies, it is important to understand the efficacy, health effects, and long-term sustainability of current dietary approaches to weight control.

This article describes various dietary approaches to weight loss: low-, very low-, and moderate-fat diets, high-protein diets, low-carbohydrate diets, and low glycemic index diets. Descriptions of each dietary strategy are followed by a review of short- and long-term efficacy data from studies published between 2005 and 2011. (See our previous review for a summary of work before 2005.)[1]

LOW-FAT DIETS

The *Dietary Guidelines for Americans* (along with My Pyramid) provides one example of a low-fat (LF) eating plan.[2] The *Dietary Guidelines* are based on evidence that eating a LF (20%–35%) diet helps manage weight, promote health, and reduce the risk of chronic disease. The guidelines include recommendations for "foods to reduce" (ie, saturated and *trans*-fat, cholesterol, sodium, added sugar, refined grains, alcohol) and "foods to increase" (ie, fruits, vegetables, whole grains, low-fat dairy and

The authors have nothing to disclose.
Center for Obesity Research and Education, Temple University, 3223 North Broad Street, Suite 175, Philadelphia, PA 19140, USA
* Corresponding author.
E-mail address: gfoster@temple.edu

Psychiatr Clin N Am 34 (2011) 813–827
doi:10.1016/j.psc.2011.08.004
0193-953X/11/$ – see front matter © 2011 Elsevier Inc. All rights reserved.

protein foods, oils) to maximize the nutrient content and health-promoting potential of the diet. Other examples of a LF diet are the Dietary Approaches to Stop Hypertension (DASH) diet and those recommended by the American Diabetes Association (ADA),[3] American Heart Association (AHA),[4] and American Cancer Society,[5] as well as commercial programs such as Weight Watchers.

Efficacy, Health Effects, and Sustainability

LF diets are the best studied of all dietary approaches to weight loss. Three large, multicenter, randomized studies—the PREMIER trial, Diabetes Prevention Program, and the Finnish Diabetes Prevention study—have demonstrated that greater weight loss is achieved in groups consuming LF diets compared to controls receiving standard lifestyle recommendations.[1] Further, they suggest that consumption of a LF, low-calorie diet, in the context of intensive group or individual counseling, has positive effects on comorbid conditions as long as it is followed. A more detailed description has been reported previously.[1]

More recent studies have reported similar findings. The Look Ahead Trial[6] was a large multicenter, randomized clinical trial that compared the effects of an intensive lifestyle intervention (ILI) to diabetes support and education (DSE) on the incidence of major cardiovascular disease (CVD) events in overweight or obese individuals with type 2 diabetes. Participants in the ILI group were assigned a calorie-restricted LF diet and received frequent behavioral therapy and extended contact. Those in the DSE group were given standard instruction on three occasions each year for eating a healthy diet and engaging in physical activity. Weight loss in the ILI group was significantly greater than in the DSE group each year over the course of 4 years, with maximal weight loss occurring at 1 year (**Table 1**). Individuals in the ILI group also displayed greater improvements in hemoglobin A_{1C} (HbA_{1C}), blood pressure, high-density lipoprotein (HDL), and triacylglycerides (TAGs) over the course of the study. Other studies prescribing LF diets with treatment phases ranging from 6 months or less to 12 months or longer have reported weight losses of approximately 6 to 11 kg after 6[7–9] and 12 months,[10,11] 4 to 5 kg after 24 to 36 months,[6,9] and 4.7% initial body weight at 48 months[6] (see **Table 1**). The Woman's Health Initiative Dietary Modification trial showed that following a LF diet without instruction for calorie restriction can help to maintain weight loss slightly better than following a diet higher in fat.[12] Taken together, these findings suggest that a LF diet is an effective weight control strategy in the short and long term as long as it is followed.

Adherence to a calorie-controlled diet appears to be one of the biggest barriers to the long-term success of weight loss maintenance. LF eating is not immune to poor long-term adherence. Researchers have investigated various strategies, from varying the percentage of fat in the diet to matching diets with food preferences, in an attempt to promote better long-term dietary adherence. One study[13] comparing weight loss and CVD risk factors in individuals consuming calorie-controlled 20% or 30% fat diets showed that although both diets produced a similar amount of weight loss after 7 months, weight loss was maintained better and CVD risk factors were reduced more after 14 months in those following the 30% fat diet. It appears that intake was more restrictive in the 20% fat diet group, making it more difficult to follow over the long term and resulting in greater weight regain. A limited number of studies have investigated the effects of matching treatment preferences with weight loss outcomes.[14–16] A recent study[15] found that whether individuals were randomized to their preferred LF diet or not (ie, standard or lacto-ovo vegetarian), they lost similar amounts of weight after 6 months; however, differences in weight regain patterns emerged after 6 months. Curiously, those who were assigned their preferred diet

Table 1
Weight loss outcomes of studies 6 months or greater in duration

Study (First Author)	Diet	Weight Loss (kg)					
		6 mo	12 mo	18 mo	24 mo	36 mo	48 mo
Look AHEAD Research Group[6]	LF (30% fat)		8.6%		6.5%	5.0%	4.7%
Jeffery et al[7]	LF (30% fat)	7	11	9			
Svetkey et al[9]	LF (DASH diet)	8	7	6	5	4	
Perri et al[10]	LF (30% fat)	10		9			
Barnard et al[21,22]	LF (ADA diet)	4[a]		3[b]			
	Vegan (10% fat)	6[a]		4[b]			
Turner-McGrievy et al[11]	LF (NCEP diet)		2		1		
	Vegan (10% fat)		5		3		
Azadbakht et al[13]	LF (30% fat)	5[c]	5[d]				
	LF (20% fat)	5[c]	1[d]				
Dansinger et al[19]	LF (Weightt Watchers)	4	3				
	Very LF Ornish diet	4	3				
	HP (Zone diet)	3	3				
	LC (Atkins diet)	3	2				
Gardner et al[20]	LF (LEARN)	3	2.5				
	Very LF Ornish diet	2	2				
	HP (Zone diet)	2	1.5				
	LC (Atkins diet)	5.5	4.5				
Foster et al[45]	LF (30% fat)	11	11		7		
	LC (Atkins diet)	12	11		6		
Brehm et al[26]	LF (25% fat)	4	4				
	MF (40% fat)	4	4				

(continued on next page)

Table 1
(continued)

Study (First Author)	Diet	Weight Loss (kg)					
		6 mo	12 mo	18 mo	24 mo	36 mo	48 mo
Shai et al[28]	LF (30% fat)	4.5	3.8	3	3		
	MF (35% fat)	4.5	4.5	4.5	4.5		
	LC (20–120 g carb/day)	6	5.3	4.8	5		
Larsen et al[36]	LF (30% fat)		2				
	HP (30% protein)		2				
Clifton et al[37]	LF (20% fat)		7[e]				
	HP (>88 g/day)		3[e]				
McAuley et al[39]	LF (30% fat)	6	4				
	HP (30% protein)	8	7				
	HF (20–50 g carb/day)	9	5				
Layman et al[41]	LF (30% fat)		7				
	HP (30% protein)		9				
Klemsdal et al[52]	LF (30% fat)	5	4				
	Low GL	6	4				
Fabricatore et al[53]	LF (30% fat)	6%[f]	5%[g]				
	Low GL	7%[f]	6%[g]				

[a] 22 weeks.
[b] 74 weeks.
[c] 7 months.
[d] 14 months.
[e] 64 weeks.
[f] 20 weeks.
[g] 40 weeks.

began regaining weight sooner (ie, 6 vs 12 months) and regained more weight (ie, 4.5% vs 2.1%) at 18 months than those who were not assigned to their preferred diet. Similar findings were recently reported for both LF and low-carbohydrate diets.[16] Borradaile and colleagues found that the group assigned their preferred diet lost less weight (–7.7 kg) than the group who did not receive their preferred diet (–9.7 kg) or who did not report a strong preference at baseline (–11.2 kg).[16] Given this seemingly counterintuitive finding, it may be useful for future studies to elaborate on "preference" (eg, is their preference based on a preferred way of eating or on an alternative to their preferred way of eating?).

VERY-LOW-FAT DIETS

Some investigators have suggested that a fat intake of 20% or less of total calories is necessary for optimal health.[17,18] Diets that provide 10% to 20% fat are defined as very low fat. The Pritikin and Ornish diets are examples of very-low-fat diets. They are primarily plant-based diets (eg, fruits, vegetables, whole grains, beans, and soy), with limited amounts of reduced fat dairy, eggs, lean meats, and fish.[17,18] Unlike LF plans that incorporate all foods, the very-low-fat diets strongly discourage consumption of foods containing high amounts of refined carbohydrate.

Efficacy, Health Effects, and Sustainability

A limited number of studies have examined the efficacy of very-low-fat diets. In our earlier review,[5] we summarized results from the Lifestyle Heart Trial showing that a very-low-fat vegetarian diet—combined with a behavior modification program including moderate aerobic activity, stress management, and smoking cessation—was effective in reducing weight and the progression of coronary atherosclerosis. Since this study was published, others have shown that participants following the Ornish diet experienced similar weight loss and improvements in CVD risk factors as participants following other popular diet strategies[19,20] (see **Table 1**). However, compared to other diets, the Ornish diet showed a trend toward higher attrition[19] and poorer adherence.[20] These findings suggest that very-low-fat diets may be more difficult to sustain over time.

More recently, Barnard and colleagues[21,22] compared weight loss in participants with type 2 diabetes who consumed either a vegan diet (ie, 10% energy from fat) or a diet based on the guidelines of the American Diabetes Association diet (ie, approximately 20%–25% fat). After 22 and 74 weeks, both diets resulted in weight loss and improved glycemic control. Reductions in weight were significantly greater in the vegan group at 22 weeks but not at 74 weeks (see **Table 1**). Dietary adherence was greater in the vegan group at 22 weeks but not at 74 weeks. Participants rated both diets as acceptable.[23] This research group also compared weight loss in individuals who consumed a vegan (ie, 10% energy from fat) and National Cholesterol Education Program (NCEP) low-fat diet (ie, 30% energy from fat) for 14 weeks and found that the vegan group had greater weight loss than the NCEP group at 1 and 2 years.[11] These studies suggest that very-low-fat diets are effective in reducing weight and, unlike the aforementioned studies, may be sustainable over the long term.

MODERATE-FAT DIETS

Given that LF diets can contain up to 35% fat, moderate fat (MF) diets are generally those that contain between 35% and 45% fat. Many people equate MF diets with Mediterranean diets but the fat content of Mediterranean diets can vary considerably. Some have reported fat contents as high as 47%[24] while others have found them to be as low as 25% fat[25]; therefore, although some Mediterranean diets can be considered moderate in fat, it should not be assumed that they all are.

Efficacy, Health Effects, and Sustainability

Previous studies have shown that weight loss was better maintained over time in individuals who followed a MF diet and suggested that it may be easier to adhere to MF diets than LF diets over the long term.[1] Recent studies that have compared MF (ie, 35%–46% fat) and LF (ie, 25%–30%) diets have reported similar[26,27] to slightly better[28] weight losses with MF diets (see **Table 1**). These diets were similar to Mediterranean diets in that they contained a high proportion of monounsaturated fatty acids (MUFAs), primarily from MUFA-rich oils, and emphasized high intake of plant foods (ie, fruits, vegetables, whole grains, legumes, and nuts) and fiber and limited amounts of saturated fat from animal foods. A meta-analysis of 16 randomized controlled trials of the effect of Mediterranean diets on body weight suggested that Mediterranean diets resulted in greater weight losses compared to a control diet, particularly when associated with energy restriction and physical activity.[29] Of the studies included in the meta-analysis that reported fat intake, only one study reported total fat intake as less than 35% fat (ie, 30% fat). Compared to LF diets, higher fat, Mediterranean style diets have also been shown to be superior in increasing HDL and reducing atherogenic index (ie, ratio of total to HDL cholesterol) and C-reactive protein in individuals with hyperlipidemia[27] or coronary heart disease.[28] They also are comparable in improving blood pressure, HDL, HbA_{1C}, and fasting glucose and insulin in individuals with type 2 diabetes.[26,28]

One study focused on the efficacy of MF diets on weight maintenance.[30,31] In this study, participants who lost at least 8% of their initial body weight on an 8-week low-energy diet were randomized to one of three ad libitum diets for 6 months: (1) MF, Mediterranean type diet (35%–45% fat with >20% MUFA); (2) LF (20%–30% fat); or (3) control (35% fat with >15% saturated fat). After 6 months, all participants regained weight with no significant differences between groups (MF, 2.5 kg; LF, 2.2 kg; control, 3.8 kg). However, body fat regain was lower in the MF and LF groups. The MF diet showed favorable effects on diabetes risk factors (ie, reduction in fasting insulin and improvements in homeostasis model assessment of insulin resistance [HOMA-IR]) and CVD risk factors (ie, reduced ratio of low-density lipoprotein [LDL] to HDL).

THE HIGH-PROTEIN DIET

There is no standard definition of a "high-protein (HP) diet"; however, intakes greater than 25% total energy or 1.6 g/kg per day of body weight can be considered high.[32] The Zone diet (30% protein, 40% carbohydrate, and 30% fat) is an example of a HP diet. The most prominent difference between a HP diet such as the Zone and a low-carbohydrate diet such as the Atkins New Diet Revolution is that a HP diet is typically low in fat.

Efficacy, Health Effects, and Sustainability

Several earlier studies have reported greater weight loss and improvements in body composition (ie, decreases in waist circumference, waist-to-hip ratio, and intra-abdominal adipose tissue and better preservation of lean body mass) in individuals prescribed HP diets than LF diets. These studies have been described in more detail previously.[1] Given that high waist-to-hip ratios and levels of intra-abdominal adipose tissue correlate positively with certain chronic conditions, interest in HP diets has grown. Findings from more recent studies are mixed. Although several studies have not found significant advantages on body weight and composition,[19, 33–36] some trials have supported previous findings that diets higher in protein have beneficial effects on weight loss[37–39] and body composition.[39–41] This appears particularly true in individuals with elevated risk of CVD and metabolic syndrome[33,42] or in individuals who combine a HP diet with resistance training[40] (see **Table 1**).

There is no clear explanation for these inconsistent results. Inadequate nutrition counseling and poor dietary adherence, particularly in longer studies, may contribute to the lack of differences between dietary groups. Poor long-term adherence has been reported in several studies comparing HP and LF diets on weight loss and body composition[19,35–37,39] and is not limited to HP diets. For example, Dansinger and colleagues[19] reported that only 25% of participants in each of four dietary groups (ie, Atkins, Zone, Weight Watchers, and Ornish) sustained a clinically meaningful adherence level. McCauley and coworkers[39] reported that, by 52 weeks, adherence to macronutrient goals declined considerably, as did Clifton and coworkers,[37] who found that by 64 weeks, macronutrient intake had shifted to a point at which the diets converged, and there was not a large enough difference in diets to be of significance. As such, data in the latter study were reanalyzed based on actual intakes of protein and 24-hour urinary urea, a marker of protein intake, instead of the assigned intervention. When actual high- and low-protein (LP) intake groups were compared, the researchers found that weight loss was greater in the HP group than in the LP group. These findings differed from those in the initial analysis in which no intergroup differences in weight were observed.

To better understand compliance and long-term changes in body composition and blood lipids, Layman and colleagues[41] compared HP and LF diets in obese but healthy adults over 12 months. This study was divided into two phases: (1) 4 months of weight loss and (2) 8 months of weight maintenance. The diets were isocaloric and equal in fat but differed in protein content. The HP group were prescribed 30% protein (providing 1.6 g protein/kg/day) while those in the LF group were prescribed 15% protein. Each group received a menu plan with meals for each day throughout the 12-month study. Participants met with a dietitian each week who reviewed diet records, answered questions, provided feedback, and measured weight. Adherence to the diet was monitored with plasma TAG, a marker of carbohydrate intake, and urinary urea.

Weight loss did not differ between groups at 4 months; however, the HP group had a greater loss of body fat compared to the LF group. At 4 months, urinary urea, as well as plasma TAG measurements, indicated that both groups were adherent to their macronutrient goals and were consistent with diet records. Adherence in the HP and LF groups also appeared to be good at 8 and 12 months, respectively. At 12 months, there were no differences in changes in weight or lean mass, but the HP group had a greater loss of fat mass. Greater reductions in weight and fat mass (ie, total and abdominal) have also been observed in studies of obese women with elevated TAG concentrations.[33,42] Noakes and colleagues[33] reported that obese women with elevated TAG concentrations who consumed a HP diet for 12 weeks lost 50% more body fat than those who consumed an isocaloric LF diet.

Layman and colleagues[41] reported that HP diets reduced TAG, HDL cholesterol, and TAG/HDL more than LF diets at 4 months. These effects were sustained at 12 months. The greater reduction in TAG with HP diets is a relatively consistent finding, observed in several studies,[42] including those of obese women with elevated TAG concentrations[33] and overweight insulin-resistant women.[39] Clifton and colleagues[42] pooled data from three clinical trials and reported that TAG concentrations decreased to a greater extent on the HP diet compared to the LF diet (ie, 29% HP vs 17% LF).

In addition, this analysis showed that patients with elevated TAG who consumed a HP diet had greater reductions in total cholesterol than those on a LF diet. These researchers also found larger reductions in LDL cholesterol in individuals with impaired glucose tolerance (IGT) who were on the HP diet. Taken together, these findings suggest that HP diets might be of some benefit to individuals with or at high risk for diabetes, dyslipidemia, CVD, and metabolic syndrome.

Weight change over the course of 2 years was evaluated in a large study[35] of 811 overweight adults randomized to one of four calorie-restricted diets: (1) 20%, 15%, and 65%, for fat, protein, and carbohydrate, respectively; (2) 20%, 25%, and 55%; (3) 40%, 15%, and 45%; or (4) 40%, 25%, and 35%. Individuals received group lifestyle modification 3 of every 4 weeks for the first 6 months and then biweekly from 6 months to 2 years. Individual counseling sessions were also provided every 8 weeks over the course of the study. Weight loss was similar at two years in participants assigned to 15% and 25% protein (3.0 kg and 3.6 kg, respectively). Adherence to protein intake targets was associated with more weight loss in the HP group. However, adherence to macronutrient goals diminished after 6 months, indicating that participants had difficulty maintaining specific macronutrient targets over time, despite intensive counseling. All diets reduced risk factors for CVD and diabetes.

Few studies have evaluated HP for weight maintenance. However, a large pan-European study, Diet, Obesity, and Genes (DIOGENES) Project, assessed the efficacy of ad libitum MF diets varying in protein and glycemic index (GI) for weight maintenance.[43] After an initial 8-week weight loss program, 773 participants were randomized to one of five LF diets: (1) LP, low-GI; (2) LP, high-GI; (3) HP, low-GI; (4) HP, high-GI; or (5) control diet (ie, moderate protein, no GI instruction). Dietary counseling was provided biweekly for the first 6 weeks and monthly thereafter. Although participants did not achieve the targeted 12% difference in protein intake between groups, those in the HP group consumed 5% more protein as a proportion of total energy than the LP group. Better weight maintenance was observed in individuals who consumed higher amounts of protein than in those who consumed smaller amounts. Weight regain was 0.9 kg less in those assigned a HP diet than those assigned a LP diet.

There has been concern regarding the overall safety of HP diets. No adverse effects have been observed for markers of kidney or liver function[28,34,36,40] or bone turnover.[33,36] However, the effects of HP diets in compromised individuals is unknown.

LOW-CARBOHYDRATE DIETS

The low-carbohydrate (LC) diet is one of the most recognized approaches to weight loss. Many versions of the LC diet exist (ie, Atkins New Diet Revolution, South Beach, Dukan diet), each with a unique interpretation of optimal LC eating. Unlike LF diets, the FDA has not established a clear definition for "low" carbohydrate. However, LC diets often consist of limited amounts of carbohydrate (20–50 g/day or about 10% of calories from carbohydrate), gradually increasing over time, and relatively high amounts of fat (approximately 60% fat), which differentiates LC diets from HP diets. LC approaches encourage consumption of controlled amounts of nutrient-dense carbohydrate containing foods (eg, low-GI vegetables, whole-grain products) and eliminate intake of refined carbohydrate. Although consumption of foods that do not contain carbohydrate (eg, meats, poultry, fish, butter, oil) is not restricted, quality rather than quantity is emphasized.

Efficacy, Health Effects, and Sustainability

In our earlier review,[1] we described findings from several short-term (<12 months) studies comparing the effects of LC and a calorie-controlled, LF diets on weight, body composition, and cardiovascular risk factors in obese adults. In summary, participants who followed a LC diet lost significantly more weight than those who adhered to a LF diet during the first 6 months of treatment. However, differences in weight loss did not persist at 1 year. A meta-analysis published in 2006[44] also found no significant differences in weight loss between diets at 1 year, suggesting that LC diets are as effective as LF diets for weight loss.

Since our last report, several studies comparing weight loss in individuals who consumed LC and LF diets from 1[19,20,39] to 2 years have been published.[28,35,45] These studies were similar in LC and LF diet prescriptions but varied in the amount of professional support they offered. Among the studies that examined weight loss over a 1-year period, two observed significantly greater weight losses with a LC diet than a LF diet at 6 months[20,39] but no significant differences in weight were observed between these two diets at 1 year in any of these studies,[19,20,39] supporting earlier findings. Adherence to the macronutrient targets of the diets decreased over time in these studies, particularly in the LC group in one study,[20] and attrition was higher in the LC group than in the LF group in another study.[19] This suggests that a LC diet may be more difficult to sustain than a LF diet over time and may explain why there were no differences in weight loss at 1 year.

Findings from studies of longer duration (ie, 2 years) are mixed. Two studies reported no differences in weight loss between LC and LF diets at 2 years,[35,45] whereas another reported greater reductions in weight at 2 years with the LC diet compared to a LF diet but similar reductions compared to a Mediterranean type diet.[28] Maximal weight loss occurred at 6 months in these studies, with weight regain beginning between 6 and 12 months. Dietary adherence findings were similar to studies shorter in duration, despite more intensive contact with study staff. The study in which better weight loss outcomes were reported with a LC diet provided participants with food and portion size guidance for the main meal of the day.[28] Taken together, these findings suggest that LF and LC diets are equally effective in reducing weight.

There have been concerns about the effects of LC diets on CVD risk and bone health. With regard to CVD risk, most studies found that LC diets decreased TAG and very-low-density lipoproteins (VLDLs) and increased HDL more than LF diets in the short term. However, these changes were not sustained in the long term, with the exception of HDL. Sustained increases in HDL were shown in two studies.[39,45] Given our current understanding, it does not appear that LC diets trigger any adverse effects on lipid variables. In addition, no differences in body composition or bone mineral density were observed between a LF and LC diet at any point in a 2-year study.[45]

LOW-GI DIET

Carbohydrates vary in the degree to which they raise blood glucose and insulin levels. The term "glycemic index" (GI) refers to a property of carbohydrate-containing food that affects the change in blood glucose after food consumption.[46] Carbohydrate-containing foods are ranked in relation to glucose or white bread, which both have a GI of 100. Thus, foods with a GI between 0 and 55 are considered low-GI foods, those with a GI of 70 or greater are considered high-GI foods, and those that fall between these two ranges are categorized as intermediate-GI foods. A variety of factors such as carbohydrate type, amount and type of fiber, degree of processing, cooking, storage, acidity, food structure, and macronutrient content can all affect GI. Glycemic load (GL) is a similar concept but takes into account both the type of carbohydrate and the amount of carbohydrate consumed.

A low-GI or low-GL diet is a unique blend of LF and LC concepts. Recommendations for this dietary approach are based not only on the GI values of foods but also on the overall nutritional content of the diet.[47] The overall goal of low-GI eating is to obtain adequate energy and nutrients without causing large spikes in insulin and blood glucose levels.

Efficacy, Health Effects, and Sustainability

There has been considerable discussion regarding whether clinicians should recommend low-GI diets to overweight and obese patients.[48,49] Findings from studies of adults, published in our earlier review,[1] suggested that there were no advantages in terms of weight loss when GI was altered and energy and macronutrient composition were held constant. Findings did suggest, however, that low-GI diets may play an important role in the prevention and treatment of metabolic and cardiovascular disease.

More recent studies of adults support previous findings. Although a number of feeding studies suggest that low-GI foods increase satiety more than high-GI foods,[50] it does not appear that the effect on appetite affects energy intake enough to impact body weight.[50] One recent study compared the effects of ad libitum low- and high-GI diets on weight loss in overweight and obese hyperinsulinemic women.[51] Two additional studies compared energy-controlled, isocaloric low-GL and high-GL diets, one in adults with at least one criterion for metabolic syndrome,[51] and the other in obese adults with type 2 diabetes.[53] The ad libitum study was a randomized crossover intervention including two 12-week periods in which women incorporated low-GI or high-GI foods into their diets.[51] A difference of 8.4 GI units (ie, 55.5 vs 63.9) differentiated the low-GI and high-GI dietary periods. Simple substitution of low-GI and high-GI foods did not reduce energy intake or lead to weight loss. In fact, weight increased during both intervention periods, with no difference between groups.

Klemsdal and coworkers[52] randomized participants with varying degrees of metabolic syndrome to either a low-GL diet or a LF diet. A 500 kcal/day deficit was recommended. Although greater reductions in weight were observed at 3 and 6 months in participants prescribed the low-GL diet, 1-year weight loss was almost identical, indicating greater weight regain in the low-GL group between 6 and 12 months. Interestingly, at 1 year the change in waist circumference was significantly greater in the LF than in the low-GL group (−5.8 cm vs −4.1 cm). Although no differences between groups were observed for systolic pressure, diastolic blood pressure was reduced more in the low-GL compared to the LF group (−4.0 mm Hg vs −1.1 mm Hg).

Given their potential to affect glucose and insulin responses, the effects of low- and high-GI/GL diets in individuals with diabetes is of particular interest. Therefore, as part of a 40-week lifestyle modification program, overweight and obese men and women with type 2 diabetes were randomized to either a 1500 kcal LF or low-GL diet.[51] Weight loss and changes in HbA_{1c} were the primary outcome measures in this study. No significant intergroup differences were observed for reductions in body weight. However, participants prescribed the low-GL diet experienced greater reductions in HbA_{1c} than those following the LF diet at 20 (−0.7% vs −0.3%) and 40 weeks (−0.8% vs −0.1%). There were no significant differences in fasting glucose, insulin, HOMA-IR, lipids, or blood pressure. Whereas other studies have not observed differences in HbA_{1c}[54,55], findings from this study suggest that low-GL diets may provide a metabolic advantage for patients with type 2 diabetes, despite the fact that they were no more effective than LF diets in reducing weight. More research is needed to better understand the metabolic and anthropometric effects of low-GI and high-GI diets in individuals with type 2 diabetes and metabolic syndrome. There is some evidence to suggest that individuals with higher insulin secretion lose more weight on a low-GL than on a high-GL diet.[56]

Only a limited number of studies have evaluated the effects of GI on weight maintenance, and findings are mixed.[43,57] One study reported no difference in body weight in individuals who had lost 6% of their initial weight and were then randomized to a high-GI/GL or low-GI/GL diet for 4 months.[57] Another study showed that weight maintenance was better in participants who followed an ad libitum low-GI diet.[43] Further, participants who consumed a low-GI, HP diet continued to lose weight after initial weight loss, whereas those who consumed a high-GI, LP diet regained weight.

SUMMARY

Various dietary strategies can effectively reduce weight, as shown by this review. Those that are coupled with behavior therapy and ongoing support tend to produce longer lasting effects. Improvements in health parameters are observed with each dietary strategy. Improvements in diabetes and CVD risk factors have been observed with diets ranging from 10% fat to 45% fat. HP diets seem to be particularly effective in reducing fat mass and TAG, especially in individuals with dyslipidemia and who are at risk for type 2 diabetes. Likewise, LC diets have been shown to be effective in decreasing TAG and VLDL and increasing HDL. Although low-GI diets do not seem to be superior to any other diet for weight loss, there is evidence to suggest that they may provide some metabolic benefit for those with type 2 diabetes.

Clearly, all of these diets have benefits but they can be realized only when they are followed. A common theme across studies is poor long-term adherence and weight regain. Dansinger and colleagues[19] found a strong association between diet adherence and clinically significant weight loss, suggesting that "sustained adherence to a diet" rather than "following a certain type of diet" is the key to successful weight management.

FUTURE DIRECTIONS FOR RESEARCH

More effective weight loss options are needed to support healthy and sustainable eating behaviors. Randomized control weight loss trials have been designed to assess which diet is best, but perhaps researchers have been asking the wrong question. The "winner take all" mentality does not serve the field or patients well. Rather than asking which is the best diet, investigators should be asking for which type of patients do certain diets work best and how can adherence be improved. Focusing efforts on developing reliable methods for facilitating long-term adherence to both sides of the energy balance equation would be worthwhile and constructive.[58] Future research might also focus more on behavioral factors that often undermine healthy eating in the long term. These studies will require large samples that will allow for examination of various behavioral and metabolic subtypes.

REFERENCES

1. Makris AP, Foster GD. Dietary approaches to the treatment of obesity. Psychiatr Clin North Am 2005;28:117–39.
2. US Department of Agriculture and US Department of Health and Human Services. Dietary guidelines for Americans, 2010. 7th edition. Washington, DC: US Government Printing Office; December 2010.
3. American Diabetes Association, Bantle JP, Wylie-Rosett J, et al. Nutrition recommendations and interventions for diabetes: a position statement of the American Diabetes Association. Diabetes Care 2008;31(Suppl 1):S61–S78.

4. American Heart Association Nutrition Committee; Lichtenstein AH, Appel LJ, Brands M, et al. Diet and lifestyle recommendations revision 2006: a scientific statement from the American Heart Association Nutrition Committee. Circulation 2006;114:82–96.

5. Kushi LH, Byers T, Doyle C, et al. The American Cancer Society 2006 Nutrition and Physical Activity Guidelines Advisory Committee. American Cancer Society guidelines on nutrition and physical activity for cancer prevention: reducing the risk of cancer with healthy food choices and physical activity. CA Cancer J Clin 2006;56:254–81.

6. Look AHEAD Research Group, Wing RR. Long-term effects of a lifestyle intervention on weight and cardiovascular risk factors in individuals with type 2 diabetes mellitus: four-year results of the Look AHEAD trial. Arch Intern Med 2010;170:1566–75.

7. Jeffery RW, Levy RL, Langer SL, et al. A comparison of maintenance-tailored therapy (MTT) and standard behavior therapy (SBT) for the treatment of obesity. Prev Med 2009;49:384–9.

8. Riebe D, Blissmer B, Greene G, et al. Long-term maintenance of exercise and healthy eating behaviors in overweight adults. Prev Med 2005;40:769–78.

9. Svetkey LP, Stevens VJ, Brantley PJ, et al. Weight Loss Maintenance Collaborative Research Group. Comparison of strategies for sustaining weight loss: the weight loss maintenance randomized controlled trial. JAMA 2008;299:1139–48.

10. Perri MG, Limacher MC, Durning PE, et al. Extended-care programs for weight management in rural communities: the treatment of obesity in underserved rural settings (TOURS) randomized trial. Arch Intern Med 2008;168:2347–54.

11. Turner-McGrievy GM, Barnard ND, Scialli AR. A two-year randomized weight loss trial comparing a vegan diet to a more moderate low-fat diet. Obesity 2007;15:2276–81.

12. Howard BV, Van Horn L, Hsia J, et al. Low-fat dietary pattern and risk of cardiovascular disease: the Women's Health Initiative Randomized Controlled Dietary Modification Trial. JAMA 2006;295:655–66.

13. Azadbakht L, Mirmiran P, Esmaillzadeh A, et al. Better dietary adherence and weight maintenance achieved by a long-term moderate-fat diet. Br J Nutr 2007;97:399–404.

14. Owen K, Pettman T, Haas M, et al. Individual preferences for diet and exercise programmes: changes over a lifestyle intervention and their link with outcomes. Public Health Nutr 2010;13:245–52.

15. Burke LE, Warziski M, Styn MA, et al. A randomized clinical trial of a standard versus vegetarian diet for weight loss: the impact of treatment preference. Int J Obes (Lond) 2008;32:166–76.

16. Borradaile KE, Halpern SD, Wyatt HR, et al. Relationship between treatment preference and weight loss in the context of a randomized controlled trial. Obesity 2011. [Epub ahead of print]. DOI:10.1038/oby. 2011.216.

17. Ornish D. Low-fat diets. N Engl J Med 1998;338:127;128–9.

18. Freedman MR, King J, Kennedy E. Popular diets: a scientific review. Obes Res 2001;9:1S–40S.

19. Dansinger ML, Gleason JA, Griffith JL, et al. Comparison of the Atkins, Ornish, Weight Watchers, and Zone diets for weight loss and heart disease risk reduction: a randomized trial. JAMA 2005;293:43–53.

20. Gardner CD, Kiazand A, Alhassan S, et al. Comparison of the Atkins, Zone, Ornish, and LEARN diets for change in weight and related risk factors among overweight premenopausal women: the A TO Z Weight Loss Study: a randomized trial. JAMA 2007;297:969–77.

21. Barnard ND, Cohen J, Jenkins DJ, et al. A low-fat vegan diet improves glycemic control and cardiovascular risk factors in a randomized clinical trial in individuals with type 2 diabetes. Diabetes Care 2006;29:1777–83.

22. Barnard ND, Cohen J, Jenkins DJ et al. A low-fat vegan diet and a conventional diabetes diet in the treatment of type 2 diabetes: a randomized, controlled, 74-wk clinical trial. Am J Clin Nutr 2009;89:1588S–1596S.

23. Barnard ND, Gloede L, Cohen J, et al. A low-fat vegan diet elicits greater macronutrient changes, but is comparable in adherence and acceptability, compared with a more conventional diabetes diet among individuals with type 2 diabetes. J Am Diet Assoc. 2009;109(2):263–72.

24. Ferro-Luzzi A, James WP, Kafatos A. The high-fat Greek diet: a recipe for all? Eur J Clin Nutr 2002;56:796–809.

25. Karamanos B, Thanopoulou A, Angelico F, et al. Nutritional habits in the Mediterranean Basin. The macronutrient composition of diet and its relation with the traditional Mediterranean diet. Multi-centre study of the Mediterranean Group for the Study of Diabetes (MGSD). Eur J Clin Nutr 2002;56:983–91.

26. Brehm BJ, Lattin BL, Summer SS, et al. One-year comparison of a high-monounsaturated fat diet with a high-carbohydrate diet in type 2 diabetes. Diabetes Care 2009;32:215–20.

27. Jenkins DJ, Chiavaroli L, Wong JM, et al. Adding monounsaturated fatty acids to a dietary portfolio of cholesterol-lowering foods in hypercholesterolemia. CMAJ 2010; 182:1961–7.

28. Shai I, Schwarzfuchs D, Henkin Y, et al. Dietary Intervention Randomized Controlled Trial (DIRECT) Group. Weight loss with a low-carbohydrate, Mediterranean, or low-fat diet. N Engl J Med 2008;359:229–41.

29. Esposito K, Kastorini CM, Panagiotakos DB, Giugliano D. Mediterranean diet and weight loss: meta-analysis of randomized controlled trials. Metab Syndr Relat Disord 2011;9:1–12.

30. Due A, Larsen TM, Mu H, et al. Comparison of 3 ad libitum diets for weight-loss maintenance, risk of cardiovascular disease, and diabetes: a 6-mo randomized, controlled trial. Am J Clin Nutr 2008;88:1232–41.

31. Sloth B, Due A, Larsen TM, et al. The effect of a high-MUFA, low-glycaemic index diet and a low-fat diet on appetite and glucose metabolism during a 6-month weight maintenance period. Br J Nutr 2009;101:1846–58.

32. Eisenstein J, Roberts SB, Dallal G, et al. High-protein weight-loss diets: are they safe and do they work? A review of the experimental and epidemiologic data. Nutr Rev 2002;1:189–200.

33. Noakes M, Keogh JB, Foster PR, et al. Effect of an energy-restricted, high-protein, low-fat diet relative to a conventional high-carbohydrate, low-fat diet on weight loss, body composition, nutritional status, and markers of cardiovascular health in obese women. Am J Clin Nutr 2005;81:1298–306.

34. Kerksick CM, Wismann-Bunn J, Fogt D, et al. Changes in weight loss, body composition and cardiovascular disease risk after altering macronutrient distributions during a regular exercise program in obese women. Nutr J 2010;9:59.

35. Sacks FM, Bray GA, Carey VJ, et al. Comparison of weight-loss diets with different compositions of fat, protein, and carbohydrates. N Engl J Med 2009;360:859–73.

36. Larsen RN, Mann NJ, Maclean E, et al. The effect of high-protein, low-carbohydrate diets in the treatment of type 2 diabetes: a 12 month randomised controlled trial. Diabetologia 2011;54:731–40.

37. Clifton PM, Keogh JB, Noakes M. Long-term effects of a high-protein weight-loss diet. Am J Clin Nutr 2008;87:23–9.

38. Meckling KA, Sherfey R. A randomized trial of a hypocaloric high-protein diet, with and without exercise, on weight loss, fitness, and markers of the metabolic syndrome in overweight and obese women. Appl Physiol Nutr Metab 2007;32:743–52.

39. McAuley KA, Smith KJ, Taylor RW, et al. Long-term effects of popular dietary approaches on weight loss and features of insulin resistance. Int J Obes (Lond) 2006;30:342–9.

40. Wycherley TP, Noakes M, Clifton PM, et al. A high-protein diet with resistance exercise training improves weight loss and body composition in overweight and obese patients with type 2 diabetes. Diabetes Care 2010;33:969–76.

41. Layman DK, Evans EM, Erickson D, et al. A moderate-protein diet produces sustained weight loss and long-term changes in body composition and blood lipids in obese adults. J Nutr 2009;139:514–21.

42. Clifton PM, Bastiaans K, Keogh JB. High protein diets decrease total and abdominal fat and improve CVD risk profile in overweight and obese men and women with elevated triacylglycerol. Nutr Metab Cardiovasc Dis 2009;19:548–54.

43. Larsen TM, Dalskov SM, van Baak M, et al. Diet, Obesity, and Genes (Diogenes) Project. Diets with high or low protein content and glycemic index for weight-loss maintenance. N Engl J Med 2010 25;363:2102–13.

44. Nordmann AJ, Nordmann A, Briel M, et al. Effects of low-carbohydrate vs low-fat diets on weight loss and cardiovascular risk factors: a meta-analysis of randomized controlled trials. Arch Intern Med 2006;166:285–93.

45. Foster GD, Wyatt HR, Hill JO, et al. Weight and metabolic outcomes after 2 years on a low-carbohydrate versus low-fat diet: a randomized trial. Ann Intern Med 2010;153: 147–57.

46. Roberts SB. High-glycemic index foods, hunger, and obesity: is there a connection? Nutr Rev 2000;58:163–9.

47. Brand-Miller J, Wolever TMS, Foster-Powell K, et al. The new glucose revolution. New York: Marlowe & Co.; 1996. p. 71-94, 173–95.

48. Pawlak DB, Ebbeling CB, Ludwig DS. Should obese patients be counseled to follow a low-glycaemic index diet? Yes. Obes Rev 2002;3:235–43.

49. Raben A. Should obese patients be counseled to follow a low-glycaemic index diet? No. Obes Rev 2002;3:245–56.

50. Ford H, Frost G. Glycaemic index, appetite and body weight. Proc Nutr Soc 2010; 69:199–203.

51. Aston LM, Stokes CS, Jebb SA. No effect of a diet with a reduced glycaemic index on satiety, energy intake and body weight in overweight and obese women. Int J Obes (Lond) 2008;32:160–5.

52. Klemsdal TO, Holme I, Nerland H, et al. Effects of a low glycemic load diet versus a low-fat diet in subjects with and without the metabolic syndrome. Nutr Metab Cardiovasc Dis 2010;20:195–201.

53. Fabricatore AN, Wadden TA, Ebbeling CB, et al. Targeting dietary fat or glycemic load in the treatment of obesity and type 2 diabetes: a randomized controlled trial. Diabetes Res Clin Pract 2011;92:37–45.

54. Wolever TM, Gibbs AL, Mehling C, et al. The Canadian Trial of Carbohydrates in Diabetes (CCD), a 1-y controlled trial of low-glycemic-index dietary carbohydrate in type 2 diabetes: no effect on glycated hemoglobin but reduction in C-reactive protein. Am J Clin Nutr 2008;87:114–25.

55. Davis NJ, Tomuta N, Schechter C, et al. Comparative study of the effects of a 1-year dietary intervention of a low-carbohydrate diet versus a low-fat diet on weight and glycemic control in type 2 diabetes. Diabetes Care 2009;32:1147–52.

56. Pittas AG, Das SK, Hajduk CL, et al. A low-glycemic load diet facilitates greater weight loss in overweight adults with high insulin secretion but not in overweight adults with low insulin secretion in the CALERIE Trial. Diabetes Care 2005;28:2939–41.
57. Philippou E, Neary NM, Chaudhri O, et al. The effect of dietary glycemic index on weight maintenance in overweight subjects: a pilot study. Obesity (Silver Spring) 2009;17:396–401.
58. Dansinger ML, Schaefer EJ. Low-fat diets and weight change. JAMA 2006;295:94–5.

Obesity and Physical Activity

John M. Jakicic, PhD*, Kelliann K. Davis, PhD

KEYWORDS
- Physical activity • Exercise • Obesity • Overweight
- Weight control

There continues to be significant public health concern about the high rates of overweight and obesity. These concerns stem from the consistent association between excess body weight and numerous chronic diseases, including heart disease, diabetes, and various forms of cancer.[1] Moreover, excess body weight has been shown to negatively influence musculoskeletal health and may limit physical function. Thus, there is a need for effective interventions to reduce body weight in those individuals who may already be overweight or obese. Physical activity can be an important component of lifestyle interventions for weight loss. Thus, it is important for clinicians, health care providers, and health-fitness professionals to recognize the influence of physical activity on body weight and to understand recommendations that can affect physical activity behavior. A conceptual model illustrating the potential pathways by which physical activity may influence energy balance and, thus, influence body weight regulation and related health outcomes is shown in **Fig. 1**.

INFLUENCE OF PHYSICAL ACTIVITY ON WEIGHT LOSS
Physical Activity With No Prescribed Reduction in Energy Intake

There have been a number of recent systematic reviews of the literature that provide a comprehensive understanding of the influence of physical activity on weight loss. For example, the Advisory Committee for the 2008 Physical Activity Guidelines for Americans reviewed the published scientific literature to summarize the influence of physical activity on change in body weight.[2] This literature review was limited to studies that examined physical activity with no prescribed change in energy intake or other dietary modification. Results of this review concluded that physical activity, performed for a minimum of 150 minutes per week at a moderate-to-vigorous intensity (e.g., brisk walking), would reduce body weight by 1% to 3%. The systematic

Disclosures: John M. Jakicic received an honorarium from JennyCraig for presentation of a scientific symposium (2010), a research grant awarded to the University of Pittsburgh from BodyMedia, Inc., and an unrestricted grant awarded to the University of Pittsburgh from Google. He is a member of the Scientific Advisory Board for Alere Wellbeing. Kelliann K. Davis declares no conflicts.
Department of Health and Physical Activity, University of Pittsburgh, Physical Activity and Weight Management Research Center, 140 Trees Hall, Pittsburgh, PA 15261, USA
* Corresponding author.
E-mail address: jjakicic@pitt.edu

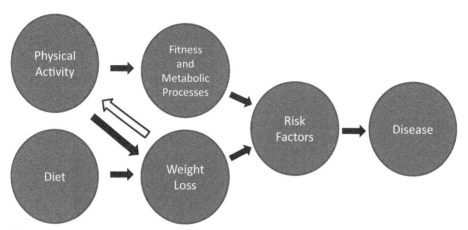

Fig. 1. Conceptual model illustrating the potential pathways by which physical activity may influence energy balance, body weight, related health outcomes.

review of the literature conducted for the recent American College of Sports Medicine position stand[3] examined the influence of physical activity on weight loss when there was no prescribed reduction in energy intake. This review concluded that, under these circumstances, performing fewer than 150 minutes of physical activity per week has minimal influence on body weight, whereas physical activity 150 minutes or more per week results in weight loss of 2 to 3 kg. Physical activity ranging from 225 to 420 minutes per week results in 5 to 7.5 kg of weight loss.

These systematic reviews suggest that physical activity, without a reduction in energy intake, can have a modest influence in decreasing body weight, with the magnitude of the reduction occurring in a dose–response manner, relative to the amount of physical activity performed. This is supported by the findings of Jakicic and co-workers[4] in a study of overweight adults (body mass index [BMI] ranging from 25.0 to <30.0 kg/m^2). Participants classified as reducing body weight by more than 3% over a period of 18 months increased physical activity by 162 minutes per week above baseline levels, whereas those participants categorized as being within 3% of their initial body weight, or gaining more than 3% of their body weight, increased physical activity above baseline levels by 78.2 and 74.7 minutes per week, respectively. The magnitude of weight loss of those classified as reducing weight by more than 3% was actually 5.4 ± 2.6 kg, corresponding with weight loss of 7.4% ± 3.6% of initial body weight.

Physical Activity Combined With Prescribed Reduction in Energy Intake

It is widely accepted that lifestyle interventions that combine an increase in physical activity with a reduction in energy intake result in the greatest weight loss in overweight and obese adults. Physical activity is beneficial because of the added weight loss attained in addition to the weight loss attained through energy restriction alone.[3] A review by Curioni and Lourenco[5] concluded that the addition of physical activity to an energy restricted diet resulted in 20% greater weight loss compared with energy restriction alone. For example, in response to a 12-week intervention, Hagan and colleagues[6] reported a reduction in body weight of 8.4% in males and 5.5% in females resulting from reduction in energy intake, with the addition of exercise to reduced energy intake producing weight loss of 11.4% and 7.5%, respectively. Wing and associates[7] reported that weight loss improved from 9.1% in response to a 24-week diet intervention to 10.4% when physical activity was added.

In a recent study of severely obese adults, Goodpaster and co-workers[8] demonstrated that the weight loss benefits of adding physical activity to an energy-restricted diet are similar to those observed in adults with lesser degrees of obesity. Weight loss resulting from 6 months of an energy restricted diet was 8.2 kg, which improved by 25% to 10.9 kg when physical activity was added to the energy-restricted diet. This added weight loss resulting from physical activity attributed to greater reductions in hepatic fat content and abdominal adiposity expressed as waist circumference. These results suggest that clinicians involved in the treatment of severe obesity should recommend physical activity as a component of the treatment plan.

Long-Term Weight Loss and Weight Loss Maintenance

Within the context of weight loss in obese adults, physical activity may be most beneficial for improving long-term weight loss and minimizing weight regain. Unick and colleagues[9] examined the treatment components that contributed to achieving 10% or more weight loss after a 24-month intervention. Although maintaining long-term contact with intervention staff and adoption of eating behaviors that contribute to weight control were significant predictors of this magnitude of weight loss at 24 months, physical activity explained more of the variability in weight loss. Physical activity was examined for participants who achieved 10% or greater weight loss at 6 months and were then able to maintain this magnitude of weight loss at 24 months compared with those participants who achieved 10% or greater at 6 months, but were unable to maintain this magnitude of weight loss at 24 months. These classifications of weight loss did not differ in the magnitude of change in physical activity from baseline to 6 months. However, the change in physical activity from baseline to 24 months was significantly greater in those who were able to maintain at least 10% weight loss at 24 months, compared with those who were not able to maintain this weight loss.

The importance of physical activity for improving long-term weight loss and minimizing weight regain is supported by the systematic review of the literature conducted for the 2009 American College of Sports Medicine Position Paper on "Appropriate Physical Activity Intervention Strategies for Weight Loss and Prevention of Weight Regain for Adults."[3] Based on the review of the literature it was concluded that more than 250 minutes per week of physical activity contributes to maintenance of lost weight, which is consistent with the results of empirical studies.[10–15]

Despite the apparent importance of physical activity for long-term weight control, physical activity does not seem to act alone to control body weight, but rather functions in synergy with appropriate levels of energy intake. Unick and associates[9] reported that both physical activity and change in eating behaviors significantly contributed to the achievement of 10% or greater weight loss after a 24-month intervention. Jakicic and colleagues[16] reported similar findings in an examination of 18-month weight loss in overweight and obese women. Similar findings were reported based on data from the National Weight Control Registry.[17] Thus, clinicians should have an appreciation of the importance of appropriate eating behaviors, as well as adequate doses of physical activity, for improving long-term weight loss in overweight and obese adults.

Physical Activity Considerations in Bariatric Surgery

Bariatric surgery has been shown to significantly reduce body weight, with the magnitude typically exceeding what can be achieved through lifestyle approaches that focus solely on reducing energy intake and increasing energy expenditure through physical activity. However, this does not imply that lifestyle behaviors, which include physical activity, should not be an aspect of the long-term care of patients who have undergone bariatric surgery. Rather, a growing body of scientific evidence supports the need for physical activity in patients after bariatric surgery.

Bond and associates[18,19] reported that physical activity contributed to improved weight loss at both 1 and 2 years after bariatric surgery. In addition, greater weight loss has been reported at 6 and 12 months after bariatric surgery among patients who participated in 150 minutes or more of exercise per week, compared with those participating for fewer than 150 minutes per week.[20] Thus, clinicians should emphasize the importance of high levels of physical activity to maximize long-term weight loss with bariatric surgery.

ALTERNATIVE TYPES OF PHYSICAL ACTIVITY

The majority of studies in the literature reporting on the influence of physical activity on body weight have included include aerobic forms of physical activity, such as walking. However, other forms of activity may be considered when prescribing physical activity to overweight and obese adults. These may include resistance exercise, aquatic exercise, or lifestyle forms of physical activity.

Resistance Exercise

A conceptual model has been proposed to explain how resistance exercise may influence body weight and body fatness.[3] This model proposes that resistance exercise can increase energy expenditure through the cost of performing resistance exercise, the influence that resistance exercise has on free-living physical activity, and the increase in resting metabolic rate that may occur from resistance exercise increasing muscle mass. However, despite this theoretical rationale, the scientific evidence suggests a modest effect of resistance exercise on body weight and body fatness,[3,21] and this may be influenced by whether the resistance exercise is accompanied by a concurrent reduction in energy intake.

A recent, systematic review of the literature has concluded that there is little to no evidence from intervention studies to support that resistance exercise, in the absence of reductions in energy intake through dietary modification, can reduce body weight.[3] This confirms the findings of an earlier review of this topic.[21] Moreover, the scientific literature is mixed on whether resistance exercise can significantly reduce body fatness in the absence of restricting energy intake. There is, however, evidence that resistance exercise can increase lean mass,[22–25] although this does not necessarily result in a decrease in absolute body fatness. Thus, relying solely on resistance exercise as a treatment modality to reduce body weight or body fatness may have limited effectiveness for overweight and obese adults. Moreover, the addition of resistance exercise to dietary modification that focuses on reducing energy intake has also been shown to have limited effectiveness in reducing body weight or total body fatness, compared with what can be achieved through dietary intervention alone.[3,21] However, there is some evidence that resistance exercise can reduce subcutaneous abdominal adiposity,[26] and this may have important clinical implications related to the reduction in health risk associated with obesity.

Aquatic Exercise

Aquatic exercise has been recommended as an alternative form of physical activity for overweight or obese individuals who have potential functional limitations.[27] However, limited data are available to support the effectiveness of this form of activity for the treatment of obesity. Nagle and co-workers[28] reported the results of one of the few published studies in this area. The intervention consisted of dietary modification to reduce energy intake, which was combined with either supervised aerobic or supervised aquatic exercise for 16 weeks. There were no differences in weight loss with aquatic exercise (-6.8 ± 3.2 kg) versus aerobic exercise (-5.6 ± 4.7 kg), with similar patterns shown in both interventions for reductions in waist circumference, waist-to-hip ratio, and body fatness. Thus, although not superior to a walking intervention, this study seems to support the use of aquatic exercise as an alternative form of activity that can be incorporated into lifestyle interventions targeting weight loss and physical activity.

Lifestyle Activity

Until recently, there has been confusion with regard to defining what is considered to be lifestyle physical activity. The American College of Sports Medicine has defined lifestyle physical activity as "any nonstructured form of physical activity performed that is not intended to constitute a structured period of exercise."[3] Examples include activity performed commuting to work versus the same form of activity done within a structured period of exercise. Given this definition, walking performed as a means of commuting to work would be considered lifestyle activity, whereas taking a structured 30 minute walk for the purpose of exercise would not be considered lifestyle activity. Levine and colleaguese[29] have termed all energy expenditure that does not result from sleeping, eating, or structured exercise as nonexercise activity thermogenesis (NEAT).

It has been suggested that an increase in NEAT of as little as 100 kcal per day may be sufficient to prevent weight gain at the population level. Alternatively, interventions targeting increases in NEAT could theoretically contribute to a negative energy balance, which would promote weight loss. A common methodology that has been examined to increase NEAT is the use of pedometers to promote additional nonstructured walking for physical activity. A systematic review of the literature has shown that promoting lifestyle forms of activity that increase steps walked by 2100 per day, as measured by a pedometer, can have decrease BMI by a modest yet significant 0.38 kg/m^2.[3]

A common public health message is to accumulate 10,000 steps per day. Daily physical activity may require approximately 6000 to 7000 steps per day (although obese individuals may take significantly fewer steps).[30] Thus, the addition of approximately 3000 to 4000 steps per day for most individuals would result in achievement of the public health goal of 10,000 steps per day. Chan and co-workers[31] reported that a 12-week pedometer campaign resulted in an increase of more than 3000 steps per day, and there was an inverse association between steps walked and reductions in waist circumference but not BMI. It is estimated that approximately 2000 steps is the equivalent of 1 mile of walking, so the addition of 3000 steps per day would be the equivalent to walking an additional 1.5 miles per day. Assuming a 20-minute walking pace, this would result in an additional 30 minutes of walking per day, which is consistent with the public health recommendation to achieve at least 30 minutes of moderate intensity physical activity per day.[1,5]

Although the effects may be modest, promoting lifestyle forms of physical activity, which may include increased walking, can contribute to decreases in either BMI or waist circumference. This approach, in combination with structured exercise, may significantly increase energy expenditure to improve weight loss in overweight and obese adults, and may contribute to prevention of further weight gain across the entire population.

FITNESS OR FATNESS: WHICH SHOULD BE THE FOCUS FOR REDUCING HEALTH RISKS IN OBESE ADULTS?

Participation in physical activity can also improve cardiorespiratory fitness in overweight and obese adults. In the context of an 18-month physical activity intervention that did not prescribe a concurrent reduction in energy intake, a dose–response relationship was reported between physical activity and improvement in cardiorespiratory fitness.[4] The observed improvement in fitness resulting from physical activity in overweight and obese adults seems to occur regardless of whether there is a reduction in body weight resulting from the intervention.[32] However, fitness does not seem to improve with weight loss achieved through dietary modification alone, without the inclusion of physical activity.[33]

Improved cardiorespiratory fitness is clinically significant in overweight and obese adults because of the inverse association between cardiorespiratory fitness and a variety of health-related outcomes. Blair and associates[34] reported that higher levels of cardiorespiratory fitness coincided with lower relative risk of all-cause mortality and age-adjusted death rates from cardiovascular disease. It has also been reported that improving fitness is associated with a lower risk of mortality,[35] with the risk of mortality decreasing 7.9% for each minute of improvement on a treadmill test. Therefore, increasing to or maintaining a sufficient level of cardiorespiratory fitness is of particular public health importance due to its role in reducing risk of all-cause mortality.

The reduced relative risk for all-cause mortality associated with greater levels of cardiorespiratory fitness continues to be observed after BMI is considered in the analysis.[34] This type of observation has spurred an interest in understanding if the health risks associated with excess body weight are a result solely of the excess body fatness that accumulates with obesity or partially or fully explained by the low level of cardiorespiratory fitness typically observed in individuals classified as overweight or obese. The majority of the evidence that supports the finding that cardiorespiratory fitness is a predictor of all-cause mortality and cardiovascular disease, independent of measures of body fatness, comes from the Aerobics Center Longitudinal Study.[36–41] The findings seem to be consistent, regardless of whether body fatness is represented as BMI[36–38,41] or a direct measure of body composition.[40,42] However, limited data are available on this topic for patients with severe obesity.

Not all studies in this area have shown that cardiorespiratory fitness completely ameliorates the health risk of fatness. Stevens and colleagues,[43] using data from the Lipids Research Clinic Study, showed that cardiorespiratory fitness reduced the risk of all-cause and cardiovascular disease mortality in overweight and obese individuals, but it did not seem to completely ameliorate the risk of fatness on these outcomes. In a prospective study of older men, McAuley and co-workers[44] reported that both cardiorespiratory fitness and BMI contributed to the risk of all-cause mortality. A recent review by Jakicic and colleagues[45] suggested that both cardiorespiratory fitness and body fatness may influence selective risk factors for cardiovascular disease and diabetes. These findings suggest that interventions for overweight and obese adults that focus on both weight loss and improvements in cardiorespiratory fitness may provide the most significant improvements in health outcomes.

CLINICAL CONSIDERATIONS FOR PHYSICAL ACTIVITY IN OVERWEIGHT AND OBESE ADULTS
Preactivity Screening

Overweight and obesity are associated with increased risk for chronic disease,[1] and this may result in some health care professionals being cautious with regard to recommending physical activity as a component of the intervention plan. However, the American College of Sports Medicine provides clear guidance on the level of prescreening that is required before initiating a physical activity program for adults with risk factors or known chronic disease.[46] Patients are classified as low, moderate, or high risk based on the presence of risk factors or known chronic disease (**Table 1**). This risk stratification is used to provide guidance to clinicians and other health care professionals with regard to the level of prescreening that is required before a patient initiates a moderate or vigorous intensity physical activity program. Moderate intensity activity is defined as an activity that is performed at 40% to 60% of maximal oxygen consumption capacity or one that ranges from 3 to 6 metabolic equivalents (METs), whereas vigorous intensity activity is an activity performed at greater than 60% of maximal oxygen consumption capacity or one that exceeds 6 METs.[46] Clinicians can refer to the compendium of physical activities for an estimate of METs required to perform a variety of physical activities.[47]

DOES PHYSICAL ACTIVITY RESULT IN INJURIES IN OVERWEIGHT AND OBESE ADULTS?

Compared with a normal weight individual, the odds are 15% to 48% greater for an overweight or obese individual to receive medical treatment for an injury. This may influence recommending physical activity for individuals who are overweight or obese. However, although data are limited on whether physical activity causes injuries in overweight and obese adults, Janney and associates[48] recently reported on the prevalence of injuries potentially caused by physical activity while participating in a structured weight loss intervention. Examination of data from 397 overweight and obese adults over a period of 18 months revealed that 32% of these individuals reported an injury that was partially or fully attributed to participation in physical activity, with the most common form of injury occurring in the lower extremity. However, only 7% of all injuries were attributed solely to participation in physical activity. Moreover, a higher initial BMI, and not volume of exercise participation, was associated with the time to first injury and the number of injuries reported over the time of the intervention. Weight loss reduced the risk of injury.

The likelihood of an injury resulting from an overweight or obese adult initiating a modest activity program as part of a comprehensive weight loss program is relatively low. Thus, if not medically contraindicated, health care professionals should recommend physical activity to these patients. Moreover, with weight loss the risk of injury decreases, which may allow for progression of activity to levels that have been recommended to enhance long-term weight loss and prevention of weight regain.

BEHAVIORAL STRATEGIES FOR PROMOTING PHYSICAL ACTIVITY

Despite the known benefits of physical activity for overweight and obese individuals, rates of long-term adherence to activity in overweight and obese adults are suboptimal. Thus, it is recommended that clinicians incorporate behavioral theories and constructs into interventions to facilitate physical activity participation in overweight and obese adults.[46] Davis and co-workers[49] have suggested that theoretical constructs from the theory of planned behavior,[50] the transtheoretical model,[51] social cognitive theory,[52] and self-determination theory[53] be incorporated into interventions targeting improvements in physical activity behavior.

Self-efficacy is an important construct that appears to be predictive of physical activity in overweight and obese adults.[49] Gallagher and colleagues[54] reported that there was a significant increase in self-efficacy for physical activity in response to a 6-month standard behavioral weight loss intervention. Moreover, after the initial 6

Table 1
Risk stratification and pre-exercise screening recommendations[46]

Risk Stratification	Asymptomatic	≤1 Cardiovascular Disease Risk Factors	≥2 Cardiovascular Disease Risk Factors	Symptomatic or Known Cardiac, Pulmonary, or Metabolic Disease	Medical Examination and Graded Exercise Test Recommended before Initiating an Exercise Program	
					For Moderate Intensity Exercise Program[a]	For Vigorous Intensity Exercise Program[b]
Low risk	X	X			No	No
Moderate risk	X	X	X		No	Yes
High risk				X	Yes	Yes

[a] Moderate intensity activity is defined as an activity performed at 40–60% of maximal oxygen consumption capacity or one that ranges from 3 to 6 metabolic equivalents (METs).
[b] Vigorous intensity activity is an activity performed at >60% of maximal oxygen consumption capacity or one that exceeds 6 METs.

months of the intervention, individuals who participated in 150 minutes or more of physical activity per week had significantly higher levels of physical activity self-efficacy than individuals who engaged in lesser amounts of physical activity. It was also reported that self-efficacy for physical activity was associated with improved weight loss at 6 months in this sample of overweight and obese adults. This suggests that interventions should target self-efficacy for physical activity to improve and maintain physical activity. This may be accomplished through engagement in mastery experiences or through engagement with others who either serve as a model for physical activity or who have a positive influence on one's engagement in physical activity.

Barrier identification seems to be another important factor to consider with regard to physical activity participation in overweight and obese adults.[55] Barriers to physical activity in overweight and obese adults have previously been reported, with lack of motivation and lack of time the most consistently reported obstacles.[55] Traditional behavioral weight loss interventions, which focus on both diet and physical activity, seem to reduce self-reported barriers to physical activity.[54] Moreover, fewer barriers to physical activity were associated with participation in 150 or more minutes per week of moderate-to-vigorous intensity physical activity. Thus, practitioners should query overweight and obese adults on their perceived barriers to physical activity and use problem-solving skills to find realistic solutions to overcoming these barriers.

Additional strategies for improving physical activity have been suggested by Davis and associates.[49] These include self-monitoring, feedback, goal setting, behavioral contracts, program tailoring, and social support for physical activity. Carpenter[56] has provided an overview of practical applications of many of these strategies to inform clinicians, health care providers, and health-fitness professionals.

SUMMARY

Physical activity seems to be an important component of lifestyle interventions for weight loss and maintenance. Although the effects of physical activity on weight loss may seem to be modest, there seems to be a dose–response relationship between physical activity and weight loss. Physical activity also seems to be a critically important behavior to promote long-term weight loss and the prevention of weight regain. The benefits of physical activity on weight loss are also observed in patients with severe obesity (BMI≥35kg/m^2) and in patients who have undergone bariatric surgery. Moreover, independent of the effect of physical activity on body weight, engagement in physical activity that results in improved cardiorespiratory fitness can contribute to reductions in health risk in overweight and obese adults. Thus, progression of overweight and obese patients to an adequate dose of physical activity needs to be incorporated into clinical interventions for weight control.

REFERENCES

1. National Institutes of Health National Heart Lung and Blood Institute. Clinical guidelines on the identification, evaluation, and treatment of overweight and obesity in adults: the evidence report. Obes Res 1998;6(Suppl 2)51S–209S.
2. US Department of Health and Human Services. Physical activity guidelines advisory committee report 2008, vol. 2009. Washington, DC: US Department of Health and Human Services; 2008.
3. Donnelly JE, Blair SN, Jakicic JM, et al. ACSM position stand on appropriate intervention strategies for weight loss and prevention of weight regain for adults. Med Sci Sports Exerc 2009;42:459–71.

4. Jakicic JM, Otto AD, Semler L, et al. Effect of physical activity on 18-month weight change in overweight adults. Obesity 2011;19:100–9.

5. Curioni CC, Lourenco PM. Long-term weight loss after diet and exercise: systematic review. Int J Obes 2005;29:1168–74.

6. Hagan RD, Upton SJ, Wong L, et al. The effects of aerobic conditioning and/or calorie restriction in overweight men and women. Med Sci Sports Exerc 1986;18:87–94.

7. Wing RR, Venditti EM, Jakicic JM, et al. Lifestyle intervention in overweight individuals with a family history of diabetes. Diabetes Care 1998;21:350–9.

8. Goodpaster BH, DeLany JP, Otto AD, et al. Effects of diet and physical activity interventions on weight loss and cardiometabolic risk factors in severely obese adults: a randomized trial. JAMA 2010;304:1795–802.

9. Unick JL, Jakicic JM, Marcus BH. Contribution of behavior intervention components to 24 month weight loss. Med Sci Sports Exerc 2010;42:745–53.

10. Jakicic JM, Marcus BH, Gallagher KI, et al.Effect of exercise duration and intensity on weight loss in overweight, sedentary women. A randomized trial. JAMA 2003;290: 1323–30.

11. Jakicic JM, Marcus BH, Lang W, et al. Effect of exercise on 24-month weight loss in overweight women. Arch Intern Med 2008;168:1550–9.

12. Jakicic JM, Winters C, Lang W, et al. Effects of intermittent exercise and use of home exercise equipment on adherence, weight loss, and fitness in overweight women: a randomized trial. JAMA 1999;282:1554–60.

13. Jeffery RW, Wing RR, Sherwood NE, et al. Physical activity and weight loss: does prescribing higher physical activity goals improve outcome? Am J Clin Nutr 2003;78: 684–9.

14. Klem ML, Wing RR, McGuire MT, et al. A descriptive study of individuals successful at long-term maintenance of substantial weight loss. Am J Clin Nutr 1997;66:239–46.

15. Schoeller DA, Shay K, Kushner RF. How much physical activity is needed to minimize weight gain in previously obese women. Am J Clin Nutr 1997;66:551–6.

16. Jakicic JM, Wing RR, Winters-Hart C. Relationship of physical activity to eating behaviors and weight loss in women. Med Sci Sports Exerc 2002;34:1653–9.

17. McGuire MT, Wing RR, Klem ML, et al. What predicts weight regain in a group of successful weight losers? J Consult Clin Psychol 1999;67:177–85.

18. Bond DS, Evans RK, Wolfe LG, et al. Impact of self-reported physical activity participation on proportion of excess weight loss and BMI among gastric bypass surgery patients. Am Surg 2004;70:811–4.

19. Bond DS, Phelan S, Wolfe LG, et al. Becoming physically active after bariatric surgery is associated with improved weight loss and quality of life. Obesity 2009;17:78–83.

20. Evans RK, Bond DS, Wolfe LG, et al. Participation in 150 minutes/week of moderate or higher intensity physical activity yields greater weight loss following gastric bypass surgery. Surg Obes Relat Dis 2007;3:526–30.

21. Donnelly JE, Jakicic JM, Pronk NP, et al. Is resistance exercise effective for weight management? Evidenced Based Preventive Medicine 2004;1:21–9.

22. Hunter GR, Bryan DR, Wetzstein CJ, et al. Resistance training and intra-abdominal adipose tissue in older men and women. Med Sci Sports Exerc 2002;34:1023–8.

23. Hunter GR, Wetzstein CJ, Fields DA, et al. Resistance training increases total energy expenditure and free-living physical activity in older adults. J Appl Physiol 2000;89: 977–84.

24. Olson TP, Dengel DR, Leon AS, et al. Changes in inflammatory biomarkers following one-year of moderate resistance exercise in overweight women. Int J Obes 2007;31: 996–1003.

25. Schmitz KH, Jensen MD, Kugler KC, et al. Strength training for obesity prevention in midlife women. Int J Obes Relat Meta Disord 2003;27:326–33.

26. Janssen I, Ross R. Effects of sex on the change in visceral, subcutaneous adipose tissue and skeletal muscle in response to weight loss. Int J Obes Relat Meta Disord 1999;23:1035–46.

27. Hergenroeder AL, Brach JS, Otto AD, et al. The influence of body mass index on self-report and performance-based measures of physical function in adult women. Cardiopulm Phys Ther J 2011;22(3):11-20.

28. Nagle EF, Robertson RJ, Jakicic JM, et al. Effects of aquatic exercise and walking in sedentary obese women undergoing a behavioral weight-loss intervention. International Journal of Aquatic Research and Education 2007;1:43–56.

29. Levine JA, Vander Weg MW, Hill JO, et al. Non-exercise activity thermogenesis: the crouching tiger hidden dragon of societal weight gain. Arterioscler Thromb Vasc Biol 2006;26:729–36.

30. Tudor-Locke C, Bassett DR. How many steps/day are enough? Preliminary pedometer indices for public health. Sports Med 2004;34:1–8.

31. Chan CB, Ryan DA, Tudor-Locke C. Health benefits of a pedometer-based physical activity intervention in sedentary workers. Prev Med 2004;39:1215–22.

32. Ross R, Dagnone D, Jones PJH, et al. Reduction in obesity and related comorbid conditions after diet-induced weight loss or exercise-induced weight loss in men. Ann Intern Med 2000;133:92–103.

33. Donnelly JE, Pronk NP, Jacobsen DJ, et al. Effects of a very-low-calorie diet and physical-training regimens on body composition and resting metabolic rate in obese females. Am J Clin Nutr 1991;54:56–61.

34. Blair SN, Kohl III H, Paffenbarger RS, et al. Physical fitness and all-cause mortality. A prospective study of healthy men and women. JAMA 1989;262:2395-401.

35. Blair SN, Kohl III H, Barlow CE, et al. Changes in physical fitness and all-cause mortality: a prospective study of healthy and unhealthy men. JAMA 1995;273: 1093–8.

36. Barlow CE, Kohl 3rd HW, Gibbons LW, et al. Physical activity, mortality, and obesity. Int J Obes Relat Metab Disord 1995;19(Suppl 4):S41-4.

37. Church TS, LaMonte MJ, Barlow CE, et al. Cardiorespiratory fitness and body mass index as predictors of cardiovascular disease mortality among men with diabetes. Arch Intern Med 2005;165:2114-20.

38. Farrell SW, Braun L, Barlow CE, et al. The relation of body mass index, cardiorespiratory fitness, and all-cause mortality in women. Obes Res 2002;10:417-23.

39. Lee S, Kuk JI, Katzmarzyk PT, et al. Cardiorespiratory fitness attenuates metabolic risk independent of subcutaneous and visceral fat in men. Diabetes Care 2005;28: 895–901.

40. Sui X, LaMonte MJ, Laditka JN, et al. Cardiorespiratory fitness and adiposity as mortality predictors in older adults. JAMA 2007;298:2507–16.

41. Wei M, Kampert JB, Barlow CE, et al. Relationship between low cardiorespiratory fitness and mortality in normal-weight, overweight, and obese men. JAMA 1999;282: 1547–53.

42. Lee CD, Blair SN, Jackson AS. Cardiorespiratory fitness, body composition, and all-cause and cardiovascular disease mortality in men. Am J Clin Nutr 1999;69: 373–80.

43. Stevens J, Cai J, Evenson KR, et al. Fitness and fatness as predictors of mortality from all causes and from cardiovascular disease in men and women in the lipid research clinics study. Am J Epidemiol 2002;156:832–41.

44. McAuley P, Pittsley J, Myers J, et al. Fitness and fatness as mortality predictors in healthy older men: the veterans exercise testing study. J Gerontol A Biol Sci Med Sci 2009;64:695 -9.

45. Jakicic JM, Mishler AE, Rogers R. Fitness, fatness, and cardiovascular disease risk and outcomes. Curr Cardiovasc Risk Rep 2011;5:113–9.

46. American College of Sports Medicine. Thompson WR, editor. ACSM's guidelines for exercise testing and prescription. 8th edition. Philadelphia: Wolters Kluwer/Lippincott Williams & Wilkins; 2009.

47. Ainsworth BE, Haskell WL, Leon AS, et al. Compendium of physical activities: classification of energy costs of human physical activities. Med Sci Sports Exerc 1993;25:71–80.

48. Janney CA, Jakicic JM. The influence of exercise and BMI on injuries and illnesses in overweight and obese individuals. Int J Behav Nutr Phys Act 2010;7:1.

49. Davis K, Jakicic JM, Otto AD. Obesity treatment: the use of exercise and behavioral strategies. In: Rios MS, Ordovas JM, Gutierrez Fuentes JA, editors. Obesity. Barcelona: Elsevier; 2011. p. 297–310.

50. Ajzen I, Madden TJ. Prediction of goal-oriented behavior: attitudes, intentions, and perceived control. J Exp Soc Psychol;22:453-74.

51. Prochaska JO, Marcus BH. The transtheoretical model: applications to exercise. In: Dishman RK, editor. Advances in exercise adherence. Champaign (IL): Human Kinetics; 1994. p. 161–80.

52. Bandura A. Social foundations of thought and action: a social cognitive theory Englewood Cliffs (NJ): Prentice-Hall; 1986.

53. Deci EL, Ryan RM. Intrinsic motivation and self-determination in human behavior. New York: Plenum; 1985.

54. Gallagher KI, Jakicic JM, Napolitano MA, et al. Psychosocial factors related to physical activity and weight loss in overweight women. Med Sci Sports Exerc 2006;38:971–80.

55. Jakicic JM, Otto AD. Physical activity recommendations in the treatment of obesity. Psychiatr Clin N Am 2005;28:141–50.

56. Carpenter RA. Physical activity and weight management. Part B: practical applications. In: Nonas CA, Foster GD, editors. Managing obesity: a clinical guide. 2nd edition. Chicago: American Dietetic Association; 2009. p. 81–99.

Behavioral Treatment of Obesity

Meghan L. Butryn, PhD[a],*, Victoria Webb, BA[b],
Thomas A. Wadden, PhD[c]

KEYWORDS

- Obesity • Weight loss • Dieting • Lifestyle • Behavioral

Weight loss treatment is recommended for adults with a body mass index (BMI) of 30 kg/m² or higher, as well as those with BMI of 25 kg/m² or higher who have weight-related comorbidities.[1] Behavioral treatment should be the first line of intervention for overweight and obese individuals.[1] This article first provides an overview of the structure and principles of behavioral weight loss treatment. Second, the short-term and long-term effectiveness of this approach is reviewed. Third, strategies for improving weight loss maintenance are described. Finally, dissemination of behavioral treatment is addressed.

STRUCTURES AND PRINCIPLES OF BEHAVIORAL TREATMENT

The lifestyle modification interventions delivered in the Diabetes Prevention Program (DPP) and Look AHEAD research studies are exemplars of behavioral treatment programs.[2,3] The intervention materials from both of these programs are in the public domain and may be used for educational or research purposes. Behavioral weight loss treatment also has been described in detail in other publications.[4–6] The structure and three key components of this approach—goal setting, self monitoring, and stimulus control—are reviewed here. Additional information about dietary and physical activity recommendations in behavioral programs can be found in the upcoming December issue of this volume.

The authors have no financial disclosures or conflicts of interest to declare. Preparation of this review was supported in part by grant K24-DK065018 to Dr Wadden.

[a] Department of Psychology, Drexel University, 245 North 15th Street, MS 626, Philadelphia, PA 19102, USA

[b] Center for Weight and Eating Disorders, University of Pennsylvania, 3535 Market Street, Philadelphia, PA 19104, USA

[c] Center for Weight and Eating Disorders, Department of Psychiatry, Perelman School of Medicine at the University of Pennsylvania, 3535 Market Street, Suite 3029, Philadelphia, PA 19104, USA

* Corresponding author.

E-mail address: mlb34@drexel.edu

Psychiatr Clin N Am 34 (2011) 841–859
doi:10.1016/j.psc.2011.08.006
0193-953X/11/$ – see front matter © 2011 Elsevier Inc. All rights reserved.

Structure of Treatment

Behavioral treatment is usually provided on a weekly basis for an initial period of 4 to 6 months. Programs that are focused on building weight loss maintenance skills may continue treatment after this period with biweekly sessions. Treatment is often provided in groups of 10 to 15 participants. Group therapy may be more effective than individual treatment. A randomized controlled trial found that group treatment induced a significantly larger initial weight loss than individual care.[7] Group treatment is cost-effective, and group sessions provide a combination of empathy, social support, and healthy competition.[8] Each session is typically scheduled to last 60 or 90 minutes. Group leaders are professionals with degrees in nutrition, psychology, or a related field. Sessions begin with private measurement of weight. Once the group convenes, each patient provides a brief report on his or her success in meeting behavioral goals. A new weight management skill is taught in each session according to a structured curriculum. Examples of skills taught include making healthy selections when eating in restaurants, using portion control, and obtaining social support for behavior changes.

Goal Setting

Behavioral treatment specifies objective goals that can be easily measured. Having objective goals allows for clear assessment of progress. Each patient has a target for average daily calorie intake, weekly minutes of physical activity, and number of days for which food records will be completed. Each week patients share with the group how successful they were in meeting these goals. Patients often report that they appreciate the accountability that results from this check-in. Amount of weight change is typically not shared with the group. However, group leaders typically advise patients to expect 0.5 to 1.0 kg per week of weight loss, with an ultimate goal of losing 10% of initial body weight. Patients also may set goals for additional specific behaviors that are expected to produce or maintain weight loss. When patients target a particular behavior to be changed, they are encouraged to operationalize the goal and carefully consider factors such as how, when, and where the behavior will be completed.

Self-Monitoring

The systematic recording of target behaviors is a cornerstone of behavioral treatment. Self-monitoring provides regular feedback about whether target behaviors are improving, deteriorating, or being maintained. As shown in **Fig. 1**, self-monitoring is strongly associated with weight loss success. Patients who monitor their eating and weight most consistently have the largest weight losses.[9–12] Throughout treatment, patients keep a weekly record of all food and beverages consumed and calculate their daily calorie intake and, in some programs, fat intake. An example of a food record is shown in **Fig. 2**. In the early phase of treatment this food record is a critical tool for identifying eating patterns that can be modified in order to reduce calorie intake. Periodically patients may be asked to monitor particular factors associated with eating behaviors such as hunger level, mood, or place of eating. Patients also record minutes of physical activity or use a pedometer to track daily number of steps.

Stimulus Control

Stimulus control principles are used to change the internal and external cues associated with targeted eating and activity behaviors.[13] Patients are taught to

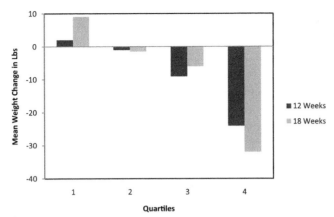

Fig. 1. Mean weight change per quartile of monitoring index (ie, frequency of recording weight and eating within a behavioral treatment program). Higher quartiles indicate more frequently engaging in self-monitoring behaviors. (*From* Baker RC, Kirschenbaum DS. Self-monitoring may be necessary for successful weight control. Behav Ther 1993;24:377–94; with permission.)

change their immediate environment (eg, in the home and workplace) so that it facilitates rather than hinders behavior change. Reducing exposure to particularly tempting high-calorie foods should reduce consumption of such foods. If, for example, a patient would like to have one serving of ice cream per week but finds it difficult to control intake of this particular food, it may be unnecessarily challenging to have a large container of ice cream in the freezer at all times. Instead, a patient may wish to buy a single serving of ice cream once per week. Increasing the availability and visibility of healthy food (eg, by placing a large bowl of fruit slices in the front of the refrigerator) should facilitate desirable eating behaviors. Physical activity also can be promoted by, for example, placing sneakers and appropriate clothing next to the bed if a patient plans to go for a walk immediately upon waking in the morning.

EFFECTIVENESS OF BEHAVIORAL TREATMENT

Participants treated with a comprehensive behavioral approach lose approximately 8 to 10 kg, equal to 8% to 10% of initial weight.[14] Approximately 80% of patients who begin treatment complete it.[14] Thus, lifestyle modification yields favorable results as judged by the criteria for success (ie, a 5%–10% reduction in initial weight) proposed by the National Institutes of Health.[1] Weight loss has more than doubled over the past 30 years as treatment duration has increased threefold.[14] Although several new components, including cognitive restructuring, have been added to the behavioral approach since 1974, the most parsimonious explanation for the larger weight losses is the longer duration of treatment. The rate of weight loss has remained constant at about 0.4 to 0.5 kg per week.

Weight loss often reaches its peak at approximately 6 months, and then weight regain often begins in the absence of weight maintenance therapy. As shown in **Fig. 3**, a metaanalysis of behavioral treatment programs that provided treatment for a range of 13 to 52 sessions found that at 1 year, 28% of individuals had a weight loss of 10% or more of baseline weight, 26% had a weight loss of 5% to 9.9%, and

Monitoring Record			
Day of Week _Thursday_____ Date _8/25____			
Time	**Food: Amount & Description**	**Calories**	
6:30 AM	Corn Flakes, 1 cup	110	
	Skim milk, ½ cup	45	
	6 medium strawberries	15	
	Orange juice, 6 fl. oz.	84	
10:00 AM	1 large peach	55	
1:00 PM	Ham sandwich		
	2 oz. ham	60	
	1 tbsp mustard	5	
	2 slices whole wheat bread	140	
	1 slice tomato	5	
	½ cup applesauce	90	
3:30 PM	¼ cup shelled pistachios	165	
6:30 PM	3 oz. chicken breast, roasted	140	
	½ cup brown rice with 1 pat of butter	145	
	½ cup chopped broccoli	25	
	1 chocolate chip cookie	50	
	Daily Total	1134	
	Type of Physical Activity	**Minutes**	
	Brisk walking	25	

Fig. 2. An example of a self-monitoring record. Participants record the times, amounts, and calories of foods consumed and the physical activity they engage in. The extra column can be used to monitor additional contextual information (eg, places, feelings).

38% had a weight loss of 4.9% or less.[15] Patients on average regain one-third of lost weight within 1 year of treatment ending, and whereas rate of weight regain may slow after that, nearly one-half of participants return to their original weight within 5 years.[5,14,16,17]

Individuals who initially succeed at weight loss in a behavioral treatment program are likely to find that their efforts are eventually challenged by profound environmental influences (eg, large portion sizes, labor-saving devices) that remain highly influential after a weight loss program has ended.[18,19] Metabolic responses to weight loss, biological preferences for palatable foods, and conservation of energy also make weight loss maintenance challenging.[20] In the context of these biological factors and the "obesogenic" environment, weight loss maintenance may require long-term vigilance with regard to eating behavior and physical activity.[21–24]

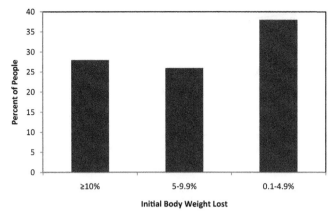

Fig. 3. Mean percentage of initial body weight lost at 1 year following involvement in a behavioral weight loss program.

IMPROVING WEIGHT LOSS MAINTENANCE

In the following section, methods of improving weight loss maintenance in behavioral treatment are addressed. Strategies that are highlighted include facilitating long-term patient-provider contact in person or via the Internet or telephone, promoting higher levels of physical activity, and combining behavioral interventions with medication.

Long-Term Patient-Provider Contact

Frequent, long-term patient-provider contact following initial weight loss is perhaps the most successful method of preventing weight regain. Such contact, typically provided in group sessions, seems to provide patients the support and motivation needed to continue to practice weight control behaviors that include regularly monitoring body weight, food intake, and physical activity.[25] Several studies conducted in the 1980s first documented the benefits of this approach.[26–28] Perri and colleagues,[28] for example, found that individuals who attended every-other-week group maintenance sessions for the year following weight reduction maintained 13.0 kg of their 13.2-kg end-of-treatment weight loss, whereas those who did not receive such therapy maintained only 5.7 kg of a 10.8-kg loss. In reviewing 13 studies on this topic, Perri and Corsica[16] found that patients who received long-term treatment, which averaged 41 sessions over 54 weeks, maintained 10.3 kg of their initial 10.7-kg weight loss. More recently, Wing and colleagues[29] showed that monthly on-site group counseling was more effective in preventing weight regain over 18 months of intervention than was an education-control group or an Internet-based intervention. Participants in the three groups regained 2.5, 4.9, and 4.7 kg, respectively, of an initial loss of approximately 19 kg. Participants in all three groups who monitored their weight weekly or more frequently were the most successful in maintaining their lost weight.[29]

The Look AHEAD study is assessing the long-term health consequences of intentional weight loss in overweight/obese patients with type 2 diabetes over up to 13.5 years of treatment with an intensive lifestyle intervention (ILI).[30] The study is providing long-term behavioral counseling based on its benefits described previously. Participants in the ILI were provided three group sessions and one individual

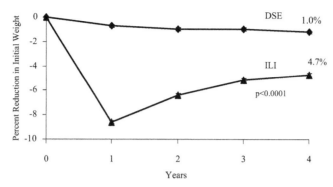

Fig. 4. Percentage change in weight for participants in the ILI and DSE groups of the Look AHEAD (Action for Health in Diabetes) trial during 4 years of follow-up. (*From* Wadden TA, Neiberg RH, Wing RR, et al. Four-Year Weight Losses in the Look AHEAD Study: Factors associated with long-term success. Obesity (Silver Spring). 2011 Jul 21. doi: 10.1038/oby.2011.230. [Epub ahead of print]; with permission.)

treatment session per month for the first 6 months, followed by two group sessions and one individual session during months 7 to 12. [3] At the end of the first year, ILI participants lost a mean of 8.6% of initial weight compared with a significantly smaller 0.7% loss for participants in an education-control group, referred to as diabetes support and education (DSE).[31,32] From years 2 to 4, ILI participants were provided one on-site meeting (of 20–25 minutes) per month with their lifestyle counselor, as well as with an additional monthly contact by telephone (5–15 minutes) or e-mail, in modeling the twice-monthly contact provided by Perri and colleagues[26–28] in their series of studies. Participants were also offered (but not required to attend) monthly open-group sessions at which they could weigh in and receive new diaries with which to monitor their weight, food intake, and physical activity. Participants also were invited (but not required) to attend two or three group refresher courses per year, each of which offered 6 to 10 weeks of treatment with which to either attempt to lose more weight or to reverse weight regain.[3]

As shown in **Fig. 4**, at the end of year 4, ILI participants had a mean weight loss of 4.7%, compared with a significantly smaller 1.0% for those in DSE.[33] This weight loss is among the largest achieved with a lifestyle intervention at 4 years, slightly larger than the loss obtained in the DPP at the same time.[34] Look AHEAD's study design prevents investigators from evaluating the benefits of the twice-monthly treatment contacts (or the other intervention components) in maintaining the weight losses achieved at the end of the first year. A third treatment arm consisting of ILI participants who received no further behavioral treatment after the first year would be necessary to test the efficacy of the weight loss maintenance therapy provided. However, the long-term patient-provider contact did seem to slow the rate of regain that is usually observed following the end of behavioral weight loss interventions. **Fig. 5** presents results of an early lifestyle intervention by Wadden and colleagues.[35] These data show that after 6 months of weight loss achieved with various dietary interventions, participants regained to their baseline weight over 4 to 5 years of follow-up.

Current evidence suggests that individuals with refractory obesity should receive patient-provider support indefinitely to facilitate the maintenance of lost weight. The

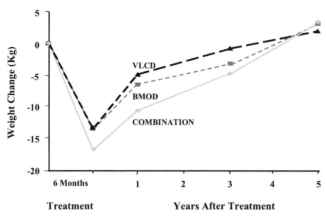

Fig. 5. Weight changes during 5 years following treatment by very low calorie diet (VLCD), behavior therapy (BMOD), or a combination of VLCD and BMOD. (*From* Wadden TA, Sternberg JA, Letizia KA, et al. Treatment of obesity by very low calorie diet, behavior therapy, and their combination: a five-year perspective. Int J Obes 1989;13(Suppl 2):39–46; with permission.)

need for such care is revealed by findings that participants regain lost weight when maintenance therapy is terminated.[16]

Long-Term Contact via Internet and Telephone

Using Internet and telephone also may facilitate extended contact with the treatment team and promote weight loss maintenance. These interventions have the potential to reach large numbers of adults and to improve cost-effectiveness of intervention. Patients may be especially interested in one of these modes of treatment delivery if they wish to have more flexibility in the time at which intervention resources are used, if arrangements for transportation and child care are difficult to arrange, or if they prefer treatment with a certain amount of anonymity.

More than a dozen randomized controlled trials have examined use of the Internet to deliver behavioral treatment to obese adults.[36] Short-term studies of these programs typically found that they were more effective than minimal treatment but less effective than face-to-face treatment.[37–41] In general, effective technology-based programs tailored information and feedback from therapists and provided structured instruction in diet, physical activity, and behavioral strategies.[36] Feedback features such as progress charts and social support features such as Web chats with other participants have been associated with greater success.[42] Systemic reviews have indicated that higher usage of Web site features is associated with larger weight losses.[43]

Several studies have examined use of the Internet specifically for weight loss maintenance with mixed results. The components of one such program, designed specifically for weight loss maintenance, are shown in **Fig. 6**. In each of the studies reviewed here, participants were randomly assigned to a weight loss maintenance intervention after initial weight loss, which was typically 7 to 10 kg. In two such studies, personal contact was more effective for weight loss maintenance than Internet treatment, consistent with many results in the weight loss literature. Harvey-Berino and colleagues[44] compared the effectiveness of 12-month maintenance

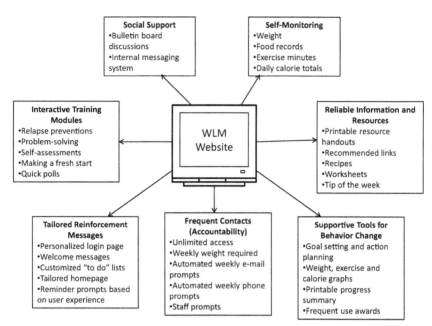

Fig. 6. Key interactive Web site features. (*From* Funk KL, Stevens VJ, Bauck A, et al. Development and implementation of a tailored self-assessment tool in an internet-based weight loss maintenance program. Clin Pract Epidemiol Ment Health 2011;7: 67–73; with permission.)

programs delivered over the Internet or face to face (with minimal or frequent contact). At end of treatment, sustained weight loss was poorer in the Internet condition than in minimal and frequent contact face-to-face conditions (5.7 kg, 10.4 kg, and 10.4 kg, respectively). Svetkey and colleagues[45] randomly assigned participants to one of three weight loss maintenance conditions: (1) an interactive Internet-based intervention that encouraged participants to monitor and submit their weight, food intake, and physical activity; (2) monthly telephone counseling, with in-person visits every fourth month; or (3) an education control group. After 30 months of maintenance treatment, weight regain in the Internet condition (5.2 kg) was significantly higher than in the personal-contact condition (4.0 kg) and not significantly different from the self-directed group (5.5 kg).

In two other studies, Internet and face-to-face weight loss maintenance treatment were found to be equally effective. Harvey-Berino and colleagues[46] conducted another comparison of a 12-month program delivered over the Internet or face to face (with minimal or frequent contact). Weight loss after 1 year of maintenance treatment did not significantly differ between groups (7.6 kg, 5.5 kg, and 5.1 kg, for the Internet, minimal face-to-face contact, and frequent face-to-face contact conditions, respectively). Wing and colleagues[29] compared a monthly Internet treatment with monthly face-to-face treatment and a quarterly newsletter control condition. After 18 months of maintenance intervention, the amount of weight gain was not significantly different in the Internet (4.7 kg) and face-to-face (2.5 kg) conditions. Weight gain was significantly less in both of these conditions than in the control group (4.9 kg).

It seems that frequent telephone contacts can help maintain weight loss in adults. Perri and colleagues[47] recently demonstrated that twice-monthly counseling delivered in 15- to 20-minute individual telephone sessions was as effective as on-site group counseling (delivered on the same schedule in 60-minute sessions) in maintaining an initial weight loss of approximately 10 kg.[26] (The initial weight loss was achieved during a 6-month run-in program that provided group lifestyle modification.) Participants in both intervention groups regained only 1.2 kg during the year of counseling compared with a significantly greater 3.7 kg for participants in an education-control group. As described earlier, Svetkey and colleagues[45] similarly demonstrated the benefits of brief individual monthly telephone counseling sessions (of 5–15 minutes) in preventing weight regain. When scheduling telephone calls, the same therapist optimally should contact the patient on each occasion. A study in which patients were contacted by staff members unknown to them failed to produce weight maintenance results superior to those of a no-contact group.[48]

Effective programs delivered via Internet or telephone should be developed as an option for adults who do not have access to face-to-face treatment, and evaluation of these programs as a method of extending treatment contact should continue.

Promoting High Levels of Physical Activity

High levels of physical activity may facilitate weight loss maintenance. A systematic review of observational and prospective evidence found that individuals who engaged in physical activity experienced less weight regain than those individuals who did not, and those individuals who engaged in the highest levels of physical activity experienced less regain than those who engaged in less physical activity.[49] A minimum of 30 to 60 minutes of activity is typically associated with a weight loss maintenance benefit. The adults enrolled in the National Weight Control Registry (NWCR), who all lost at least 13.6 kg and maintained that weight loss for at least 1 year, have reported engaging in very high levels of physical activity—the equivalent of walking 28 miles per week.[50] Assessment of NWCR participants with accelerometers confirmed that they engaged in an average of 290 minutes per week of sustained (ie, bouts of 10 minutes or more) moderate to vigorous physical activity.[51] Prospective analysis of maintenance of intentional weight loss in the Nurses' Health Study II found that, compared with women who remained sedentary, women who engaged in 30 or more minutes per day of physical activity were more likely to limit their weight regain to 30% or less.[52]

Among the limited number of studies that have used experimental designs to examine the relationship between physical activity level and weight loss maintenance, the pattern of results has been less clear.[21,28,53–56] In several studies, experimental condition did not produce differences in weight loss maintenance. However, across groups, participants who reported exercising the most typically experienced the greatest weight loss maintenance. For example, Wadden and colleagues[54] found that a 1-year program of supervised exercise training did not result in better weight loss maintenance than a program of diet alone, but the participants who reported exercising regularly during follow-up had less weight regain than those who did not report exercising. Maintenance of physical activity seemed challenging for these participants. Of those who originally received on-site exercise training, only 50% reported exercising regularly during the last 4 months of the 1-year follow-up.

Jakicic and colleagues[57] randomly assigned women to behavioral weight loss intervention groups that varied according to targeted physical activity energy expenditure (1000 vs 2000 kcal per week) and intensity (moderate vs vigorous). All participants also reduced calorie intake. Weight loss at 2 years did not differ between conditions. Participants generally did not sustain the prescribed differences in physical activity, which may have contributed to the lack of differences in weight loss among group. As shown in **Fig. 7**, level of physical activity was associated with weight

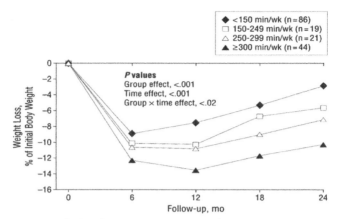

Fig. 7. Percentage weight loss by minutes per week of physical activity. (*From* Jakicic JM, Marcus BH, Lang W, et al. Effect of exercise on 24-month weight loss maintenance in overweight women. Arch Intern Med 2008;168:1550–9; with permission.)

loss maintenance across treatment conditions. A high level of physical activity was needed to achieve weight loss maintenance: individuals who maintained a weight loss of 10% or more had increased their physical activity since baseline by, on average, 275 minutes per week.

Jeffery and colleagues[24] conducted a similar study that yielded comparable results. Participants who were randomly assigned to complete a high level of physical activity (equivalent to approximately 75 minutes per day of brisk walking) experienced significantly greater weight loss maintenance at 18 months than those told to complete a lower level of physical activity. However, most participants were unable to sustain this high level of physical activity after 18 months, so group differences were no longer apparent by 30 months. As shown in **Fig. 8**, the subset of participants who were able to sustain a high level of physical activity (ie, expending at least 2500 kcal per week with exercise) maintained significantly larger weight losses at 30 months than those participants who engaged in a lower level of physical activity.

Based on the available evidence, The American College of Sports Medicine[58] concluded that adults who wish to minimize weight regain should engage in the equivalent of 60 minutes per day of brisk walking.[23,59–61] Additional experimental research must be conducted to learn more about how physical activity can promote weight loss maintenance. Given the limitations of the available research, there is a particular need for studies that have sufficient statistical power, long periods of follow-up, and objective assessment of physical activity. Behavioral therapy also may need to be refined or supplemented with strategies that promote long-term adherence to prescribed levels of physical activity.

Combining Behavioral and Pharmacologic Approaches

The long-term use of weight loss medications could provide another option for improving the maintenance of lost weight.[62,63] This approach recognizes that obesity is a chronic disorder that requires long-term pharmacologic treatment in the same manner that type 2 diabetes or hypertension requires chronic pharmacologic intervention to achieve optimal control of these conditions. The long-term prescription of weight loss medications represents a marked change in their use, which previously was limited to only 6 to 12 weeks.[63]

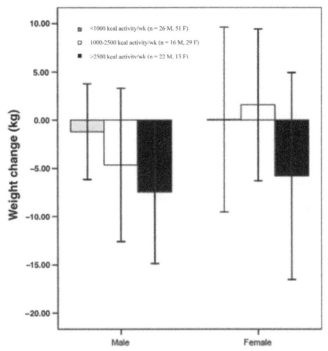

Fig. 8. Weight changes by physical activity level at 30 months. Main effect of sex, $P = .04$; main effect of exercise group, $P = .003$; sex × exercise group interaction, $P = .29$ (not significant). Error bars are ± 1 standard deviation. (*From* Tate DF, Jeffery RW, Sherwood NE, et al. Long-term weight losses associated with prescription of higher physical activity goals. Are higher levels of physical activity protective against weight regain? Am J Clin Nutr 2007;85:954–9; with permission.)

Adding weight loss medication to comprehensive behavioral treatment significantly improves the induction of weight loss, as demonstrated by several studies.[11,64] The combination of medication plus lifestyle modification is also more effective than lifestyle modification alone (ie, with placebo) in maintaining weight loss originally achieved with diet and exercise alone. Hill and colleagues,[65] for example, found that in patients who had lost an average of 10 kg during a diet run-in period, those who were assigned to receive orlistat (a lipase inhibitor) plus lifestyle modification regained only 32% of their weight loss in the following year compared with a significantly greater gain of 56% in those treated by placebo plus lifestyle intervention. Orlistat-treated patients also maintained significantly greater reductions in low-density lipoprotein cholesterol.

Several factors currently limit pharmacotherapy's use to improve the maintenance of lost weight, the most critical of which is that only one medication—orlistat—is approved by the US Food and Drug Administration (FDA) for long-term administration. This medication is only modestly effective, producing only a 3- to 4-kg greater weight loss than placebo.[62] Sibutramine, a serotonin-norepinephrine reuptake inhibitor, facilitated the maintenance of a 10-kg weight loss at 2 years.[66] However, the drug was removed from the market in November 2010 because of findings that it increased cardiovascular morbidity and mortality in patients who had a prior history of cardiovascular disease.[67] Rimonabant, a cannabinoid inverse agonist, was removed from the market in Europe (and never approved in the United States) because of its association with symptoms of depression and suicidal ideation.[68,69] This removal appropriately led other manufacturers to discontinue development of their cannabinoid agents, despite success in maintaining lost weight.[70] In 2010, the FDA declined to approve any of the three weight loss medications that it reviewed. These included lorcaserin, a selective serotonin 2C receptor agonist,[71] the combination of phentermine and topirimate,[72] and the combination of bupropion and naltrexone.[73] The sponsors of these three medications are still seeking approval by FDA. The next weight loss medication to be reviewed by FDA is likely to be liraglutide, a glucagon-like peptide–1 inhibitor, which is approved by the FDA for the treatment of type 2 diabetes.[74]

The long-term treatment of obesity with the combination of lifestyle modification and pharmacotherapy remains of interest to investigators; however, numerous factors have limited progress in this area. These factors include the general lack of reimbursement for weight loss medications (requiring payment out of pocket), as well as patients' unrealistic treatment expectations, which can cause them to stop taking medication when they stop losing weight.[75] Thus, advances are required in the medications themselves, in the FDA's perceptions of weight loss agents, in health care payers reimbursement policies, and in patients' weight loss expectations before pharmacological therapy can significantly improve the long-term management of obesity.

DISSEMINATION OF BEHAVIORAL TREATMENT

Intensive behavioral treatment, as provided in the DPP[33] and Look AHEAD[3] is successful but can be time-consuming, costly, and unavailable to most overweight or obese individuals. Such programs typically are offered in academic medical centers and as a result are rarely accessible to rural populations. ILIs also use registered dietitians, psychologists, and other professionals who have expertise in the behavioral treatment of obesity. Yet there is not a sufficient number of these providers to treat all of the individuals who need lifestyle modification. Thus investigators are currently exploring ways to adapt these approaches to reach a larger proportion of overweight and obese individuals.

Primary Care Practice

Several trials have evaluated the feasibility of providing lifestyle modification in a primary care-based setting. Ashley and colleagues[76] randomly assigned overweight women to a dietitian-led intervention, a dietitian-led intervention with meal replacements, or a primary care office intervention with meal replacements. Participants in the primary care group attended brief every-other-week visits with their primary care physician or nurse, following the LEARN manual.[4] After 1 year of treatment, completers in the primary care group lost 4.3% of initial weight versus 4.1% in the dietitian-led group. However, participants in the dietitian-led group that incorporated meal replacements lost 9.1%, significantly more than both of the other groups. Another study randomly assigned physicians to provide a tailored weight loss intervention or standard treatment to 144 African American female patients.[77,78] The tailored intervention consisted of 6 brief monthly counseling sessions with the physician. At month 6, the tailored group lost significantly more weight than the standard group (−2.0 kg vs +0.2 kg), but there was no difference between groups at the 12- or 18-month follow-up assessments. In a third study, participants were randomly assigned to receive quarterly visits with their primary care physician, along with weight loss materials, or these visits plus eight additional primary care physician visits with a medical assistant trained to deliver brief weight loss counseling.[79] The participants who received the additional counseling, compared with those who did not, lost significantly more weight at 6 months (4.4 kg vs 0.9 kg) but regained their weight between month 6 and month 12 (ie, after counseling visits were discontinued).

Results of these and other studies indicate that whereas primary care settings offer an option for disseminating behavioral weight loss treatment, the benefits generally are modest.[80] There are several barriers to implementing lifestyle interventions in primary care, including a lack of physician time, training, and reimbursement. These factors explain physicians' reluctance to add an intensive weight management to an already busy practice.

Community Settings

Community centers and workplaces offer additional venues for weight management. Ackermann and colleagues[81] successfully adapted the DPP to be delivered by YMCA staff in a group format. Participants randomly assigned to the treatment group received 16 sessions modeled on the original DPP protocol. At 6 months, participants in the intervention lost 6.0% of initial weight compared with a loss of 2.0% in control participants who received advice only. This significant difference was still present at 12 months. Cost per participant in the study was estimated to be $275 to $325, which was substantially lower than the estimated cost of $1400 per participant during the first year of the original DPP.[82] Another study similarly adapted components of the DPP to be delivered to residents of rural communities.[47] All of the obese women in the study first participated in a 6-month weight loss intervention through their local cooperative extension service (CES) office, and were then randomized to receive telephone counseling, face-to-face counseling, or newsletters twice monthly for an additional year. Counseling during both the induction and maintenance phases was conducted by trained CES staff. Women lost an average of 10.0 kg after the 6-month weight loss program. Thereafter, those in the telephone and face-to-face groups regained less weight (1.2 kg in both) than the newsletter group (3.7 kg) during the extended treatment phase. Both of these studies demonstrate that community organizations may be viable options for adapting weight interventions loss.

Worksites also may provide a suitable setting for weight management programs, given the amount of time people spend at work as well as employers' potential motivation to improve the health of their employees. Workplace programs can include multiple components such as changes to the work environment, social support and/or competitions, and healthy messaging throughout the worksite.[83] A recent systematic review of worksite programs found a net loss of 1.3 kg after 6 to 12 months of intervention.[83] Inclusion of structured sessions and behavioral counseling seemed to improve programs' efficacy. The costs of such interventions are usually lower than the ILIs provided in academic settings and may prove cost-effective for employers by reducing medical expenditures and increasing employee productivity.

Commercial Weight Loss Programs

Commercial weight loss programs offer behavioral weight management to the general public. These programs are diverse and may include behavioral and dietary counseling (in-person or via telephone or the Internet), prepackaged meals, and/or group support. The three largest commercial providers are Weight Watchers, Jenny Craig, and Nutrisystem. Weight Watchers offers a point system dietary plan in combination with group meetings or a Web-based monitoring program. Jenny Craig customers choose from in-person or telephone-delivered individual counseling, in addition to prepackaged meals. Nutrisystem also offers a prepackaged (home-delivered) meal plan. The company does not provide personal counseling but online self-monitoring tools are available on the Web site.

Randomized controlled trials of these three major commercial interventions have revealed that they produce greater weight loss than control groups.[84–88] A large trial that randomized participants to Weight Watchers or to self-help found that the Weight Watchers group lost significantly more weight than the self-help group at both 1 year (4.3 kg vs 1.3 kg) and 2 years (2.9 kg vs 0.2 kg).[85] A recent randomized controlled trial sponsored by Jenny Craig randomly assigned women to usual care (ie, two in-person counseling sessions and monthly contacts), face-to-face counseling at a Jenny Craig center, or telephone-based Jenny Craig counseling.[87] Women in the face-to-face group lost a mean of 10.1 kg at 1 year and maintained an average weight loss of 7.4 kg at 2 years. Those in the telephone-based group lost a mean of 8.5 kg at 1 year and sustained a loss of 6.2 kg at 2 years. Participants in the usual care group lost 2.4 kg at 1 year and maintained a loss of 2.0 kg at 2 years. Both counseling groups were superior to usual care but did not differ significantly from each other. One trial has tested Nutrisystem. At 3 months, participants who were prescribed the Nutrisystem diet lost significantly more than those in a diabetes support and education group (7.1% vs 0.4%).[88] Results of all these trials are generally encouraging. However, the authors note that the trials typically provided participants with additional on-site support and free products, which are not offered to regular consumers. Moreover, access to commercial weight loss programs may be limited by the costs involved.

Technology-Based Interventions

As discussed earlier in this article, investigators are increasingly studying methods to provide effective behavioral weight loss programs via the Internet. One example of a more wide-scale Internet-based intervention is Shape Up Rhode Island, a statewide team-based competition that encouraged weight loss and increased physical activity.[89] The 16-week program consisted of online self-monitoring, free community events and workshops, and free pedometers. The 2007 campaign enrolled 4717 adults. The 3311 participants who completed 12 or more weeks lost an average of 3.2 kg. Additional studies are under way to test the efficacy of smart phones, social networking, and Web sites for weight loss, especially in young adults.[90] As these types of technology become more accessible and popular, there are more possibilities for interventions with broad public health impact.

Conclusions

Weight losses achieved in primary care and community settings are usually modest compared with the results from academic-based ILIs such as the DPP[33] and Look AHEAD.[3] However, innovative programs potentially can provide weight loss to a larger number of obese and overweight individuals and at a lower cost. Thus, such programs are likely to have a more positive net effect on our nation's weight and health than traditional, academically-based programs with their limited reach.

SUMMARY

This review has shown that behavioral treatment is effective in inducing a 10% weight loss, which is sufficient to significantly improve health. Weight loss maintenance is challenging for most patients. Long-term outcomes have the potential to be improved through various methods including prolonging contact between patients and providers (either in the clinic or via Internet or telephone), facilitating high amounts of physical activity, or combining lifestyle modification with pharmacotherapy. Innovative programs also are being developed to disseminate behavioral approaches beyond traditional academic settings.

ACKNOWLEDGMENTS

The authors thank Stephanie Kerrigan and Caroline Moran for their assistance in manuscript preparation.

REFERENCES

1. Clinical guidelines on the identification, evaluation, and treatment of overweight and obesity in adults: executive summary. Expert panel on the identification, evaluation, and treatment of overweight in adults. Am J Clin Nutr 1998;68:899–917.
2. The diabetes prevention program (DPP): description of lifestyle intervention. Diabetes Care 2002;25:2165–71.
3. The Look AHEAD Research Group. The look AHEAD study: A description of the lifestyle intervention and the evidence supporting it. Obesity (Silver Spring) 2006;14: 737–52.
4. Brownell KD. The LEARN Program for Weight Management. Dallas (TX): American Health Publishing Company; 2000.
5. Wing RR. Behavioral weight control. In: Wadden TA, Stunkard AJ, editors. Handbook of obesity treatment. New York: The Guilford Press; 2002:301–16.
6. Wadden TA, Butryn ML. Behavioral treatment of obesity. Endocrinol Metab Clin North Am 2003;32:981–1003.
7. Renjilian DA, Perri MG, Nezu AM, et al. Individual versus group therapy for obesity: effects of matching participants to their treatment preferences. J Consult Clin Psychol 2001;69:717–21.
8. Wadden TA, Foster GD. Behavioral treatment of obesity. Med Clin North Am 2000; 84:441–61, vii.
9. Butryn ML, Phelan S, Hill JO, et al. Consistent self-monitoring of weight: a key component of successful weight loss maintenance. Obesity (Silver Spring) 2007;15: 3091–6.
10. Boutelle KN, Kirschenbaum DS. Further support for consistent self-monitoring as a vital component of successful weight control. Obes Res 1998;6:219–24.
11. Wadden TA, Berkowitz RI, Womble LG, et al. Randomized trial of lifestyle modification and pharmacotherapy for obesity. N Engl J Med 2005;353:2111–20.
12. Baker RC, Kirschenbaum DS. Self-monitoring may be necessary for successful weight control. Behav Ther 1993;24:377–94.
13. Foster GD. Clinical implications for the treatment of obesity. Obesity (Silver Spring) 2006;14:182S–5S.
14. Wadden TA, Butryn ML, Wilson C. Lifestyle modification for the management of obesity. Gastroenterology 2007;132:2226–38.
15. Christian JG, Tsai AG, Bessesen DH. Interpreting weight losses from lifestyle modification trials: using categorical data. Int J Obes 2010;34:207–9.
16. Perri MG, Corsica JA. Improving the maintenance of weight lost in behavioral treatment of obesity. In: Wadden TA, Stunkard AJ, editors. Handbook of obesity treatment. New York: Guilford; 2002:357–79.
17. Curioni CC, Lourenço PM. Long-term weight loss after diet and exercise: a systematic review. Int J Obes 2005;29:1168–74.
18. Lowe MR. Self-regulation of energy intake in the prevention and treatment of obesity: is it feasible? Obes Res 2003;11(Suppl):44S–59S.

19. Drewnowski A, Rolls BJ. How to modify the food environment. J Nutr 2005;135: 898–9.

20. Rosenbaum M, Hirsch J, Gallagher DA, et al. Long-term persistence of adaptive thermogenesis in subjects who have maintained a reduced body weight. Am J Clin Nutr 2008;88:906–12.

21. Jakicic JM, Marcus BH, Gallagher KI, et al. Effect of exercise duration and intensity on weight loss in overweight, sedentary women: a randomized trial. JAMA 2003;290: 1323–30.

22. Catenacci VA, Ogden LG, Stuht J, et al. Physical activity patterns in the national weight control registry. Obesity (Silver Spring) 2008;16:153–61.

23. Tate DF, Jeffery RW, Sherwood NE, et al. Long-term weight losses associated with prescription of higher physical activity goals. Are higher levels of physical activity protective against weight regain? Am J Clin Nutr 2007;85:954–9.

24. Jeffery RW, Wing RR, Sherwood NE, et al. Physical activity and weight loss: does prescribing higher physical activity goals improve outcome? Am J Clin Nutr 2003;78: 684–9.

25. Wing RR, Hill JO. Successful weight loss maintenance. Annu Rev Nutr 2001;21: 323–41.

26. Perri MG, Shapiro RM, Ludwig WW, et al. Maintenance strategies for the treatment of obesity: an evaluation of relapse prevention training and posttreatment contact by mail and telephone. J Consult Clin Psychol 1984;52:404–13.

27. Perri MG, McAdoo WG, McAllister DA, et al. Enhancing the efficacy of behavior therapy for obesity: effects of aerobic exercise and a multicomponent maintenance program. J Consult Clin Psychol 1986;54:670–5.

28. Perri MG, McAllister DA, Gange JJ, et al. Effects of four maintenance programs on the long-term management of obesity. J Consult Clin Psychol 1988;56:529–34.

29. Wing RR, Tate DF, Gorin AA, et al. A self-regulation program for maintenance of weight loss. N Engl J Med 2006;355:1563–71.

30. Ryan DH, Espeland MA, Foster GD, et al. Look AHEAD (action for health in diabetes): design and methods for a clinical trial of weight loss for the prevention of cardiovascular disease in type 2 diabetes. Control Clin Trials 2003;24:610–28.

31. Look AHEAD Research Group. Reduction in weight and cardiovascular disease risk factors in individuals with type 2 diabetes: one-year results of the look AHEAD trial. Diabetes Care 2007;30:1374–83.

32. Wadden TA, West DS, Neiberg RH, et al. One-year weight losses in the look AHEAD study: factors associated with success. Obesity (Silver Spring) 2009;17:713–22.

33. The Look AHEAD Research Group. Long term effects of lifestyle intervention on weight and cardiovascular risk factors in individuals with type 2 diabetes: four year results of the look AHEAD trial. Arch Intern Med 2010;170:1566–75.

34. Knowler WC, Barrett-Connor E, Fowler SE. Reduction in the incidence of type 2 diabetes with lifestyle intervention or metformin. N Engl J Med 2002;346:393–403.

35. Wadden TA, Sternberg JA, Letizia KA, et al. Treatment of obesity by very low calorie diet, behavior therapy, and their combination: a five-year perspective. Int J Obes 1989;13:39–46.

36. Saperstein SL, Atkinson NL, Gold RS. The impact of Internet use for weight loss. Obes Rev 2007;8:459–65.

37. Tate DF, Wing RR, Winett RA. Using Internet technology to deliver a behavioral weight loss program. JAMA 2001;285:1172–7.

38. Tate DF, Jackvony EH, Wing RR. Effects of Internet behavioral counseling on weight loss in adults at risk for type 2 diabetes: a randomized trial. JAMA 2003;289:1833–6.

39. Tate DF, Jackvony EH, Wing RR. A randomized trial comparing human e-mail counseling, computer-automated tailored counseling, and no counseling in an Internet weight loss program. Arch Intern Med 2006;166:1620–5.

40. Harvey-Berino J, West D, Krukowski R, et al. Internet delivered behavioral obesity treatment. Prev Med 2010;51:123–8.

41. Digenio AG, Mancuso JP, Gerber RA, et al. Comparison of methods for delivering a lifestyle modification program for obese patients. Ann Intern Med 2009;150:255–62.

42. Krukowski RA, Harvey-Berino J, Ashikaga T, et al. Internet-based weight control: the relationship between web features and weight loss. Telemed J E Health 2008;14:775–82.

43. Neve M, Morgan PJ, Jones PR, et al. Effectiveness of web-based interventions in achieving weight loss and weight loss maintenance in overweight and obese adults: a systematic review with meta-analysis. Obes Rev 2010;11:306–21.

44. Harvey-Berino J, Pintauro S, Buzzell P, et al. Does using the Internet facilitate the maintenance of weight loss? Int J Obes Relat Metab Disord 2002;26:1260.

45. Svetkey LP, Stevens VJ, Brantley PJ, et al. Comparison of strategies for sustaining weight loss: the weight loss maintenance randomized controlled trial. JAMA 2008;299:1139–48.

46. Harvey-Berino J, Pintauro S, Buzzell P, et al. Effect of Internet support on the long-term maintenance of weight loss. Obes Res 2004;12:320–9.

47. Perri MG, Limacher MC, Durning PE, et al. Extended-care programs for weight management in rural communities: the treatment of obesity in underserved rural settings (TOURS) randomized trial. Arch Intern Med 2008;168:2347–54.

48. Wing RR, Jeffery RW, Hellerstedt WL, et al. Effect of frequent phone contacts and optional food provision on maintenance of weight loss. Ann Behav Med 1996;18:172–6.

49. Fogelholm M, Kukkonen-Harjula K. Does physical activity prevent weight gain: a systematic review. Obes Rev 2000;1:95–111.

50. Klem ML, Wing RR, McGuire MT, et al. A descriptive study of individuals successful at long-term maintenance of substantial weight loss. Am J Clin Nutr 1997;66:239–46.

51. Catenacci VA, Grunwald GK, Ingebrigtsen JP, et al. Physical activity patterns using accelerometry in the national weight control registry. Obesity (Silver Spring) 2011;19:1163–70.

52. Mekary RA, Feskanich D, Hu FB, et al. Physical activity in relation to long-term weight maintenance after intentional weight loss in premenopausal women. Obesity (Silver Spring) 2010;18:167–74.

53. Weinstock RS, Dai H, Wadden TA. Diet and exercise in the treatment of obesity: effects of 3 interventions on insulin resistance. Arch Intern Med 1998;158:2477–83.

54. Wadden TA, Vogt RA, Foster GD, et al. Exercise and the maintenance of weight loss: 1-year follow-up of a controlled clinical trial. J Consult Clin Psychol 1998;66:429–33.

55. Wing RR, Venditti E, Jakicic JM, et al. Lifestyle intervention in overweight individuals with a family history of diabetes. Diabetes Care 1998;21:350–9.

56. Leermakers EA, Perri MG, Shigaki CL, et al. Effects of exercise-focused versus weight-focused maintenance programs on the management of obesity. Addict Behav 1999;24:219–27.

57. Jakicic JM, Marcus BH, Lang W, et al. Effect of exercise on 24-month weight loss maintenance in overweight women. Arch Intern Med 2008;168:1550–9 [discussion: 1559–60].

58. Donnelly J, Blair SN, Jakicic JM, et al. Appropriate physical activity intervention strategies for weight loss and prevention of weight regain for adults. Med Sci Sports Exerc 2009;41:450–71.

59. Ewbank PP, Darga LL, Lucas CP. Physical activity as a predictor of weight maintenance in previously obese subjects. Obes Res 1995;3:257–63.

60. Jakicic JM, Winters C, Lang W, et al. Effects of intermittent exercise and the use of home exercise equipment on adherence, weight loss, and fitness in overweight women: a randomized controlled trial. JAMA 1999;282:1554–60.

61. Schoeller DA, Shay K, Kushner RF. How much physical activity is needed to minimize weight gain in previously obese women? Am J Clin Nutr 1997;66:551–6.

62. Bray GA. Drug treatment of the overweight patient. Gastroenterology 2007;132: 2239–52.

63. Yanovski SZ, Yanovski JA. Obesity. N Engl J Med 2002;346:591–602.

64. Phelan S, Wadden TA. Combining behavioral and pharmacological treatments for obesity. Obes Res 2002;10:560–74.

65. Hill JO, Hauptman J, Anderson JW, et al. Orlistat, a lipase inhibitor, for weight maintenance after conventional dieting: a 1-y study. Am J Clin Nutr 1999;69: 1108–16.

66. James WP, Astrup A, Finer N, et al. Effect of sibutramine on weight maintenance after weight loss: s randomised trial. Lancet 2000;356:2119–25.

67. James WP, Caterson ID, Coutinho W, et al. Effect of sibutramine on cardiovascular outcomes in overweight and obese subjects. N Engl J Med 2010;363:905–17.

68. Pi-Sunyer FX, Aronne LJ, Heshmati HM, et al. Effect of rimonabant, a cannabinoid-1 receptor blocker, on weight and cardiometabolic risk factors in overweight or obese patients: RIO-North America: a randomized controlled trial. JAMA 2006;295:761–75.

69. Jones D. End of the line for cannabinoid receptor 1 as an anti-obesity target? Nat Rev Drug Discov 2008;7:961–2.

70. Wadden TA, Fujioka K, Toubro S, et al. A randomized trial of lifestyle modification and taranabant for maintaining weight loss achieved with a low-calorie diet. Obesity (Silver Spring) 2010;18:2301–10.

71. Smith SR, Weissman NJ, Anderson CM, et al. Multicenter, placebo-controlled trial of lorcaserin for weight management. N Engl J Med 2010;363:245–56.

72. Gadde KM, Allison DB, Ryan DH, et al. Effects of low-dose, controlled-release, phentermine plus topiramate combination on weight and associated comorbidities in overweight and obese adults (CONQUER): a randomised, placebo-controlled, phase 3 trial. Lancet 2011;377:1341–52.

73. Wadden TA, Foreyt JP, Foster GD, et al. Weight loss with naltrexone SR/bupropion SR combination therapy as an adjunct to behavior modification: the COR-BMOD trial. Obesity (Silver Spring) 2011;19:110–20.

74. Astrup A, Rössner S, Van Gaal L, et al. Effects of liraglutide in the treatment of obesity: a randomised, double-blind, placebo-controlled study. Lancet 2009;374:1606–16.

75. Wadden TA, Womble LG, Sarwer DB, et al. Great expectations: I'm going to lose 25% of my weight no matter what you say. J Consult Clin Psychol 2003;71:1084–9.

76. Ashley JM, St Jeor ST, Schrage JP, et al. Weight control in the physician's office. Arch Intern Med 2001;161:1599–604.

77. Martin PD, Rhode PC, Dutton GR, et al. A primary care weight management intervention for low-income African-American women. Obesity (Silver Spring) 2006; 14:1412–20.

78. Martin PD, Dutton GR, Rhode PC, et al. Weight loss maintenance following a primary care intervention for low-income minority women. Obesity (Silver Spring) 2008;16: 2462–7.

79. Tsai AG, Wadden TA, Rogers MA, et al. A primary care intervention for weight loss: results of a randomized controlled pilot study. Obesity (Silver Spring) 2010;18: 1614–8.

80. Tsai AG, Wadden TA. Treatment of obesity in primary care practice in the United States: a systematic review. J Gen Intern Med 2009;24:1073–9.
81. Ackermann RT, Finch EA, Brizendine E, et al.Translating the Diabetes Prevention Program into the community. The DEPLOY Pilot Study. Am J Prev Med 2008;35: 357–63.
82. Ackermann RT, Marrero DG. Adapting the Diabetes Prevention Program lifestyle intervention for delivery in the community: the YMCA model. Diabetes Educ 2007;33: 69, 74–5, 77–8.
83. Anderson LM, Quinn TA, Glanz K, et al. The effectiveness of worksite nutrition and physical activity interventions for controlling employee overweight and obesity: a systematic review. Am J Prev Med 2009;37:340–57.
84. Heshka S, Greenway F, Anderson JW, et al. Self-help weight loss versus a structured commercial program after 26 weeks: a randomized controlled study. Am J Med 2000;109:282–7.
85. Heshka S, Anderson JW, Atkinson RL, et al. Weight loss with self-help compared with a structured commercial program: a randomized trial. JAMA 2003;289:1792–8.
86. Rock CL, Pakiz B, Flatt SW, et al. Randomized trial of a multifaceted commercial weight loss program. Obesity (Silver Spring) 2007;15:939–49.
87. Rock CL, Flatt SW, Sherwood NE, et al. Effect of a free prepared meal and incentivized weight loss program on weight loss and weight loss maintenance in obese and overweight women: a randomized controlled trial. JAMA 2010;304:1803–10.
88. Foster GD, Borradaile KE, Vander Veur SS, et al. The effects of a commercially available weight loss program among obese patients with type 2 diabetes: a randomized study. Postgrad Med 2009;121:113–8.
89. Wing RR, Pinto AM, Crane MM, et al. A statewide intervention reduces BMI in adults: Shape Up Rhode Island results. Obesity (Silver Spring) 2007;17:991–5.
90. National Heart, Lung, and Blood Institute. Trials use technology to help young adults achieve healthy weights. National Institutes of Health. http://public.nhlbi.nih.gov/newsroom/home/GetPressRelease.aspx?id=2744. Published November 29, 2010. Accessed May 9, 2011.

Motivational Interviewing for Weight Loss

Vicki DiLillo, PhD[a],*, Delia Smith West, PhD[b]

KEYWORDS
- Weight management • Motivational interviewing
- Behavioral interventions • Lifestyle counseling

Weight loss interventions have improved over the years, although sustained weight management remains a challenge for overweight individuals and practitioners alike.[1] One approach that has been proposed to enhance the efficacy of behavioral weight loss treatment is motivational interviewing (MI). Although the application of MI in this context is relatively new, emerging research isolating the unique contributions of MI to weight loss treatment[2] suggests that this approach has utility as part of a comprehensive multicomponent behavioral obesity intervention. Therefore, an introduction to MI and the evidence supporting the approach is warranted for practitioners in applied settings who seek to promote weight loss among their patients.

AN OVERVIEW OF MOTIVATIONAL INTERVIEWING

MI is a patient-centered, directive approach to counseling for behavior change that emphasizes individual autonomy and a collaborative relationship between patient and provider.[3,4] MI strives to help patients move toward behavior change by assisting them in the process of identifying, articulating, and strengthening personally relevant reasons for change and addressing ambivalence about the change. The counseling strategy was initially implemented in the context of problem drinking and has since been successfully adapted to a wide range of challenging behavior problems including weight loss.[5–8] This approach seeks to promote behavior change using an empathic, interactive style that supports self-determination, enhances self-efficacy, and underscores individual control for behavior change. MI differs from a traditional patient education–based approach, which tends to provide advice and information, often in a didactic or prescriptive manner.

A defining characteristic of the MI counseling approach is the collaborative style of the health promotion encounter in which the provider elicits from the patient

Neither Dr DiLillo nor Dr West has anything to disclose.
[a] Department of Psychology, Ohio Wesleyan University, 61 South Sandusky Street, Delaware, OH 43015, USA
[b] Department of Health Behavior, Fay W. Boozman College of Public Health, University of Arkansas for Medical Sciences, 4301 West Markham Street #820, Little Rock, AR 72205, USA
* Corresponding author.
E-mail address: vgdilill@owu.edu

Psychiatr Clin N Am 34 (2011) 861–869
doi:10.1016/j.psc.2011.08.003
0193-953X/11/$ – see front matter © 2011 Elsevier Inc. All rights reserved.

autonomous, personally relevant reasons for behavior change and builds the health promotion message around these goals and concerns. The collaborative relationship between patient and provider does not place the provider in the role of "expert" whose job it is to "fix" the patient by disseminating information on what the patient "should do" or dispensing unsolicited advice. Rather, the provider views the patient as an individual with expertise in his or her own behavior that is critical to the success of the behavior change effort. Consistent with this approach, the provider actively seeks the patient's input and direction throughout the encounter.

Another hallmark of the MI approach is the elicitation and reinforcement of change talk, or statements made by the patient suggesting personal investment in changing current behavior. Emerging research suggests that change talk predicts actual behavior change.[9] Therefore, significant emphasis is placed on the exploration, enhancement, and elaboration of change talk using techniques such as open-ended questioning, reflective listening, and offering periodic strategic summaries using terms and phrases that patients themselves have generated. A key MI strategy for generating change talk involves framing the targeted lifestyle behavior changes into the context of broader life goals and personal values that the patient holds.

In contrast to some other counseling styles, MI explicitly takes a nonconfrontational approach to the resistance to behavior change that sometimes arises. Within MI, resistance is conceptualized as a function of the patient-provider relationship rather than as a characteristic of an uncooperative or difficult patient who "just does not want to change." More important, MI views resistance as a sign that a provider has been pushing for behavior change rather than allowing the impetus for change to come from the patient, and this impasse should serve as a signal to the provider to change his or her behavior. MI recommends that providers alter their behavior to sidestep resistance by engaging in reflective listening that mirrors both sides of the ambivalence about change and then refocusing on the elicitation of change talk. This technique is referred to as "rolling with resistance" and is another hallmark feature of MI. Arguing or persuading a patient into behavior change is not consistent with MI (and likely not effective).

WHAT IS THE EVIDENCE SUPPORTING MOTIVATIONAL INTERVIEWING FOR WEIGHT LOSS?

Well-designed research evaluating the efficacy of MI in the context of behavioral weight control tests whether MI, as a distinct intervention offered as an adjunct to a behavioral weight loss intervention, confers any advantages to weight loss outcomes over and above the behavioral intervention alone. Perhaps of particular interest is a small but growing body of research on the efficacy of MI delivered by health care providers to promote weight loss. There are also studies of multicomponent weight management programs that include MI or MI-based strategies as part of an integrated weight loss program. For example, both the Look AHEAD Lifestyle intervention and the Diabetes Prevention Program Lifestyle Balance program demonstrated impressive weight losses, averaging 8% and 7%, respectively.[10,11] Although weight loss outcomes and associated health benefits documented in these studies are compelling, the isolated contributions from MI cannot be disentangled from the other components in the overall treatment package.

UNIQUE CONTRIBUTIONS OF MI TO WEIGHT LOSS OUTCOMES

Studies that provide insight into the unique weight loss enhancements that may be achieved with the addition of MI to behavioral obesity treatment methods have used a randomized controlled study design to directly compare behavioral approaches augmented by MI to the same behavioral approach without MI. There are a limited number of such studies, but they tend to provide support for the efficacy of MI in enhancing weight loss outcomes. For example, West and colleagues[5] investigated the impact of adding a series of individually delivered MI sessions to a group behavioral weight loss intervention for overweight and obese women with type 2 diabetes. All women were offered a group-based multidisciplinary behavioral weight loss intervention, and study participants were randomized to receive either an additional 5 individual MI counseling sessions or to receive 5 health education sessions (attention placebo control). Results indicated that women who received the MI sessions lost significantly more weight than those in the control condition at the 6-month assessment, and this superior weight loss was maintained through follow-up at both 12 and 18 months. The weight loss advantage was modest (approximately 2 kg of additional weight loss than was achieved with the behavioral program alone), but this advantage was present after only 2 MI sessions. Furthermore, the enhanced weight loss among those receiving MI was mediated by enhanced adherence to specific behavioral recommendations, such as greater self-monitoring and better group attendance.

Carels and colleagues[12] demonstrated a similar benefit of adding MI to a behavioral weight loss program using a stepped care model that provided the MI to individuals who encountered a weight loss plateau. Participants were randomized to receive a comprehensive group-based behavioral weight loss program or to receive the group-based program augmented with MI sessions if they began to struggle with achieving the targeted weight losses. Among participants who struggled and hit a weight loss plateau during the 20-session program, those who were offered MI ultimately lost significantly more weight than their counterparts who hit a plateau but did not receive MI. The authors suggest that this stepped care approach to MI may be particularly well-suited to those individuals who are struggling in a more traditional behavioral weight loss program.

Another small study investigated the utility of adding an MI component to a guided self-help weight loss program.[13] All participants received a total of 8 sessions, 6 of which were self-help materials adapted from the LEARN behavioral weight loss program.[14] Participants were randomized to receive either 2 additional sessions that explored motivational issues using MI techniques or 2 additional sessions that featured a more traditional persuasive approach that emphasized the benefits of weight loss. MI counseling was delivered by clinical psychology graduate students. Although the high overall attrition rates, small sample size, and very limited follow-up period preclude definitive conclusions, the addition of MI to the guided self-help seemed to confer some weight loss advantages in this study. Attrition trended ($P = $ .059) toward being lower in the condition that received the MI in addition to the guided self-help compared with those who were offered the more traditional approach to motivation. Further, effect size calculations indicated a small to medium advantage in terms of body mass index reduction for the MI condition. An effect of this magnitude is consistent with other published reports of MI in weight loss.[2]

Not all studies investigating the addition of MI to a behavioral weight loss program have shown clear benefit. With a design similar to that of West and colleagues,[5] Befort and colleagues[15] examined the efficacy of augmenting a culturally targeted group behavioral weight loss program for African American women with MI in comparison with the group program plus a health education attention control. The authors found no MI-related advantage in terms of either program adherence or weight loss. Women in the MI group, however, did report higher satisfaction with individual sessions than participants in the health education group.

The impact of varying levels of MI exposure on weight loss outcomes was explored in a randomized trial that compared a minimal versus enhanced MI-based intervention for weight loss delivered primarily online.[16] All participants in this study were provided an initial face-to-face meeting that incorporated MI strategies and then were offered a self-directed, 16-week behavioral weight loss program featuring content adapted for online use from the intervention implemented in the Diabetes Prevention Project.[17] Half the participants were randomized to attend a weekly MI-based leader-facilitated online chat group (enhanced MI) while the other half of the sample did not have the option to participate in these additional chats. Both groups lost significant weight from baseline; the minimal intervention group lost 5.2 ± 4.7 kg and the enhanced group lost 3.7 ± 4.5 kg. These intervention-related weight losses were not statistically different between the groups. Use of the additional chats by the enhanced group was lower than anticipated, averaging 8 of the 16 available groups. The failure to make full use of available MI-inspired chats may have decreased the potential utility of the intervention. The MI components were delivered by a graduate student with 3 days of training in MI, which raises questions about the skill level of the treatment delivery. This issue of what constitutes adequate training to provide highest quality MI intervention is of strong interest, and definitive standards or guidance are not available at this time.[18] However, the findings that both groups did equally well and that intervention engagement (as evidenced by behaviors such as completion of online self-monitoring logs, posting on message boards, and Web site visits) was related to weight loss in both conditions suggests that delivery of MI from professionals with modest training presents no harm, even if it may not offer specific additive benefit. This conclusion should be reassuring to those implementing MI in applied settings.

Inconclusive outcomes in some studies raise concerns that greater attention to the training and supervision of MI counselors is warranted. Sufficient expertise in MI methods and appropriate ongoing supervision of MI applications are likely necessary for MI to produce the maximum impact on weight loss and treatment engagement outcomes. The studies that do provide evidence for a positive effect of MI on weight loss seem to be ones in which MI was delivered by individuals with greater counseling experience and more MI training.[5,12]

On balance, evidence to date suggests that MI is a promising, well-received intervention that may enhance weight loss among certain populations. A recent metaanalysis of the extant literature in this area reaches a similar conclusion.[2] Given the limited number of weight loss studies that have evaluated MI as an isolated adjunct to standard intervention as well as the lack of uniform results, more research is indicated in order to fully explore how MI may be most effective in boosting weight loss, particularly among men who are often underrepresented in the existing weight management research.

MOTIVATIONAL INTERVIEWING FOR WEIGHT MAINTENANCE

The challenges associated with weight maintenance have prompted researchers to examine MI-based strategies integrated into behavioral programs specifically targeted at weight loss maintenance. For example, the PRIDE trial randomized a cohort of overweight women with urinary incontinence who had completed a 6-month group behavioral weight loss intervention to two different group-based weight maintenance approaches as part of a larger trial.[19] One group of participants was provided a 12-month comprehensive skills-focused maintenance program that is typical of the standard behavioral weight management approach; the other group was randomized to receive a novel 12-month motivation-focused intervention that offered a variety of strategies for enhancing and maintaining motivation for sustaining behaviors associated with weight loss (eg, physical activity, self-monitoring). The motivation-focused group maintained as much weight loss over a period of 1 year as the traditional skills-focused group. These results suggest that the motivational intervention could serve as a feasible weight maintenance approach to complement the traditional skills refinement programs that are also effective. However, the motivational intervention implemented in this study does not allow the isolation of the unique and specific effects of MI per se, and the results do not indicate that the motivational approach is superior to the traditional approach.

MI may help individuals maintain weight losses achieved after gastric bypass. Stewart and colleagues[20] examined the efficacy of an intervention that combined MI and cognitive behavioral strategies to promote sustained weight loss in a group of patients who had undergone bariatric surgery at least 18 months prior to study enrollment and who were struggling with postsurgical weight gain. Although weight loss outcomes were not formally assessed as part of this pilot study, qualitative feedback suggested that participants learned new maintenance skills and experienced both enhanced motivation and weight loss as a result of the intervention. Future studies focusing on MI for weight maintenance in postsurgical populations would benefit from the addition of objective outcomes such as clinic-assessed weight and measures of adherence.

MI DELIVERED IN HEALTH CARE SETTINGS

One appealing aspect of MI is the potential for the intervention to be delivered by a range of health care providers in clinical settings to target weight loss among their patients. For example, in one study based in a primary care setting, the delivery of MI-based dietary counseling (in person and over the phone) was more effective for promoting weight loss among those at high risk for type 2 diabetes than was the distribution of written materials conveying comparable dietary information.[21] After the intervention, participants in the MI-based counseling group weighed significantly less (mean difference of 1.3 kg) than those in the control group. Further, a significantly greater proportion of those participants who received MI counseling (23.6%) reached the predefined goal of 5% weight loss than did those provided with written materials (7.2%). Similarly, another study demonstrated that overweight and obese individuals who received weight loss counseling from a physician who used MI-consistent techniques were more likely to return to clinic having lost weight than those who received advice to lose weight from a primary care physician who used more MI-inconsistent behaviors.[22]

In a family medicine clinic, McDoniel and colleagues[23] investigated the effects of a technology-delivered weight loss intervention provided to obese patients. In this study, all patients received 2 MI sessions delivered by exercise physiologists plus a series of automated e-mailed newsletters designed to promote weight loss. Additionally, patients were randomized to one of two groups. One group received a standard written nutrition plan and self-monitoring journal. The other group was provided with a smart phone that allowed detailed self-monitoring and provided personalized feedback with a nutrition program tailored to the patient's resting metabolic rate and individual energy expenditure. Both groups lost 3 kg or more over the 12-week intervention, but there were no significant differences between groups. The authors concluded that an MI-based intervention in and of itself is effective in inducing weight loss and that additional technology may not add benefit. However, given that all participants received both MI sessions and nutritional information, it is not possible to disentangle potential independent effects of MI in this study. Further, there was no control group to offer more definitive evidence of a significant effect of the MI intervention alone.

Brief MI strategies also have been implemented as part of a worksite intervention. Groenveld and colleagues[24] used MI in an attempt to help lower the cardiovascular risk of male workers in the construction industry. Participants were randomized to either a usual care condition, which consisted of brief communication from a physician about their individual risk for cardiovascular disease, or an MI condition, in which participants were offered 7 MI contacts from a nurse or physician over 6 months. As part of the MI intervention, participants could elect to focus on smoking cessation or weight loss–enhancing behaviors (diet and physical activity). Participants who elected to focus on diet and physical activity lost weight (relative to baseline) at both 6 and 12 months, but the loss was not significantly greater than that of patients in other groups. Process evaluations indicated that although the interventionists used many MI-consistent strategies, they did not reach a level of skill that would be considered MI-proficient by standard MI quality control measures. This lesser proficiency may account for the lack of superior efficacy and points to the importance of skilled MI delivery when considering the potential magnitude of additive benefit achieved with MI.

ISSUES RELATED TO TRAINING

The amount of training necessary to ensure adequate MI skill development among practitioners seeking to promote weight loss is not clear at this time. Standard recommendations are to obtain formal MI training and receive performance feedback to cultivate adequate MI skills. Providers may find that obtaining MI training enhances their interactions with patients beyond the scope of weight loss per se, given the range of behavior change targets that seem to benefit from an MI approach. Evidence of benefits for using MI to address such common issues as smoking cessation,[25] medication adherence,[26,27] and preventive screening behaviors[28,29] argues for acquiring MI proficiency to promote adherence with a broad range of treatment recommendations.

Practitioners interested in developing proficiency in MI skills should begin by becoming familiar with MI's basic principles through participation in a workshop led by a certified trainer. Although this initial training is key for understanding the fundamentals of MI,[30] additional practice and supervision that includes regular feedback is critical to the development of proficiency in the delivery of MI-based interventions.[31] This approach to training can facilitate the development and refinement of MI skills and provides the practitioner personalized feedback about strengths and areas for improvement. Although it may be impractical for practitioners to obtain this level of MI training, a more limited exposure to an MI approach can foster the collaborative, patient-centered spirit of MI and improve counseling interactions.

COST-EFFECTIVENESS

One question that remains to be thoroughly explored is whether MI strategies for the promotion of weight loss are cost-effective. Although MI has been shown to be cost-effective for addressing some other health-related behaviors such as relapse prevention for smoking among low-income pregnant women[32] and alcohol-related risk behavior among adolescents,[33] no studies to date have addressed the cost-effectiveness of an isolated intervention for MI in the context of behavioral weight control. That being said, treatment packages for weight loss that incorporate MI strategies more diffusely such as the Diabetes Prevention Project have been shown to be cost-effective because of the pronounced impact that successful weight loss has on a variety of health-related outcomes.[34] These encouraging findings underscore the need for well-designed research that investigates the cost-effectiveness of MI as an isolated component of behavioral weight control strategies.

TRANSLATIONAL RESEARCH

Finally, there is continued need for additional high-quality translational research to explore more fully the parameters of applied contexts in which MI is efficacious and with which populations MI may be most helpful for the long-term management of weight. Many of the relevant studies to date were designed as highly controlled efficacy trials targeting specific populations with MI delivered by highly trained individuals. As a result, additional studies focused on the feasibility and utility of MI for weight loss in more real-world settings with more representative patient populations are warranted.

SUMMARY

MI is a patient-centered directive counseling style that aims to facilitate patients' likelihood of making behavior change through the exploration and strengthening of personal motivations. Hallmarks of MI include a collaborative relationship between patient and practitioner, a focus on the elicitation and enhancement of change talk, a nonconfrontational style, and a concerted effort to minimize resistance. MI has been applied to a variety of health-related behaviors, and a growing body of research suggests that this approach may be useful in the context of behavioral weight management.

Although results are not uniform, the majority of research suggests that MI delivered as an independent component in addition to a behavioral weight loss program can augment weight loss and likely exerts its beneficial effects through enhancement of treatment engagement and adherence to behavioral recommendations. Furthermore, preliminary research suggests that MI may be helpful in promoting weight maintenance after an initial loss has been achieved.

Given that behavioral weight management is a relatively new application of MI, a variety of issues merit further investigation. Of particular interest are issues related to the type and extent of provider training necessary to ensure adequate skill development, cost-effectiveness of MI, and translational research to determine the feasibility and effectiveness of incorporating MI strategies into real-world weight loss settings.

REFERENCES

1. Wadden TA, Butryn ML, Wilson C. Lifestyle modification for the management of obesity. Gastroenterology 2007;132:2226–38.
2. Armstrong M, Mottershead T, Ronksley P, et al. Motivational interviewing to improve weight loss in overweight and/or obese patients: a systematic review and meta-analysis of randomized controlled trials. Obes Rev 2011;12:709–23.
3. Miller WR, Rollnick S. Motivational interviewing: preparing people for change. 2nd edition. New York: Guilford Press; 2002.
4. Miller WR, Rollnick S. Motivational interviewing: preparing people to change addictive behavior. New York: Guilford Press; 1991.
5. West DS, Gore SA, DiLillo V, et al. Motivational interviewing improves weight loss in women with type 2 diabetes. Diabetes Care 2007;30:1081–7.
6. Smith DE, Heckemeyer CM, Kratt PP, et al. Motivational interviewing to improve adherence to a behavioral weight control program for older obese women with NIDDM: a pilot study. Diabetes Care 1997;20:52–4.

7. Dunn C, DeRoo L, Rivara FP. The use of brief interventions adapted from motivational interviewing across behavioral domains: a systematic review. Addiction 2001;96: 1725–42.

8. Burke B, Arkowitz H, Menchola M. The efficacy of motivational interviewing: a meta-analysis of controlled clinical trials. J Consult Clin Psychol 2003;71:843–61.

9. Moyers TB, Martin T, Houck J, et al. From in-session behaviors to drinking outcomes: a causal chain for motivational interviewing. J Consult Clin Psychol 2009;77:1113–24.

10. Look AHEAD Research Group. Long term effects of lifestyle intervention on weight and cardiovascular risk factors in individuals with type 2 diabetes: four year results of the Look AHEAD trial. Arch Intern Med 2010;170:1566–75.

11. Diabetes Prevention Program Research Group. Reduction in the incidence of type 2 diabetes with lifestyle intervention or metformin. N Engl J Med 2002;346:393–403.

12. Carels RA, Darby L, Cacciapaglia HM, et al. Using motivational interviewing as a supplement to obesity treatment: a stepped-care approach. Health Psychol 2007; 26:369–74.

13. DiMarco I, Klein D, Clark V, et al. The use of motivational interviewing techniques to enhance the efficacy of guided self-help behavioral weight loss treatment. Eat Behav 2009;10:134–6.

14. Brownell K. The LEARN program for weight management. 10th edition. Dallas (TX): American Health Publishing Company; 2004.

15. Befort C, Nollen N, Ellerbeck E, et al. Motivational interviewing fails to improve outcomes of a behavioral weight loss program for obese African-American women: a pilot randomized trial. J Behav Med 2008;31:367–77.

16. Webber KH, Tate DF, Bowling JM. A randomized comparison of two motivationally enhanced Internet behavioral weight loss programs. Behav Res Ther 2008;46: 1090–5.

17. Diabetes Prevention Program Research Group. The Diabetes Prevention Program (DPP): description of lifestyle intervention. Diabetes Care 2002;25:2165–71.

18. Madson MB, Loignon A, Lane C. Training in motivational interviewing: a systematic review. J Subst Abuse Treat 2009;36:101–9.

19. West DS, Gorin AA, Subak LL, et al. A motivation-focused weight loss maintenance program is an effective alternative to a skill-based approach. Int J Obes (Lond) 2011;35:259–69.

20. Stewart K, Olbrisch ME, Bean M. Back on track: confronting post-surgical weight gain. Bariatric Nursing and Surgical Patient Care 2010;5:179–85.

21. Greaves CJ, Middlebrooke A, O'Loughlin L, et al. Motivational interviewing for modifying diabetes risk: a randomised controlled trial. Br J Gen Pract 2008;58:535–40.

22. Pollack KI, Alexander SC, Coffman CJ, et al. Physician communication techniques and weight loss in adults: Project CHAT. Am J Prev Med 2010;39:321–8.

23. McDoniel SO, Wolskee P, Shen J. Treating obesity with a novel hand-held device, computer software program, and Internet technology in primary care: the SMART motivational trial. Patient Educ Couns 2010;79:185–91.

24. Groeneveld IF, Proper KI, van der Beek AJ, et al. Sustained body weight reduction by an individual-based lifestyle intervention for workers in the construction industry at risk for cardiovascular disease: results of a randomized controlled trial. Prev Med 2010; 51:240–6.

25. Lai D, Cahill K, Qin Y, et al. Motivational interviewing for smoking cessation. Cochrane Database Syst Rev 2010;1:CD006936.

26. Schmaling K, Blume A, Afari N. A randomized controlled pilot study of motivational interviewing to change attitudes about adherence to medications for asthma. J Clin Psychol Med Settings 2001;8:167–72.

27. Dilorio C, Resnicow K, McDonnell M, et al. Using motivational interviewing to promote adherence to antiretroviral medications: a pilot study. J Assoc Nurses AIDS Care 2003;14:52–62.

28. Costanza ME, Luckmann R, White MJ, et al. Moving mammogram-reluctant women to screening: a pilot study. Ann Behav Med 2009;37:343–9.

29. Chacko MR, Wiemann CM, Kozinetz CA, et al. Efficacy of a motivational behavioral intervention to promote chlamydia and gonorrhea screening in young women: a randomized controlled trial. J Adolesc Health 2010;46:152–61.

30. Miller WR, Mount KA. A small study of training in motivational interviewing: does one workshop change clinician and client behavior? Behav Cogn Psychother 2001;29: 457–71.

31. Miller WR, Yahne CE, Moyers TB, et al. A randomized trial of methods to help clinicians learn motivational interviewing. J Consult Clin Psychol 2004;72:1050–62.

32. Ruger J, Weinstein M, Hammond S, et al. Cost-effectiveness of motivational interviewing for smoking cessation and relapse prevention among low-income pregnant women: a randomized controlled trial. Value Health 2008;11:191–8.

33. Neighbors C, Barnett N, Rohsenow D, et al. Cost-effectiveness of a motivational intervention for alcohol-involved youth in a hospital emergency department. J Stud Alcohol Drugs 2010;71:384–94.

34. Herman WH, Hoerger TJ, Brandle M. Diabetes Prevention Program Research Group. The cost-effectiveness of lifestyle modification or metformin in preventing type 2 diabetes in adults with impaired glucose tolerance. Ann Intern Med 2005;142:323–32.

Drug Treatment of Obesity

George A. Bray, MD, MACP*, Donna H. Ryan, MD

KEYWORDS
- Obesity • Diet • Drugs • Treatment

The prevalence of obesity now exceeds 30% of US adults,[1] but may be leveling off at an unacceptably high level. Over two thirds of Americans are overweight,[1] and excessive weight is a problem for children and adolescents as well.[2] The fundamental problem is the result of a small, but prolonged, positive energy balance, in which energy from food exceeds energy needed for everyday living.[3,4]

REALITIES IN TREATING AN OBESE PATIENT

One of the key messages for obese patients is that when caloric intake is reduced below that needed for daily energy expenditure, there is a predictable rate of weight loss.[3] Men generally lose weight faster than women of similar height and weight on any given diet, because men have more lean body mass and therefore higher energy expenditure. Similarly, older patients have a lower metabolic expenditure and as a rule lose weight more slowly than do younger persons with similar adherence to weight loss programs. Thus, adherence to any program is an essential component of success.

MODEL FOR ADDRESSING THE PROBLEM

If obesity is the result of a prolonged small difference between energy intake and energy expenditure, then losing body fat requires reversing this imbalance. The relationship between energy intake and expenditure is shown at the top of **Fig. 1**. Below this are various strategies that can be used to treat this imbalance.

MECHANISMS UNDERLYING DRUG THERAPY OF OBESITY

Currently available medications to treat obesity work in the brain and on the gut.[3,5] A number of neurotransmitter systems, including monoamines, amino acids, and neuropeptides, are involved in modulating food intake. Serotonin $5-HT_{2C}$ receptors modulate fat and caloric intake. Mice that cannot express the $5-HT_{2C}$ receptor are obese and have increased food intake. Sibutramine blocks serotonin and norepinephrine reuptake. Lorcaserin, a drug in clinical trial, works directly on serotonin-2C

Disclosure: See last page of article.
Pennington Biomedical Research Center, Louisiana State University System, 6400 Perkins Road, Baton Rouge, LA 70808, USA
* Corresponding author.
E-mail address: George.Bray@pbrc.edu

Psychiatr Clin N Am 34 (2011) 871–880
doi:10.1016/j.psc.2011.08.013
0193-953X/11/$ – see front matter © 2011 Elsevier Inc. All rights reserved.

Energy Balance Model and Sites of Drug Action in the Host

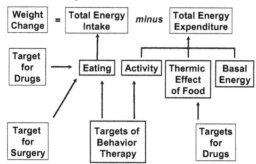

Fig. 1. A model for energy balance and treatment of obesity. The top shows that changes in energy stores are the result of changes in either intake or/and energy expenditure. The other boxes show ways in which these 2 components of the system can be altered therapeutically.

receptors in the brain. These receptors may work through modulation of downstream melanocortin-4 receptors.[6]

α_1-Receptors also modulate feeding.[5] Some α_1-receptor drugs that are used to treat hypertension produce weight gain, indicating that this receptor is clinically important. In contrast, stimulation of α_2-receptors increases food intake, and a polymorphism in the α_{2a}-adrenoceptor is associated with reduced metabolic rate in humans. Activation of β_2-receptors in the brain reduces food intake, and β-blocker drugs can increase body weight.

Other drugs act in the periphery.[5] Blockade of intestinal lipase with orlistat will produce weight loss. Glucagon-like peptide-1 (GLP-1) released from intestinal L-cells acts on the pancreas and brain to reduce food intake. Amylin is secreted from the pancreas and can reduce food intake.

DRUGS APPROVED BY THE US FOOD AND DRUG ADMINISTRATION FOR THE TREATMENT OF OBESITY

Several drugs are currently approved in the United States to treat obesity **(Table 1).**

Sympathomimetic Drugs

The sympathomimetic drugs—benzphetamine, diethylpropion, phendimetrazine, and phentermine—are grouped together because they act like norepinephrine and were tested before 1975. One of the longest of the clinical trials of drugs in this group lasted 36 weeks and compared placebo treatment with continuous phentermine or intermittent phentermine.[3,5] Both continuous and intermittent phentermine therapy produced more weight loss than did placebo. In 1 survey of bariatric physicians, use of these sympathomimetic amines was found to be more frequent than sibutramine or orlistat, and they were often used for longer than approved by the US Food and Drug Administration (FDA).[7]

Safety

Sympathomimetic drugs produce insomnia, dry mouth, asthenia, and constipation. They are scheduled by the Drug Enforcement Agency, suggesting the US government's

Table 1		
Drugs approved by the US FDA that produce weight loss		
Generic Name	**Trade Names**	**Usual Dose**
Drugs approved by the FDA for the Long-term treatment of obesity (12 months)		
Orlistat (may have GI side effects)	Xenical	120 mg 3 times a day
Drugs approved by the US FDA for short-term treatment of obesity (12 weeks); sympathomimetic drugs; approved for use for only a short time		
Diethylpropion[a]		
Tablets	Tenuate	25 mg 3 times a day
Extended release	Tenuate	75 mg in morning
Phentermine HCl[a]		
Capsules	Phentridol Teramine Adipex-P	15–37.5 mg in the morning
Tablets	Tetramine Adipex-P	
Extended release	Ionamin	15 or 30 mg/d in the morning
Benzphetamine[b]	Didrex	25 to 150 mg/d in single or divided doses
Phendimetrazine[b]		
Capsules, extended release	Adipost Bontril Melfial Prelu-2 X-trozine	105 mg once daily
Tablets	Bontril Obezine	35 mg 2–3 times a day

[a] Drug Enforcement Agency Schedule IV.
[b] Drug Enforcement Agency Schedule III.
Adapted from Bray GA. A guide to obesity and the metabolic syndrome: origins and treatment. Boca Raton (FL): CRC Press; 2011; with permission.

view that they may be abused. Sympathomimetic drugs can also increase blood pressure. If a physician decides to use any of these drugs more than 3 months in succession, it is appropriate to obtain written, informed consent from the patient.

Orlistat

Orlistat is a potent and selective inhibitor of pancreatic lipase that reduces intestinal digestion of fat. It is available as a prescription drug, and at half the dose as an over-the-counter preparation. A number of long-term clinical trials with orlistat have been published using uncomplicated obese patients and obese patients with diabetes. A 4-year, double-blind, randomized, placebo-controlled trial with orlistat in 3304 overweight patients, 21% of whom had impaired glucose tolerance,[8] achieved a weight loss during the first year of more than 11% below baseline in the orlistat-treated group compared with 6% below baseline in the placebo-treated group. Over the remaining 3 years of the trial, there was a small regain in weight, such that by the end of 4 years, the orlistat-treated patients were 6.9% below baseline, compared with 4.1% for those receiving placebo. There was a reduction of 37% in the conversion of patients from impaired glucose tolerance to diabetes.

Orlistat has also been studied in adolescents. In 539 adolescents, orlistat (120 mg 3 times per day) decreased body mass index (BMI) by 0.55 kg/m^2 in the drug-treated group compared with an increase of +0.31 kg/m^2 in the placebo group.[9] In a meta-analysis of trials with orlistat, the weighted mean weight loss in the placebo group was 2.40 ± 6.99 kg, and the weight loss in those treated with orlistat was 5.70 ± 7.28 kg, for a net effect of 2.87 (95% confidence interval [CI], −3.21 to −2.53).[10]

Safety

Orlistat is not absorbed to any significant degree, and its side effects are thus related to the blockade of triglyceride digestion in the intestine.[3,5] Fecal fat loss and related gastrointestinal (GI) symptoms are common initially, but they subside as patients learn to use the drug. Orlistat can cause small but significant decreases in fat-soluble vitamins. Levels usually remain within the normal range, but a few patients may need vitamin supplementation. Because it is impossible to tell which patients need vitamins, it is wise to provide a multivitamin routinely with instructions to take it before bedtime. Orlistat does not seem to affect the absorption of other drugs, except acyclovir. Rare cases of severe liver injury have been reported with the use of orlistat, only 1 of which occurred in the United States, and 13 elsewhere over 10 years, at a time when an estimated 40 million people took orlistat.[11] A causal relationship has not been established, but patients who take orlistat should contact their health care provider if itching, jaundice, pale color stools, or anorexia develop.

DRUGS THAT HAVE BEEN USED TO TREAT OBESITY BUT ARE NOT APPROVED BY THE FDA FOR THIS PURPOSE

Several drugs approved for purposes other than weight loss have been used for the treatment of obesity, including metformin, fluoxetine, bupropion, topiramate, and zonisamide.[3] Physicians who decide to try these agents are using them off-label and would be well advised to do so only with signed informed consent from the patient.[12]

Antidiabetic Drugs that Lower Body Weight

Metformin

Metformin is a biguanide that is approved by the FDA for the treatment of diabetes mellitus, and has a good safety profile.[5] This drug reduces hepatic glucose production, decreases intestinal glucose absorption from the GI tract, and enhances insulin sensitivity. One mechanism for the reduction in hepatic glucose production by metformin may depend on the phosphorylation of a nuclear binding protein [cAMP response element binding (CREB) binding protein (CBP) at Ser436) AMPK]. This disrupts a number of other signals, including a master transcription factor, peroxisome proliferator activated receptor-γ coactivator 1A, which in turn leads to the suppression of hepatic glucose output.[13]

Most of the clinical literature on metformin deals with its use in treatment and prevention of diabetes.[14–16] Only a relatively few studies have focused on weight loss with metformin.[3,5,17] In 1 French trial, called BIGPRO, metformin was compared with placebo in a 1-year, multicenter study involving 324 middle-aged subjects with upper body adiposity and the insulin resistance syndrome (metabolic syndrome). The subjects treated with metformin lost significantly more weight (1–2 kg) than the placebo group, and the study concluded that metformin may have a role in the primary prevention of type 2 diabetes.[18,19] In a meta-analysis of weight loss of 3 studies with metformin, Avenell and colleagues[20] reported a nonsignificant weight loss at 12 months of −1.09 kg (95% CI, −2.29 to 0.11 kg). A meta-analysis of 3 studies with metformin in children and adolescents also found a nonsignificant loss of body weight (-0.17 kg; 95% CI, -0.62 to 0.28).[17]

The longest and best study of metformin on body weight comes from the Diabetes Prevention Program.[21,22] During the first 2.8 years of the double-blind, placebo-controlled trial, the metformin-treated group lost 2.9 kg (-2.5%) of their body weight versus -0.42 kg in the placebo group ($P<.001$). The degree of weight loss was related to the adherence to metformin. Those who were the most adherent lost -3.5 kg at 2 years, compared with a small weight gain of 0.5 kg in those who were assigned to but never took metformin. This differential weight loss persisted throughout the 8 years of follow-up with highly adherent patients remaining 3 to 4 kg below baseline and those who were not adherent being no different from placebo.[22]

Metformin has been used to reduce weight gain in people treated with antipsychotic drugs. In a systematic review, Bushe and associates[23] found that metformin may have some value in reducing or preventing weight gain and change in metabolic parameters during treatment with antipsychotic medications.

Pramlintide

Pramlintide is a modified form of amylin, a peptide secreted from the β-cell of the pancreas along with insulin. Pramlintide has been approved by the FDA for treatment of diabetes and in clinical trials produced weight loss. Leptin is a secretory product, primarily from adipocytes, that can act as a negative feedback signal to the brain and inhibit food intake. In clinical trials leptin produced disappointing weight loss.[24] The combination of leptin with pramlintide, however, produced additive weight loss in a 6-month clinical trial that may offer promise for the future,[25] although further studies have not been undertaken.

Exenatide

Exenatide (Exendin-4) is a 39 amino acid peptide that is produced in the salivary gland of the Gila monster lizard. It has 53% homology with GLP-1, but it has a much longer half-life. Exenatide has been approved by the FDA for treatment of type 2 diabetics who are inadequately controlled while being treated with either metformin or sulfonylureas. In human beings, exenatide reduces fasting and postprandial glucose levels, slows gastric emptying, and decreases food intake by 19%.[26] A systematic review of incretin therapy in type 2 diabetes[27] showed a weight loss of 2.37 kg for all GLP-1 analogs versus control, 1.44 kg for exenatide versus placebo injection, and 4.76 kg for exenatide vs insulin (the latter which often leads to weight gain). A 24-week, multicenter, randomized, placebo-controlled, clinical trial of exenatide enrolled diabetics poorly controlled with either metformin or sulfonylurea with a HbA_{1c} between 6.6 and 10.0% and a BMI between 25.0 and 39.9 kg/m^2. The decrease in caloric intake by exenatide (378 $\pm$ 58 kcal/d) was not significantly different from placebo (295 $\pm$ 58 kcal/d). Weight loss was significantly greater and HbA_{1c} and blood pressure were reduced more in the exenatide treated patients.[28] The side effects of exenatide in humans are headache, nausea, and vomiting that are lessened by gradual dose escalation.[29] The interesting feature of this weight loss is that it occurred without prescribing lifestyle modification, diet, or exercise. A 26-week, randomized, controlled trial of exenatide produced a 2.3-kg weight loss compared with a gain of 1.8 kg in the group receiving the glargine form of insulin.[30]

Liraglutide

Liraglutide is another GLP-1 agonist that has a 97% homology to GLP-1. This molecular change extends the circulating half-life from 1 to 2 minutes to 13 hours.

Liraglutide reduces body weight. In a 20-week, multicenter European clinical trial, Astrup and co-workers[31] reported that daily injections of liraglutide at 1.2, 1.8, 2.4, or 3.0 mg produced weight losses of 4.8, 5.5, 6.3, and 7.2 kg, respectively, compared with 2.8 kg in the placebo-treated group and 4.1 kg in the orlistat-treated comparator group. In the group treated with 3.0 mg/d, 76% achieved at least a 5% weight loss compared with 30% in the placebo group. Blood pressure was significantly reduced, but there was no change in lipids. The prevalence of prediabetes was reduced by liraglutide. In a head-to-head comparison, liraglutide and exenatide produced similar amounts of weight loss (3.24 kg with liraglutide vs 2.87 kg with exenatide).[32] In poorly controlled type 2 diabetics on maximally tolerated doses of metformin and/or sulfonylurea, liraglutide reduced mean HbA_{1c} significantly more than did exenatide (−1.12% vs −0.79%).[32] Liraglutide has been approved by the European Medicines Agency and the US FDA for the treatment of diabetes.

OTHER DRUGS THAT PRODUCE WEIGHT LOSS
Bupropion

Bupropion is a norepinephrine and dopamine reuptake inhibitor that is approved for the treatment of depression and for smoking cessation. These neurotransmitters are involved in the regulation of food intake. Gadde and colleagues[33] reported a clinical trial in which 50 obese subjects were randomized to bupropion or placebo for 8 weeks, with a blinded extension for responders to 24 weeks. The dose of bupropion was increased to a maximum of 200 mg twice daily in conjunction with a calorie-restricted diet. After 8 weeks, the 18 subjects in the bupropion group who remained in the study had lost −6.2% of body weight compared with −1.6% loss for the 13 subjects in the placebo group who were still in the study ($P<.0001$). After 24 weeks, the 14 responders to bupropion lost −12.9% of initial body weight, of which 75% was fat loss as determined by dual energy x-ray absorptiometry.[33]

In a study with uncomplicated and nondepressed obese subjects, 327 subjects were randomized to placebo, bupropion 300 mg/d, or bupropion 400 mg/d, in equal proportions.[34] All patients were prescribed a hypocaloric diet that included the use of liquid meal replacements. At 24 weeks, 69% of those randomized remained in the study, and body weight was reduced by −5.0%, −7.2%, and −10.1% for the placebo, bupropion 300 mg/d, and bupropion 400 mg/d groups, respectively ($P<.0001$). The placebo group was randomized to the 300- or 400-mg group at 24 weeks, and the trial was extended to week 48. By the end of the trial, the dropout rate was 41%, and the weight losses in the bupropion 300-mg and bupropion 400-mg groups were −6.2% and −7.2% of initial body weight, respectively.[34]

Topiramate

Topiramate is an anticonvulsant drug that is approved for use in certain types of epilepsy and for the treatment of migraine headache.[5] It was shown to reduce food intake, but was not developed clinically because of the side effects at the doses selected for trials. Topiramate was found to induce weight loss in clinical trials for epilepsy treatment. Weight losses of −3.9% of initial weight at 3 months and −7.3% of initial weight at 1 year were seen. In a 6-month, placebo-controlled, dose-ranging study,[35] 385 subjects were randomized to 5 groups: Topiramate at 64, 96, 192, or 384 mg/d, or placebo. These doses were gradually increased over 12 weeks and were tapered off in a similar manner at the end of the trial. Weight loss from baseline to 24 weeks was −5.0%, −4.8%, −6.3%, −6.3%, and −2.6% in the 5 groups, respectively. The most frequent adverse events were paresthesias (tingling or prickly feelings in skin), somnolence, and difficulty with concentration, memory, and attention.

DRUGS REVIEWED IN 2010 BY FDA ADVISORY PANELS
Combination of Topiramate and Phentermine

Some of the side effects of topiramate seem to be reduced when it is combined with phentermine. This pairing has been tried in clinical trials in 1 of 3 combinations: 3.75, 7.5, or 15 mg/d of phentermine combined, respectively, with 23, 46, or 92 mg/d of topiramate. This drug combination was reviewed by a panel at the FDA in 2010. The Advisory Panel voted against approval of the drug because of concerns about side effects. Additional evaluation is underway. A clinical trial with this combination included individuals with 3 or more comorbidities (diabetes, impaired fasting glucose, hypertension, dyslipidemia, and elevated waist circumference) and BMI of 27 to 45 kg/m².[36] The LEARN Manual provided the behavioral program for this trial. Two doses of topiramate and phentermine were used (mid and high dose) against a placebo. At the start, the medication was titrated over 4 weeks to reduce side effects from topiramate. A total of 2487 patients were randomized, 994 to placebo, 498 to the mid dose, and 995 to the higher dose. At 56 weeks, weight loss was −1.4, −8.1, and −10.2 kg for those assigned to placebo, mid dose, and high dose, respectively. The percentage of those losing at least 5% was 21%, 62%, and 70% for placebo, mid dose, and high dose, respectively. The percentage losing at least 10% was 7%, 37%, and 48% for the same groups, respectively.[36] At the end of 1 year, there were significant improvements in all risk factors in the high-dose group, and all but diastolic blood pressure and low-density lipoprotein cholesterol in the middle dose group. The most common adverse events were dry mouth, paraesthesia, constipation, insomnia, dizziness, and dysgeusia. As for depression and anxiety, 4% of patients assigned to placebo, 4% assigned to phentermine 7.5 mg plus topiramate 46 mg, and 7% assigned to phentermine 15 mg plus topiramate 92 mg had depression-related adverse events; 3%, 5%, and 8%, respectively, had anxiety-related adverse events.

Combination of Bupropion and Naltrexone

As noted, bupropion reduces food intake by acting on adrenergic and dopaminergic receptors in the hypothalamus. Naltrexone is an opioid receptor antagonist with minimal effect on weight loss on its own. The rationale for combining bupropion with naltrexone is that naltrexone might block inhibitory influences of opioid receptors activated by β-endorphin, which is released in the hypothalamus and stimulates feeding, while allowing α-melanocyte stimulating hormone, which reduces food intake.[37] With this rationale, the combination of bupropion and naltrexone was tested to validate the concept and then to show long-term effects. Bupropion was used at a dose of 360 mg/d, halfway between the doses described. Naltrexone has been tested at 16, 32, and 48 mg/d in a dose-ranging study, but the later trials have used doses of 32 and 48 mg/d.

The clinical program designed to establish the use of this combination consists of 4 main trials, called Contrave Obesity Research (COR) trials. COR-I used both 16 and 32 mg/d of naltrexone with 360 mg/d of bupropion; COR II used a single 32-mg/d dose of naltrexone with 360 mg/d of bupropion, with re-randomization to 32 or 48 mg/d of naltrexone + bupropion for nonresponders at week 28. The other 2 trials are COR-diabetes and COR-BMod, which examined the effect of the drug combination in diabetics and for maintenance of weight loss. Contrave is the name of the combination of bupropion and naltrexone. This drug combination was reviewed by a FDA Advisory Panel in December 2010, and the panel recommended approval. However, the letter from the FDA indicated that a preapproval trial of drug safety would be required. The company is currently reviewing options for potential uses of this combination.

In a 52-week, multicenter, randomized, placebo-controlled trial the participants were predominantly younger women whose body weight was nearly 100 kg.[37] The combination of bupropion (360 mg/d) and naltrexone at 16 or 32 mg/d produced greater weight loss and decrease in waist circumference than placebo. The decrease in blood triglycerides, high-density lipoprotein cholesterol, glucose, and insulin improved with the degree of weight loss. Only with weight losses of 10% or more did blood pressure and pulse show a significant decrease. Nausea, constipation, and headache were among the more prominent side effects.[38] There was no evidence of increased suicidal thoughts. The failure of blood pressure to fall until there was significant weight loss is a concern, and approval of the drug will probably hinge on a cardiovascular outcomes study.

Lorcaserin

Lorcaserin has been evaluated in clinical trials, including 1 large study,[32] which demonstrated modest weight loss and acceptable tolerability and toxicity. However, when reviewed by the FDA Advisory Panel in 2010, it was revealed that preclinical toxicology studies in animals showed increased risk for several types of tumors. The company is evaluating the data and ways in which it might answer the FDA's concerns.

SUMMARY

Both diet and medications are useful in the treatment of the obese patient. Weight loss of about 10% below baseline can be achieved with both, and there is no evidence that the composition of the diet, by itself, has any influence on weight loss. Presently only 1 drug is approved for long-term treatment of overweight patients, and its effectiveness is limited to palliation of the chronic disease of obesity. Combinations of medications and antidiabetic drugs that produce weight loss are being evaluated.

DISCLOSURES

Dr George Bray is an occasional consultant to Takeda Global Research and Nutrition Advisory Board, and a member of Herbalife.

Dr Ryan has served over the last 20 years as a paid advisor to many industrial entities that make medications or provide commercial products for weight loss. She has not accepted remuneration for these activities since January 2008. Prior paid affiliations include Abbott, Ajinomoto, Amylin, Arena, GSK, Merck, Novo Nordisk, Orexigen, NutriSystem, Sanofi Aventis, Shionogi, Takeda, Vivus, and Weight Watchers. She received income from speaking engagements in the last 12 months from the Cleveland Clinic Educational Foundation, American Gastroenterology Association, American Association for the Advancement of Science, Medical Exchange International, Cardiometabolic Health Congress, and Medical Foundation of Spain. She has no other conflicts to report.

REFERENCES

1. Flegal KM, Carroll MD, Ogden CL, et al. Prevalence and trends in obesity among US adults, 1999–2008. JAMA 2010;303:235–41.
2. Ogden CL, Carroll MD, Curtin LR, et al. Prevalence of high body mass index in US children and adolescents, 2007–2008. JAMA 2010;303:242–9.

3. Bray GA. A guide to obesity and the metabolic syndrome: origins and treatment. Boca Raton (FL): CRC Press; 2011.

4. Bray GA. The low-fructose approach to weight control. Pittsburgh: Dorrance Publishing; 2009.

5. Bray GA, Greenway FL. Pharmacological treatment of the overweight patient. Pharmacol Rev 2007;59:151–84.

6. Lam DD, Pryzdzial MJ, Ridley SH, et al. Serotonin 5-HT2C receptor agonist promotes hypophagia via downstream activation of melanocortin 4 receptors. Endocrinology 2008;40:1323–8.

7. Hendricks EJ, Rothman RB, Greenway FL. How physician obesity specialists use drugs to treat obesity. Obesity (Silver Spring) 2009;17:1730–5.

8. Torgerson JS, Hauptman J, Boldrin MN, et al. XENical in the prevention of diabetes in obese subjects (XENDOS) study: a randomized study of orlistat as an adjunct to lifestyle changes for the prevention of type 2 diabetes in obese patients. Diabetes Care 2004;27:155–61. Erratum in: Diabetes Care 2004;27:856.

9. Chanoine JP, Hampl S, Jensen C, et al. Effect of orlistat on weight and body composition in obese adolescents: a randomized controlled trial. JAMA 2005;293:2873–83. Erratum in: JAMA 2005;294:1491.

10. Rucker D, Padwal R, Li SK, et al. Long term pharmacotherapy for obesity and overweight: updated meta-analysis. BMJ 2007;335:1194–9.

11. US Food and Drug Administration. Questions and answers: Orlistat and severe liver injury. Available at: www.fda.gov/Drugs/DrugSafety/PostmarketDrugSafetyInformation forPatientsandProviders /ucm213040.htm. Accessed May 27, 2010.

12. Snow V, Barry P, Fitterman N, et al. Pharmacologic and surgical management of obesity in primary care: a clinical practice guideline from the American College of Physicians. Ann Intern Med 2005;142:525–31.

13. He L, Sabet A, Djedjos S, et al. Metformin and insulin suppress hepatic gluconeogenesis through phosphorylation of CREB binding protein. Cell 2009;137:635–46.

14. Setter SM, Iltz JL, Thams J, et al. Metformin hydrochloride in the treatment of type 2 diabetes mellitus: a clinical review with a focus on dual therapy. Clin Ther 2003;25:2991–3026.

15. Crandall JP, Knowler WC, Kahn SE, et al. The prevention of type 2 diabetes. Nat Clin Pract Endocrinol Metab 2008;4:382–93.

16. Gillies CL, Abrams KR, Lambert PC, et al. Pharmacological and lifestyle interventions to prevent or delay type 2 diabetes in people with impaired glucose tolerance: systematic review and meta-analysis. BMJ 2007;334:299.

17. Park MH, Kinra S, Ward KJ, et al. Metformin for obesity in children and adolescents: a systematic review. Diabetes Care 2009;32:1743–5.

18. Fontbonne A, Charles MA, Juhan-Vague I, et al. The effect of metformin on the metabolic abnormalities associated with upper-body fat distribution. BIGPRO Study Group. Diabetes Care 1996;19:920–6.

19. Fontbonne A, Diouf I, Baccara-Dinet M, et al. Effects of 1-year treatment with metformin on metabolic and cardiovascular risk factors in non-diabetic upper-body obese subjects with mild glucose anomalies: a post-hoc analysis of the BIGPRO1 trial. Diabetes Metab 2009;35:385–91.

20. Avenell A, Broom J, Brown TJ, et al. Systematic review of the long-term effects and economic consequences of treatments for obesity and implications for health improvement. Health Technol Assess 2004;8:1–182.

21. Knowler WC, Barrett-Connor E, Fowler SE, et al. Reduction in the incidence of type 2 diabetes with lifestyle intervention or metformin. N Engl J Med 2002;346:393–403.

22. Knowler WC, Fowler SE, Hamman RF, et al. 10-year follow-up of diabetes incidence and weight loss in the Diabetes Prevention Program Outcomes Study. Lancet 2009;374:1677–86.

23. Bushe CJ, Bradley AJ, Doshi S, et al. Changes in weight and metabolic parameters during treatment with antipsychotics and metformin: do the data inform as to potential guideline development? A systematic review of clinical studies. Int J Clin Pract 2009;63:1743–61.

24. Heymsfield SB, Greenberg AS, Fujioka K, et al. Recombinant leptin for weight loss in obese and lean adults: a randomized, controlled, dose-escalation trial. JAMA 1999; 282:1568–75.

25. Ravussin E, Smith SR, Mitchell JA, et al. Enhanced weight loss with pramlintide/metreleptin: an integrated neurohormonal approach to obesity pharmacotherapy. Obesity (Silver Spring) 2009;17:1736–43.

26. Edwards CM, Stanley SA, Davis R, et al. Exendin-4 reduces fasting and postprandial glucose and decreases energy intake in healthy volunteers. Am J Physiol Endocrinol Metab 2001;281:E155–61.

27. Amori RE, Lau J, Pittas AG. Efficacy and safety of incretin therapy in type 2 diabetes: systematic review and meta-analysis. JAMA 2007;298:194–206.

28. Heine RJ, Van Gaal LF, Johns D, et al. Exenatide versus insulin glargine in patients with suboptimally controlled type 2 diabetes: a randomized trial. Ann Intern Med 2005 143:559–69.

29. Apovian C, Bergenstal R, Cuddihy R, et al. Effects of exenatide combined with lifestyle modification in patients with type 2 diabetes. Am J Med 2010;123:468.e9–17.

30. Fineman MS, Shen LZ, Taylor K, et al. Effectiveness of progressive dose-escalation of exenatide (exendin-4) in reducing dose-limiting side effects in subjects with type 2 diabetes. Diabetes Metab Res Rev 2004;20:411–7.

31. Astrup A, Rössner S, Van Gaal L, et al. Effects of liraglutide in the treatment of obesity: a randomised, double-blind, placebo-controlled study. Lancet 2009;374:1606–16.

32. Smith SR, Weissman NJ, Anderson CM, et al. Multicenter, placebo-controlled trial of lorcaserin for weight management. N Engl J Med 2010;363:245–56.

33. Gadde KM, Parker CB, Maner LG, et al. Bupropion for weight loss: an investigation of efficacy and tolerability in overweight and obese women. Obes Res 2001;9:544–51.

34. Anderson JW, Greenway FL, Fujioka K, et al. Bupropion SR enhances weight loss: a 48-week double-blind, placebo- controlled trial. Obes Res 2002;10:633–41.

35. Bray GA, Hollander P, Klein S, et al. A 6-month randomized, placebo-controlled, dose-ranging trial of topiramate for weight loss in obesity. Obes Res 2003;11:722–33.

36. Gadde KM, Allison DB, Ryan DH, et al. Effects of low-dose, controlled-release, phentermine plus topiramate combination on weight and associated comorbidities in overweight and obese adults (CONQUER): a randomised, placebo-controlled, phase 3 trial. Lancet 2011;377:1341–52.

37. Greenway FL, Whitehouse MJ, Guttadauria M, et al. Rational design of a combination medication for the treatment of obesity. Obesity (Silver Spring) 2009;17:30–9.

38. Greenway FL, Fujioka K, Plodkowski RA, et al. Effect of naltrexone plus bupropion on weight loss in overweight and obese adults (COR-I): a multicentre, randomised, double-blind, placebo-controlled, phase 3 trial. Lancet 2010;376:595–605.

Surgical Treatments for Obesity

Marion L. Vetter, MD, RD[a],*, Kristoffel R. Dumon, MD[b],
Noel N. Williams, MBBCh, MCh[b]

KEYWORDS

- Bariatric surgical procedures • Gut hormones
- Gastric banding • Complications • Enteroendocrine factors

The twin epidemics of obesity and diabetes threaten the health and well-being of millions of Americans. As these conditions rise in tandem, bariatric surgery has become an increasingly popular treatment option. In the United States alone, over 220,000 bariatric surgery procedures were performed in 2009.[1] At present, bariatric surgery is the only therapy that produces mean long-term weight losses of 15% or more of initial weight.[2]

Bariatric surgery is currently indicated as a treatment option for individuals with a body mass index (BMI) of 40 kg/m² or greater, or of 35 kg/m² of greater in the presence of comorbidities (including type 2 diabetes, hypertension, and sleep apnea) who have failed to achieve clinically significant weight loss with lifestyle modification with or without adjunct pharmacotherapy.[3] These guidelines, developed by the National Institutes of Health in 1991, have recently been challenged in light of emerging data on outcomes of bariatric surgery in mild to moderately obese individuals. Trials are currently underway to determine the safety and efficacy of bariatric surgery in individuals with a BMI of 30 to 40 kg/m².

TYPES OF PROCEDURES

Bariatric procedures were initially classified as restrictive, malabsorptive, or combined, based on their purported mechanism of inducing weight loss.[4] Restrictive procedures induce early satiety by decreasing the volume of the stomach, but do not alter the anatomy of the small or large bowel. In contrast, malabsorptive procedures significantly shorten the length of the small intestine to decrease nutrient absorption.

[a] Department of Medicine, University of Pennsylvania School of Medicine, 3400 Spruce Street, 4 Silverstein, Philadelphia, PA 19104, USA
[b] Department of Surgery, University of Pennsylvania School of Medicine, 3400 Spruce Street, 4 Silverstein, Philadelphia, PA 19104, USA
* Corresponding author. Center for Weight and Eating Disorders, 3535 Market Street, Suite 3108, Philadelphia, PA 19104.
E-mail address: marion.vetter@uphs.upenn.edu

Psychiatr Clin N Am 34 (2011) 881–893
doi:10.1016/j.psc.2011.08.012
0193-953X/11/$ – see front matter © 2011 Elsevier Inc. All rights reserved.

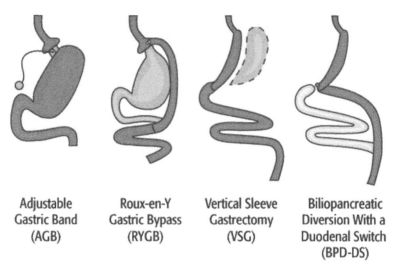

Adjustable	Roux-en-Y	Vertical Sleeve	Biliopancreatic
Gastric Band	Gastric Bypass	Gastrectomy	Diversion With a
(AGB)	(RYGB)	(VSG)	Duodenal Switch
			(BPD-DS)

Fig. 1. Bariatric and metabolic surgical operations. (*Image credit*: Walter Pories, MD, FACS. *From* NIDDK, Weight-information network. Bariatric surgery for severe obesity. Available at: http://win.niddk.nih.gov/publications/gastric.htm. Accessed January 25, 2010.)

Combined procedures involve restriction of the stomach and bypass of the small bowel. Recent evidence suggests that the mechanisms of weight loss are far more complex than initially thought, and likely involve alterations in multiple hormonal and neural pathways. Combined and purely restrictive procedures currently account for 49.0% and 48.6% of surgeries performed worldwide, respectively, followed by malabsorptive procedures (2.0%; **Fig. 1**).[5]

Restrictive Procedures

Adjustable gastric banding
The laparoscopic adjustable silicone gastric band (AGB) has become increasingly popular since it was approved in 2001 by the Food and Drug Administration and is now the most commonly performed restrictive procedure worldwide.[6] An inflatable silicone band is placed around the fundus of the stomach to create a 30-cc pouch (about the size of an egg). Saline can be added or removed through a subcutaneous port to adjust the diameter of the band. Gut anatomy remains intact, and the rate of gastric emptying is not altered.[7] Complications include band erosions or slippage, esophageal dilation, port problems, wound infection, and gastric reflux.[2] Approximately 22% of patients who undergo gastric banding require a revision or repeat surgery.[2]

Sleeve gastrectomy
Sleeve gastrectomy (SG) is a relatively new restrictive procedure in which approximately 75% of the stomach is removed, including virtually all of the hormonally active gastric fundus.[2] This procedure was initially developed as the first stage of a 2-part operation, but increasing evidence suggests that SG induces weight loss comparable with other bariatric surgeries (including gastric bypass), and SG is now being performed alone.[8–11] The SG is conceptually a restrictive procedure, but the removal of endocrine-rich gastric tissue and an accelerated rate of gastric emptying[12,13] may account for its superior efficacy compared with

other restrictive procedures. Complications include postoperative leakage and vomiting owing to overeating.

Malabsorptive Procedures

Biliopancreatic diversion with duodenal switch

Biliopancreatic diversion (BPD) involves a partial gastrectomy to create a 150- to 200-cc gastric sleeve, which is anastomosed to the distal 250 cm of small intestine. The excluded portion of the small intestine that serves as the conduit for bile and pancreatic juices is attached 100 cm proximal to the ileocecal valve. In the duodenal switch variation, the antrum of the stomach, the pylorus, and a short portion of the duodenum are left intact, and vagal nerve activity is preserved to decrease the risk of dumping syndrome.[14] This condition occurs when undigested nutrients are rapidly delivered to the small bowel, causing nausea, bloating, cramping, diarrhea, and vomiting.[2] Despite the impressive amount of weight loss, BPD is associated with a significant number of complications, including leaks and ulceration at the site of anastomosis, chronic loose stools, protein malnutrition, vitamin deficiencies, and anemia.[2] BPD is usually reserved for patients with BMIs greater than 50 kg/m^2 and accounts for only 2% of bariatric operations performed in the United States.[14]

Combined Procedures

Roux-en-Y gastric bypass

The Roux-en-Y gastric bypass (RYGB) remains the most common bariatric procedure performed worldwide and is considered the "gold standard" treatment for extreme obesity.[14–16] The stomach is divided to create a gastric pouch roughly 30 cc in volume, and the distal jejunum is attached to the pouch. The proximal jejunum is reattached 75 to 150 cm below the gastrojejunal anastomosis, resulting in bypass of 95% of the stomach, the entire duodenum, and most of the jejunum.[14] Although malabsorption may occur transiently after surgery, the remaining small bowel undergoes adaptation to compensate for the shortened segment, such that clinically significant malabsorption does not usually occur.[4] The majority of RYGB are now performed laparoscopically.[16] Complications of RYGB include leaks at the site of anastomosis, acute gastric dilatation, ulceration, wound hernias, vomiting, and the dumping syndrome.[2]

WEIGHT LOSS WITH DIFFERENT PROCEDURES

Comparison of bariatric data has been difficult owing to the lack of standardization in reporting weight loss.[2,15–17] In the surgical literature, weight loss is typically expressed as percentage of excess weight lost (EWL), in which excess weight is defined as total preoperative weight minus ideal weight. The percentage of excess weight loss is defined as [(weight loss/excess weight) × 100].[18] Percentage change in total weight and percentage change in BMI have also been reported.[15–18] In the largest meta-analysis to date, Buchwald and colleagues[19] evaluated the effect of bariatric surgery on weight loss in 135,246 patients. An overall loss of 55.9% of excess weight was reported for all procedures, although individual rates associated with each procedure varied. On average, bariatric surgery has been found to result in a 10- to 15-kg/m^2 reduction in BMI and a weight loss of 30 to 50 kg.[16,18] Two randomized, controlled trials reported greater weight loss with RYGB than AGB.[20,21] A recent trial that included 250 participants randomly assigned to RYGB or AGB reported a mean percent EWL of 68.4% and 45.4%, respectively, at 4 years after surgery.[21] These

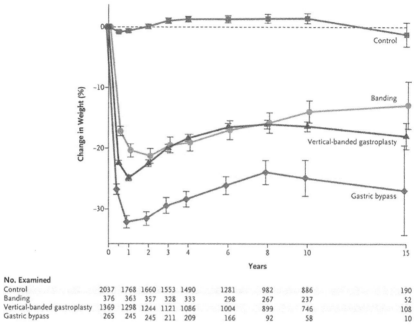

No. Examined

Control	2037	1768	1660	1553	1490	1281	982	886		190
Banding	376	363	357	328	333	298	267	237		52
Vertical-banded gastroplasty	1369	1298	1244	1121	1086	1004	899	746		108
Gastric bypass	265	245	245	211	209	166	92	58		10

Fig. 2. Mean percent weight change over a 15-year period in the control group and surgery group, according to the method of bariatric surgery. Bars indicate 95% confidence intervals. (*Reprinted from* Sjöström L, Lindroos AK, Peltonen M, et al. Lifestyle, diabetes, and cardiovascular risk factors 10 years after bariatric surgery. N Engl J Med 2004;351:2683–93; with permission.)

results were confirmed in an earlier, smaller, randomized trial that provided 5 years of follow-up; mean EWL at that time was 66.6% in participants who underwent RYGB compared with 47.5% in those who underwent AGB.[20]

Given that SG is a relatively new procedure, there are few published studies comparing it with other bariatric surgeries. In a randomized trial, AGB resulted in an EWL of 41.4% and 48% at 1 and 3 years, respectively, versus 57.5% and 66% for SG.[22] Comparable weight loss was reported at 3 months in 1 small, randomized, trial that compared SG and RYGB.[8] A second randomized trial reported greater percent EWL with SG than RYGB at 12 months (69.7% vs 60.5%, respectively; $P = .05$).[9]

Maximal weight loss is typically achieved by 12 to 18 months after the procedure.[15] However, recent evidence suggests that some patients regain a significant amount of weight several years after surgery, as observed in the Swedish Obese Subjects Study, a prospective cohort study that included 4047 obese participants who underwent a variety of bariatric surgery procedures or nonsurgical, conventional weight management. **Fig. 2** shows that mean total weight loss decreased from 32% at 1 year to 25% at 10 years in the RYGB group, from 25% to 18% in patients who underwent gastroplasty (a restrictive procedure that is rarely performed anymore), and from 20% to 13% at 10 years in the gastric banding group.[23] Despite this weight regain, all 3 procedures were associated with far greater weight loss at 10 years than a control intervention.

Table 1			
Improvement in comorbidities and mortality associated with various bariatric procedures			
	Restrictive (AGB)	Malabsorptive (BPD)	Combined (RYGB)
EWL, %	48	70	62
Resolution of comorbid conditions, %			
Type 2 diabetes	48	98	84
Hypertension	38	81	75
Hyperlipidemia (improved)	71	100	94
Sleep apnea	95	95	87
Operative mortality rate, %	0.1	1.1	0.5

Mean values from a meta-analysis of 22,094 patients.[18]

Weight regain has also been reported after SG. For 6 years, Himpens and colleagues[22] followed 53 patients who underwent SG (11 of whom underwent an additional duodenal switch procedure at a later stage because of significant weight regain).[22] Of the 30 patients who underwent SG alone, EWL at 3 years was 77.5%, but decreased to 53.3% at 6 years.

IMPROVEMENT IN COMORBIDITIES AND MORTALITY

Patients who undergo bariatric surgery frequently experience remission or significant improvements in several comorbid conditions. In a recent meta-analysis that included 3188 participants with type 2 diabetes, 78.1% achieved remission (defined as the ability to maintain normoglycemia after all diabetes medications were discontinued), and another 8.5% were improved.[19] Comparable rates of remission and improvement were reported in an earlier meta-analysis (by the same authors) that included data from 22,094 patients.[18] In the latter report, hypertension was found to resolve in 61.7% of patients, hyperlipidemia improved in 70%, and obstructive sleep apnea resolved in 85.7%, examining across procedures. Individual rates of remission are reported for each procedure in **Table 1**.

The Swedish Obese Subjects study observed a significant reduction in overall mortality among participants who underwent bariatric surgery compared with matched obese controls in the conventional treatment group.[24] The unadjusted hazard ratio was 0.76 ($P = .04$). The observed reduction in the rate of death remained significant after adjustment for gender, age, and risk factors ($P = .01$). A reduction in mortality was also reported in a recent retrospective cohort study that included 9949 patients who had undergone gastric bypass surgery, compared with a control group that did not undergo surgery.[25] The adjusted long-term mortality from any cause decreased by 40% in the surgery group, as compared with the control group (37.6 vs 57.1 deaths per 10,000 person-years; $P<.001$). Cause-specific mortality in the surgery group decreased by 56% for coronary artery disease, by 92% for diabetes, and by 60% for cancer.

SAFETY AND COMPLICATIONS

Perioperative and postoperative complications are generally low after bariatric surgery procedures, although open procedures (performed using a traditional incision) carry a higher risk than laparoscopic procedures.[26] A recent prospective observational study that included 4776 patients who underwent RYGB or AGB at 10 clinical sites across the United States reported a 30-day death rate of 0.3%[26] (no deaths occurred with AGB). At least 1 complication occurred in 4.3% of patients within 30 days of surgery. Common early complications include deep venous thrombosis, venous thromboembolism, infection, and anastomotic leaks.[2] Late complications include incisional hernias, gallstones, failure to lose weight, and the dumping syndrome (which is specific to RYGB). Vitamin and mineral deficiencies can also occur if individuals are not compliant with supplements after surgery, with deficiencies of B_{12} and iron occurring most frequently.[2] The overall mortality rates for each procedure are provided in **Table 1**.

LIMITATIONS IN THE QUALITY OF EVIDENCE

Few high-quality, randomized, controlled trials have been performed to evaluate the safety and efficacy of bariatric surgery.[2] The majority of studies are uncontrolled case series and low-quality cohort studies, which are limited by incomplete reporting of data.[2,15,16] In 1 meta-analysis,[16] one quarter of these studies did not report whether consecutive patients were studied, and fewer than 50% reported on the percentage of original patients included in follow-up data. In light of the limited evidence and the generally poor quality of trials, caution is advised when evaluating the comparative safety and effectiveness of bariatric procedures.

BARIATRIC SURGERY FOR MILD TO MODERATE OBESITY

The dramatic improvement in comorbid conditions as a consequence of weight loss induced by bariatric surgery has fostered a growing interest in lowering the criteria for surgery to include individuals with BMIs less than 35 kg/m². The majority of studies in mild to moderately obese individuals have been limited to the AGB.[27–29] O'Brien and colleagues[27] found, in a randomized trial that included 80 participants with a BMI of 30 to 35 kg/m², that those who underwent AGB maintained a loss of 87% of excess weight at 2 years, compared with 22% in the nonsurgical group. In a follow-up study performed by the same investigators,[28] 60 participants with type 2 diabetes and a BMI of 30 to 40 kg/m² were randomly assigned to AGB versus lifestyle modification. Surgical and conventional therapy groups lost a mean of 20.7% and 1.7%, respectively, at 2 years. Remission of diabetes (defined as a fasting blood glucose level < 126 mg/dL and hemoglobin A1c level $<6.2\%$) was achieved by 22 (73%) in the surgical group and 4 (13%) in the control group. Given these findings and those from other studies, in December 2010 a US Food and Drug Administration advisory panel endorsed the expanded use of gastric banding in individuals with a BMI of 30 to 35 kg/m².[30] Randomized trials are currently underway to compare the effects of different bariatric procedures to intensive nonoperative management on efficacy and safety in individuals with a BMI range of 25 to 40 kg/m².[31] Two case series have also been published of bariatric procedures in individuals with a BMI of less than 30 kg/m².[32,33]

NOVEL GASTROINTESTINAL PROCEDURES

The field of bariatric surgery has rapidly evolved since the advent of laparoscopic surgery in the late 1980s. Although AGB and RYGB are frequently performed using conventional laparoscopic techniques, experience using robotic laparoscopy has grown. Robotic laparoscopic gastric banding appears to be as safe as the conventional laparoscopic procedure,[34] and emerging clinical data appear to support its role in RYGB as well.

Clinical trials are also currently underway to evaluate the safety, efficacy, and feasibility of several innovative, minimally invasive procedures that may expand treatment options for obesity. These include endoscopic approaches, endoluminal surgery, and natural orifice transluminal endoscopic surgery.

Endoluminal Surgery

Endoluminal approaches are performed entirely through the gastrointestinal tract using flexible endoscopy. Current approaches are primarily restrictive, and include suturing, stapling, or the insertion of an inflatable intragastric balloon to reduce stomach volume.[35] More recently, malabsorptive endoluminal procedures have also been developed. The duodenojejunal bypass sleeve, a 60-cm plastic sleeve that bypasses the proximal small intestine, extends into the jejunum and induces malabsorption. Human data on endoluminal approaches as a primary modality for weight loss are limited.

Natural Orifice Transluminal Endoscopic Surgery

Natural orifice transluminal endoscopic surgery is an experimental operative procedure that combines endoscopic and laparoscopic techniques to access the abdominal cavity through natural orifices such as the mouth, vagina, rectum, or bladder.[36] Incisions are made internally, which results in improved cosmesis ("scarless"), and fewer external incision-related complications such as pain, hernias, and external wound infections.[35]

THE EFFECT OF BARIATRIC SURGERY ON ENTEROENDOCRINE FACTORS

AGB and RYGB result in distinctly different effects on the secretion of orexigenic (ie, appetite-inducing) and anorexigenic (ie, appetite-reducing) gut peptides that interact with appetitive centers in the brain to regulate energy homeostasis.[4] These neuroendocrine factors are secreted by the gut mucosa in response to ingested nutrients, neural signals, and nutrient sensing. They include the satiety factors, glucagon-like peptide-1 (GLP-1) and peptide YY (PYY), as well as the orexigenic hormone, ghrelin. Many of these peptides also influence glycemic control by modulating insulin secretion. Several key peptides that regulate satiety and appetite are thought to have a blunted response in obese individuals and may be improved after surgery.[37]

Because AGB leaves the gastrointestinal tract intact and does not significantly alter the rate of gastric emptying, changes in gut hormones occur in response to weight loss only, and are less pronounced than changes after malabsorptive or combined procedures. RYGB excludes the proximal gut and expedites nutrient delivery to the distal ileum, resulting in the enhanced secretion of the enteroendocrine factors described below.[9] Similar changes in the secretion of gut peptides are observed after BPD.[38] Although SG is a restrictive procedure, gastric emptying is accelerated, and 2 investigators have reported comparable changes in gut peptides in response to RYGB and BPD.[8,9] Changes in the secretion of gut peptides associated with the individual procedures are shown in **Table 2**.

Ghrelin

Ghrelin, secreted primarily by the gastric fundus and proximal small intestine, enhances appetite and is associated with the anticipatory response to food ingestion.[39,40] Systemic levels of ghrelin rise before a meal and fall after food ingestion.[39] Weight loss by any means increases ghrelin levels, suggesting that ghrelin is a key mediator of the

Table 2				
Overview of altered secretion of gut peptides in response to different bariatric procedures				
	Type of Bariatric Surgery			
Hormone	**AGB**	**BPD**	**RYGB**	**SG**
Ghrelin	Increases	Decreases	Decreases	Decreases
GLP-1	No change	Increases	Increases	Increases
PYY	No change	Increases	Increases	Increases

long-term regulation of body weight.[41] Paradoxically, circulating ghrelin levels are decreased in obese persons.[42]

Suppression of ghrelin has been postulated as a potential mechanism for the generalized loss of hunger that is associated with RYGB, as observed by Cummings and other investigators.[43–45] However, other investigators have reported no change[46] or minimal changes in ghrelin,[40] despite substantial weight loss. In contrast, others have reported increased ghrelin after RYGB.[47] Different operative techniques may account for the inconsistent findings in ghrelin after gastric bypass.[41] Because ghrelin secretion may be mediated in part via the vagus nerve, circulating levels may be affected by the integrity of the nerve after surgery and the amount of intact residual ghrelin-producing tissue in the fundus.

In contrast with procedures that bypass segments of the intestine, ghrelin levels increase after weight loss with restrictive procedures that leave the fundus and the vagal nerve intact.[48] The elevated ghrelin levels observed after restrictive procedures may explain the smaller weight losses associated with AGB compared with RYGB. Because most of the fundus is removed in SG, ghrelin levels are suppressed after this procedure.[8,9]

GLP-1

GLP-1, a potent satiety signal and insulin secretagogue, is secreted by the L-cells of the distal ileum in response to ingested nutrients and neural signals arising from the proximal gut.[49] Circulating levels rise in the short term upon eating and decline over the course of the meal. Known as the "ileal brake," GLP-1 inhibits gastrointestinal motility, decreases gastrointestinal secretions, and slows gastric emptying to regulate the transit of nutrients through the gut. GLP-1 also binds to receptors in the brainstem, hypothalamus, and periphery to induce satiety. Peripheral infusion of GLP-1 significantly enhances satiety and reduces food intake in both normal weight and obese individuals.[50] Basal levels of GLP-1 are decreased in obesity, and the postprandial response is blunted.[50]

Multiple studies after RYGB and BPD have demonstrated a markedly enhanced GLP-1 response.[51–54] This increase seems to be independent of weight loss, as demonstrated by a study by Laferrère and colleagues[53] that compared postprandial GLP-1 levels in subjects who had undergone RYGB with those of matched obese controls who had lost an equivalent amount of weight on a hypocaloric diet. Supraphysiologic GLP-1 levels were seen in the post-RYGB patients, whereas a nonsignificant increase was observed in the controls. Moreover, GLP-1 levels remain persistently elevated after RYGB.[52] Enhanced GLP-1 levels may promote weight loss after RYGB by several mechanisms. GLP-1 suppresses gastrointestinal motility and delays gastric emptying, which induces subsequent reductions in food intake.[55]

Additionally, GLP-1 acts as a satiety factor and may play a role in early meal termination.

In contrast, AGB does not alter GLP-1 levels, in part because the rate of gastric emptying is not altered.[56] Korner and colleagues[57] showed that postprandial GLP-1 increased 3-fold after RYGB, but remained unchanged after gastric banding. Because SG is a relatively new procedure, fewer studies have evaluated its effect on gut peptides. Significant increases in GLP-1 were reported after SG in 2 small studies,[8,10] which is consistent with increased nutrient delivery to the distal ileum as a consequence of accelerated gastric emptying.

PYY

PYY is a satiety signal that is co-secreted with GLP-1 from the L-cells of the distal ileum in response to nutrients. PYY inhibits food intake and delays gastric emptying through interaction with neuropeptide Y-receptor subtypes in both the peripheral and central nervous system.[58] Intravenous administration of PYY_{3-36} (a cleaved molecule of PYY) increases satiety and decreases food intake in humans.[58] Like GLP-1, basal and postprandial levels of PYY levels are decreased in obese individuals.[59]

Procedures that expedite nutrient delivery to the distal ileum, such as RYGB, result in an exaggerated PYY response to nutrient ingestion. Korner and colleagues[57] reported a 10-fold postprandial increase in PYY in individuals who had undergone RYGB, compared with a much smaller increase in lean and obese, nonoperated controls. To control for the effects of weight loss, Valderas and colleagues[10] measured the postprandial PYY response in participants who achieved equivalent weight loss (~15%) after RYGB, SG, or lifestyle modification. The PYY area under the curve increased significantly 2 months after RYGB and SG, but was unchanged in participants who lost an equivalent amount of weight through a hypocaloric diet. In a longer duration, randomized trial, Karamanakos and colleagues[9] found that SG and RYGB resulted in comparable elevation of PYY for the first 6 months after surgery. However, PYY secretion decreased significantly by 12 months after SG, whereas the response was maintained months after RYGB. The authors postulated that physiologic adaptation of the gastric remnant over time may account for the decreased secretion of PYY after SG.

In contrast with the procedures described, the PYY response to nutrient ingestion remains blunted after AGB.[57] This observation is not surprising, because AGB does not alter the rate of gastric emptying.[7] The additive effect of the enhanced PYY and GLP-1 response may contribute to the enhanced satiety and earlier meal termination seen after RYGB and SG. Data consistent with this hypothesis were provided by a study in which poor responders to RYGB (weight loss <25%) were found to have a lesser PYY and GLP-1 response than those who had a good response (weight loss >30%).[60]

SUMMARY

Bariatric surgery is currently the most effective and durable treatment option for extreme obesity. Restrictive procedures, such as AGB and SG, limit gastric capacity and, thus, food intake while leaving the gastrointestinal tract intact. Malabsorptive procedures, such as BPD, shorten the length of the intestine to decrease nutrient absorption. Combined procedures, such as RYGB, include restriction and gastrointestinal rearrangement. Procedures that bypass segments of the gut are associated with greater weight loss and greater improvements in comorbid conditions than is gastric banding. This may be due, in part, to the differential effects of gastrointestinal rearrangement on the secretion of orexigenic and anorexigenic gut peptides that regulate appetite, glucose homeostasis, and body weight. Bariatric surgery is generally associated with low rates of perioperative and postoperative morbidity and mortality, although rigorous comparative safety data are lacking. High-quality, long-term, randomized, controlled trials are needed to compare the efficacy, safety, and cost effectiveness of the various bariatric surgery procedures with each other, as well as with intensive nonsurgical weight loss interventions.

REFERENCES

1. Taylor K. Bariatric surgery fact sheet. American Society for Metabolic & Bariatric Surgery web site. Available at: http://www.asbs.org/Newsite07/media/asmbs_fs_surgery.pdf. Accessed February 23, 2011.
2. Colquitt JL, Picot J, Loveman E, et al. Surgery for obesity. Cochrane Database Syst Rev 2009;2:CD003641.
3. National Institutes of Health. Gastrointestinal surgery for severe obesity. National Institutes of Health Consensus Development Conference Statement. Am J Clin Nutr 1992;55:615S–9S.
4. Cummings DE, Overduin J, Shannon MH, et al. Hormonal mechanisms of weight loss and diabetes resolution after bariatric surgery. Surg Obes Rel Dis 2005;1:358–68.
5. Buchwald H, Oien DM. Metabolic/bariatric surgery worldwide 2008. Obes Surg 2009;19:1605–11.
6. Schneider BE, Mun EC. Surgical management of morbid obesity. Diabetes Care 2005;28:475–80.
7. de Jong JR, van Ramshorst B, Gooszen HG, et al. Weight loss after laparoscopic adjustable gastric banding is not caused by altered gastric emptying. Obes Surg 2009;19:287–92.
8. Peterli R, Wölnerhanssen B, Peters T, et al. Improvement in glucose metabolism after bariatric surgery: comparison of laparoscopic Roux-en-Y gastric bypass and laparoscopic sleeve gastrectomy: a prospective randomized trial. Ann Surg 2009; 250:234–41.
9. Karamanakos SN, Vagenas K, Kalfarentzos F, et al. Weight loss, appetite suppression, and changes in fasting and postprandial ghrelin and peptide-YY levels after Roux-en-Y gastric bypass and sleeve gastrectomy: a prospective, double-blind study. Ann Surg 2008;247:401–7.
10. Valderas JP, Irribarra V, Rubio L, et al. Effects of sleeve gastrectomy and medical treatment for obesity on glucagon-like peptide-1 levels and glucose homeostasis in non-diabetic subjects. Obes Surg 2011;21:902–9.
11. Valderas JP, Irribarra V, Boza C, et al. Medical and surgical treatments for obesity have opposite effects on peptide YY and appetite: a prospective study controlled for weight loss. J Clin Endocrinol Metab 2010;95:1069–75.
12. Braghetto I, Davanzo C, Korn O, et al. Scintigraphic evaluation of gastric emptying in obese patients submitted to sleeve gastrectomy compared to normal subjects. Obes Surg 2009;19:1515–21.
13. Melissas J, Koukouraki S, Askoxylakis J, et al. Sleeve gastrectomy: a restrictive procedures? Obes Surg 2007;17:57–62.
14. Rubino F. Bariatric surgery: effects on glucose homeostasis. Curr Opin Clin Nutr Metab Care 2006;9:497–507.
15. Shah M, Simha V, Garg A. Review: long-term impact of bariatric surgery on body weight, comorbidities, and nutritional status. J Clin Endocrinol Metab 2006;91:4223–31.

16. Maggard M, Shugarman LR, Suttorp M, et al. Meta-analysis: surgical treatment of obesity. Ann Intern Med 2005;142:547–559.
17. Ferchak CV, Meneghini LF. Obesity, bariatric surgery, and type 2 diabetes: a systematic review. Diabetes Metab Res Rev 2004;20:438–45.
18. Buchwald H, Avidor Y, Braunwald E, et al. Bariatric surgery: a systematic review and meta-analysis. JAMA 2004;292:1724–37.
19. Buchwald H, Estok R, Fahrback K, et al. Weight and type 2 diabetes after bariatric surgery: systematic review and meta-analysis. Am J Med 2009;122:248–56.
20. Angrisani L, Lorenzo M, Borrelli V. Laparoscopic adjustable gastric banding versus Roux-en-Y gastric bypass: 5-year results of a prospective randomized trial. Surg Obes Relat Disord 2007;3:127–32.
21. Nguyen NT, Slone JA, Nguyen XM, et al. A prospective randomized trial of laparoscopic gastric bypass versus laparoscopic adjustable gastric banding for the treatment of morbid obesity: Outcomes, quality of life, and costs. Ann Surg 2009;250: 631–41.
22. Himpens J, Dobbeleir J, Peeters G. Long-term results of laparoscopic sleeve gastrectomy for obesity. Ann Surg 2010;252:319–24.
23. Sjöström L, Lindroos AK, Peltonen M, et al. Lifestyle, diabetes, and cardiovascular risk factors 10 years after bariatric surgery. N Engl J Med 2004;351:2683–93.
24. Sjöström L, Narbro K, Sjöström D, et al. Effects of bariatric surgery on mortality in Swedish obese subjects. N Engl J Med 2007;357:741–52.
25. Adams TD, Gress RE, Smith SC, et al. Long-term mortality after gastric bypass surgery. N Engl J Med 2007;357:753–61.
26. Longitudinal Assessment of Bariatric Surgery (LABS) Consortium; Flum DR, Belle SH, King WC, et al. Perioperative safety in the longitudinal assessment of bariatric surgery. N Engl J Med 2009;361:445–54.
27. O'Brien PE, Dixon JB, Laurie C, et al. Treatment of mild to moderate obesity with laparoscopic adjustable gastric banding or an intensive medical program: a randomized trial. Ann Intern Med 2006;144:625–33.
28. Dixon JB, O'Brien PD, Playfair J, et al. Adjustable gastric banding and conventional therapy for type 2 diabetes: a randomized controlled trial. JAMA 2008;299: 316–23.
29. Sultan S, Parikh M, Youn H, et al. Early U.S. outcomes after laparoscopic adjustable gastric banding in patients with a body mass index less than 35 kg/m^2. Surg Endosc 2009;23:1569–73.
30. U.S. Food and Drug Administration. FDA expands use of banding system for weight loss. Available at: http://www.fda.gov/NewsEvents/Newsroom/PressAnnouncements/ucm245617.htm. Accessed March 17, 2011.
31. Lautz D, Halperin F, Goebel-Fabbri A, et al. The great debate: medicine versus surgery. What is best for the patient with type 2 diabetes? Diabetes Care 2011;34:763–70.
32. Cohen RV, Schiavon CA, Pinheiro JS, et al. Duodenal-jejunal bypass for the treatment of type 2 diabetes in patients with BMI of 22–34 kg/m^2: a report of 2 cases. Surg Obes Relat Dis 2007;3:195–7.
33. Chiellini C, Rubino F, Castagneto M, et al. The effect of bilio-pancreatic diversion on type 2 diabetes in patients with BMI < 35 kg/m^2. Diabetologia 2009;52:1027–30.
34. Edelson PK, Dumon KR, Sonnad SS, et al. Conventional laparoscopic gastric banding: a comparison of 407 cases. Surg Endosc 2010;25:1402–8.
35. Coté GA, Edmundowicz SA. Emerging technology: endoluminal treatment of obesity. Gastrointest Endosc 2009;70:991–9.

36. Targarona EM, Maldonado EM, Marzol JA, et al. Natural orifice transluminal endoscopic surgery: the transvaginal route moving forward from cholecystectomy. World J Gastrointest Surg 2010;2:179–86.

37. Vollmer K, Holst JJ, Baller B, et al. Predictors of incretin concentrations in subjects with normal, impaired, and diabetic glucose intolerance. Diabetes 2008;57:678–87.

38. Guidone C, Manco M, Valera-Mora E, et al. Mechanisms of recovery from type 2 diabetes after malabsorptive bariatric surgery. Diabetes 2006;55:2025–41.

39. Cummings DE, Overduin J. Gastrointestinal regulation of food intake. J Clin Invest 2007;117:13–23.

40. Cummings DE, Purnell JO, Fravo RS, et al. A preprandial rise in plasma ghrelin suggests a role in meal initiation in humans. Diabetes 2001;50:1714–9.

41. Cummings DE, Shannon MH. Ghrelin and gastric bypass: is there a hormonal contribution to surgical weight loss? J Clin Endocrinol Metab 2003;88:2999–3002.

42. Tschöp M, Weyer C, Tataranni PA, et al. Circulating ghrelin levels are decreased in human obesity. Diabetes 2001;50:707–9.

43. Cummings DE, Weigle DS, Frayo RS, et al. Human plasma ghrelin levels after diet-induced weight loss and gastric bypass surgery. N Engl J Med 2002;346:1623–30.

44. Geloneze B, Tambascia MA, Pilla VF, et al. Ghrelin: a gut-brain hormone: effect of gastric bypass surgery. Obes Surg 2003;13:17–22.

45. Fruhbeck G, Diez-Caballero A, Gil MJ, et al. Plasma ghrelin concentrations following bariatric surgery depend on the functional integrity of the fundus. Int J Obesity 2004;14:606–12.

46. Faraj M, Havel PJ, Phelis S, et al. Plasma acylation-stimulating protein, adiponectin, leptin, and ghrelin before and after weight loss induced by gastric bypass surgery in morbidly obese subjects. J Clin Endocrinol Metab 2003;88:1594–602.

47. Holdstock C, Engstrom BE, Obrvall M, et al. Ghrelin and adipose tissue regulatory peptides: effect of gastric bypass surgery in obese humans. J Clin Endocrinol Metab 2003;88:3177–83.

48. Nijhuis J, van Dielen FM, Buurman WA, et al. Ghrelin, leptin, and insulin levels after restrictive surgery: a 2 year follow-up study. Obes Surg 2004;14:783–7.

49. Strader AD, Woods SC. Gastrointestinal hormones and food intake. Gastroenterology 2005;128:175–91.

50. Holst JJ. The physiology of glucagon-like peptide-1. Physiol Rev 2007;1409–39.

51. Laferrère B, Teixeira J, McGinty J, et al. Effect of weight loss by gastric bypass surgery versus hypocaloric diet on glucose and incretin levels in type 2 diabetes. J Clin Endocrinol Metab 2008;93:2379–85.

52. Laferrère B, Tran H, Egger J, et al. The increase in GLP-1 levels and incretin effect after Roux-en-Y gastric bypass surgery (RYGBP) persists up to 1 year in patients with type 2 diabetes mellitus (T2DM). Obesity 2007;15:7 (Abstr).

53. Laferrère B, Heshka S, Wang K, et al. Incretin levels and effect are markedly enhanced 1 month after Roux-en-Y gastric bypass surgery in obese patients with type 2 diabetes. Diabetes Care 2007;30:1709–16.

54. Naslund E, Gryback P, Backman L, et al. Distal small bowel hormones: correlation with fasting antroduodenal motility and gastric emptying. Dig Dis Sci 1998;43:945–52.

55. Cummings DE, Overduin J, Shannon MH, et al. Hormonal mechanisms of weight loss and diabetes resolution after bariatric surgery. Surg Obes Rel Dis 2005;1:358–68.

56. Horowitz M, Collins PJ, Catteron BE, Harding PE, Watts JM, Shearman DJ. Gastric emptying after gastroplasty for morbid obesity. Br J Surg 1984;71:435–7.
57. Korner J, Bessler M, Inabnet W, et al. Exaggerated glucagons-like peptide-1 and blunted glucose-dependent insulinotropic peptide secretion are associated with Roux-en-Y gastric bypass but not adjustable gastric banding. Surg Obes Relat Dis 2007;3:597–601.
58. Ballantyne GH. Peptide YY (1-36) and peptide YY (3-36): Part II. Changes after gastrointestinal surgery and bariatric surgery. Obes Surg 2006;16:795–803.
59. Le Roux CW, Batterham RL, Aylwin SJ, et al. Attenuated peptide YY release in obese subjects is associated with reduced satiety. Endocrinology 2006;147:3–8.
60. Le Roux CW, Welbourn R, Werling M, et al. Gut hormones as mediators of appetite and weight loss after Roux-en-Y gastric bypass. Ann Surg 2007;246:780–5.

Obesity: A Public Health Approach

Nicole L. Novak, MSc[a],*, Kelly D. Brownell, PhD[b]

KEYWORDS
- Obesity prevention • Public health • Public policy
- Legislation

Public attention has turned to obesity, and for good reason. Fully 1.5 billion people worldwide are considered overweight or obese.[1] In the United States twice as many adults are overweight as are not.[2] Being obese is associated with numerous health problems including cardiovascular disease, type 2 diabetes mellitus, sleep-disordered breathing, and certain cancers.[3–6] The economic impact of obesity is also great: the direct costs account for 5% to 7% of health care costs in the United States.[7]

Although obesity is a major public health issue, [8–10] prevention has only recently begun to receive significant attention. For years the US government stood in the way of global progress on the issue by merely issuing platitudes, focusing only on individual education, and supporting policies that protected food industry interests.[11–13]

More recently the federal government has begun to take the lead on policy approaches to obesity prevention. There are many examples of this new attitude, including the development of the Interagency Working Group on Food Marketed to Children, the White House Task Force on Childhood Obesity, the Let's Move! Campaign, obesity prevention efforts from the US Department of Agriculture (USDA), new scrutiny of food labeling practices by the Food and Drug Administration, and legal action by the Federal Trade Commission to document food marketing practices directed at children. There is also considerable activity at state and local levels. These initiatives represent important steps toward effective obesity prevention policy, but they still must compete with public dialogue fueled by the food industry framing obesity as a matter of personal and parental responsibility and individual-level changes.

A large body of evidence illustrates that the current obesity epidemic has social, economic, and political causes and that change must be made on a population level.

Funding support: The Rudd Foundation.
Financial disclosures: The authors have nothing to disclose.
[a] Department of Psychology, Rudd Center for Food Policy and Obesity, Yale University, 309 Edwards Street, New Haven, CT 06511, USA
[b] Departments of Psychology and Epidemiology and Public Health, Rudd Center for Food Policy and Obesity, Yale University, 309 Edwards Street, New Haven, CT 06511, USA
* Corresponding author.
E-mail address: nicole.novak@yale.edu

By viewing obesity as first and foremost a medical problem, the nation has sidestepped the need for changes in the environment and instead has focused on the individual, attributing weight gain to poor habits and lack of willpower. This article compares medical and public health models as they relate to obesity and ends by proposing public policy changes the authors believe may help advance the field.

MEDICAL AND PUBLIC HEALTH PERSPECTIVES ON OBESITY

Traditionally, public discourse on obesity has centered on a medical or disease model. In this framework, obesity is seen primarily as a disease or condition that arises in certain individuals as a result of genetic predisposition, dietary choices, and sedentary behavior. Regarding obesity as an individual-level problem implies an individual-level remedy, either through treatment or education in which overweight or obese persons are expected to turn to lifestyle changes, medications, or surgery to shed excess weight and overcome their condition. Certainly obesity has medical consequences, and once diet worsens and activity declines there is a predictable pathophysiology. But these tendencies alone do not indicate that biological factors are the cause of stampeding rises in prevalence around the world.

Medical and behavioral approaches to treating obesity are arduous and often unsuccessful. Even with the most effective behavioral and pharmacological treatments, patients typically lose 8% to 12% of initial body weight but often regain much or all of their lost weight.[14] Even for those who succeed in maintaining large weight losses, the effort is considerable and unyielding. The National Weight Control Registry, which is made up of people who report successfully maintaining weight losses of 30 pounds or more for 1 year or more, finds that successful maintainers exercise with moderate intensity for about 1 hour each day and report average intake of 1400 kcal per day,[15] which is substantially more exercise and fewer calories than the average American is accustomed to. These maintainers also seem vigilant about monitoring their weight. Forty-four % of Registry members weigh themselves at least once per day, and another 31% report doing so once a week. These data suggest that even for individuals who are able to lose weight, maintaining weight loss requires persistent effort and attention.

In contrast to the medical focus on treating obesity in individuals, public health aims to prevent obesity in populations. Rather than prescribing dramatic changes for a small number of individuals, public health aims to make improvements that will affect large groups of people.[16] Within public health there are a range of approaches to improving the well-being of a population. A high-risk approach aims to identify and intervene on subsections of the population that are more likely to suffer from a particular condition. An example would be screening programs to identify and treat individuals at risk for diabetes or high blood pressure. In contrast, the population approach aims to benefit all parts of a population by making changes that affect everyone. Public sanitation is a prime example of a population-level public health impact; clean water and sanitary services prevent the spread of infectious disease for the entire population. Other classic population-level public health interventions include the iodization of salt supplies to prevent goiter or the fluoridation of water to prevent tooth decay. Changing the default source of water or salt addressed the root causes of key diseases, decreasing the risk for the entire population.

Treatment is important in any nation's approach to the problem, and it is important that treatment be delivered in conditions free of bias and stigma.[17–18] Obese individuals face a serious medical condition and deserve effective, compassionate help. Such help can reduce risk in some individuals, can improve quality of life, and should be considered a basic right.

Treatments can be seen as providing help for individuals with obesity but not for addressing prevalence. For every person successfully treated and therefore removed from the obese population, many thousands enter it because of environmental conditions that push people toward calorie-dense foods and sedentary lifestyles. Prevention must be the priority for reducing the impact of obesity on individuals and nations.

RESPONSES TO OBESITY

Individual responsibility is woven deeply into the nation's response to the obesity problem, and to most treatments. Behavioral treatment teaches overweight individuals to change eating and exercise habits without addressing the environment that fosters the behavior, and medications are targeted at mechanisms, such as hunger and satiety, thought to be deficient in overweight individuals. Diet advertisements on television and in magazines suggest repeatedly that the individual must take charge and that the right pill, device, or book will enable them to do so. Individuals, therefore, are blamed if they fail to lose weight. These individuals are stigmatized as being weak or undisciplined and are discriminated against in a variety of domains.[19-21]

Even governmental agencies with public health roles such as the USDA and the Department of Health and Human Services have traditionally focused on the individual. Most obesity prevention efforts have focused on education, imploring members of the public to change their diet and exercise habits without addressing the economic and social structures (some driven by government itself) that push people toward poor diet and sedentary lifestyle. This stance is typified by the words of former Secretary of the US Department of Health and Human Services Tommy Thompson, who urged the nation "to spread the gospel of personal responsibility."[22]

However, the assumption that obesity results from personal irresponsibility is not supported by data. At the same time that rates of obesity have been increasing, the United States has shown stable or improving trends across a variety of other behaviors such as seat belt use, protected sex, alcohol consumption, and tobacco use.[2,23] Something about the environment undermines the ability of people to act responsibly with regard to their weight.

EVIDENCE THAT ENVIRONMENT MATTERS

A wide range of studies supports the premise that the food and physical activity environment have a substantial impact on body weight. Laboratory experiments demonstrate that animals are adept at maintaining a steady body weight until they are placed in a situation in which hyperpalatable, high-fat, high-sugar food is consistently available to them. Under these conditions, laboratory animals overeat and can gain great amounts of weight, even when nutritionally balanced food is available.[24] In people, cross-country and migration studies also reveal the impact of environment on body weight. Migration evidence suggests that when individuals move from countries with less obesity to countries with more, weight gain is common.[25-27]

Of particular interest are the Pima Indians of the southwestern United States, who suffer high rates of obesity and diabetes.[28-30] In 1994, Ravussin and colleagues[30] investigated whether obesity in the Pimas might be related to lifestyle factors rather than genetics alone by comparing the Pima Indians now living in Arizona to a population of Pima ancestry in northwestern Mexico separated several hundred years ago from the American Pimas. Those in Mexico lived a more traditional lifestyle with a diet comprised of less animal fat, more complex carbohydrates, and more physical activity than the lifestyle of the American Pimas.

The data showed that the Pimas living in Mexico had a mean body mass index (BMI) of 24.9 kg/m^2, which was significantly lower than that of the American Pimas, who had a mean BMI of 33.4 kg/m^2, well within the obese range. The Mexican Pimas had significantly lower cholesterol levels and diabetes than the American Pimas. This study is a compelling demonstration of the critical role that environment plays in body weight.

This association between Western industrialized environments and body weight has been demonstrated in several populations. People of African (Benin) descent in the United States are heavier than those in less industrialized West Africa, whereas people living in the Caribbean are in between.[31] Rates of obesity among Mexican Americans are far higher than among people in Latin America or Haiti.[32] Peruvian residents in South America have lower total cholesterol, blood pressure, and BMI in men and higher rates of physical activity in women compared with Peruvian immigrants in California.[33] Even within the same country, lifestyle is related to body weight. South Indians in urban settings are heavier than those in rural settings.[34]

To place genetics and environment in context, it seems that with the exception of rare genetic syndromes, obesity is likely to occur in the absence of a healthy environment. An individual's genetics may make some individuals more vulnerable to environmental changes than others, but with two-thirds of the population overweight, it seems that most people are genetically susceptible to obesity. It is difficult to ignore the relationship between living in the particular environments and having a heavier body weight. The environment is causing the obesity crisis.

ENVIRONMENTAL CONTRIBUTORS TO OBESITY
Food Environment

The current food environment so effectively promotes heavy consumption of foods high in sugar, fat, sodium, and calories that it is not an overstatement to call it toxic. Unhealthy foods can be found virtually anywhere, not only at fast food and other restaurants, convenience stores, and vending machines, but at gas stations, museums, bookstores, train stations, airports, and hospitals. Healthier foods, especially fresh fruits and vegetables, are more expensive and less available. In some neighborhoods, particularly lower income areas, full-service grocery stores with a wide selection of produce may not exist. In addition, preparation of many healthful foods requires more time and knowledge than eating out or obtaining less healthy but conveniently prepared foods.

Increasingly, Americans are eating meals away from home, and when they do they eat more and worse food than when eating at home. In 2008 Americans spent 49% of their food budget on food eaten away from home compared with 33% in 1970.[35] On average, each meal eaten outside the home increases that day's consumption by 134 kcal and decreases diet quality by reducing fruit, vegetable, and whole grain consumption and increasing saturated fat and added sugar.[36] Restaurant portions grew markedly in the 1980s and 1990s and continue to far exceed recommended serving sizes.[37] Sodas, sold originally in 6.5-oz bottles, now commonly are found in 20-oz containers, triple their original size. Experimental studies indicate that portion size directly influences consumption and that nearly all consumers will eat more when given larger portions.[38]

The advertisement and promotion of unhealthy foods overwhelms that for healthy foods, with massive advertising targeting children. It is estimated that children view 5500 food advertisements per year, with 95% of those advertising restaurant and fast food, sugared cereals, sugary drinks, and other unhealthy foods.[39] In 2010, Coca-Cola spent

$758 million on United States advertising, McDonalds spent $1.3 billion, and Burger King spent $392 million.[40] In contrast, the budget for the development and promotion of the USDA "My Plate" food guide released in 2011 is $2 million per year.[41]

Food companies have defended their marketing practices, claiming that advertisements affect only brand choice (eg, whether a child wants Lucky Charms vs Fruity Pebbles; Coke vs Pepsi), but do not create demand for classes of foods such as soft drinks or sugared cereals. However, a growing body of evidence demonstrates that food marketing has done more than merely persuade people, particularly children, to like one brand over another. Children's preferences for foods, and their requests to parents for those foods, increase with exposure to food marketing. These increases occur both at the brand level and at the category level. Exposure to advertising also increases children's consumption of the advertised foods, often subconsciously.[42]

Cost is another factor pushing people toward unhealthy food choices. Because unhealthy foods tend to be highly processed and made of relatively inexpensive ingredients (refined grains and oils), they are often far less expensive than healthy foods that cost more per calorie and tend to have shorter shelf lives.[43–44] The cost disparity between healthy and unhealthy food may be exacerbated by the USDA's practice of subsidizing grain production but not fruit and vegetable production.[45]

The food environment has a marked impact on dietary choices. It is estimated that people make over 200 food-related decisions each day but only recall making less than 10% of those decisions.[46] This leaves the overwhelming majority of dietary choices vulnerable to the influence of the marketing, sizing, convenience, appearance, and pricing of the foods and beverages around them. A promising opportunity to improve public health is to intervene on these conditions to shift the balance away from obesity-promoting foods and toward healthier options.

Environment for Physical Activity

Whereas the food environment has pushed Americans to consume more energy, physical activity levels have remained low. The Surgeon General recommends 30 minutes of moderate activity 5 days per week, yet more than 33% of Americans report being completely sedentary.[47] More people have sedentary jobs than ever before; it has been estimated that work-related energy expenditure has dropped by over 100 kcal per day since 1960.[48] In addition, commuting and taking short trips by vehicle has increased, whereas walking and biking to work have decreased. In 1969, 40% of children walked to school; by 2001 only 12% did.[49] Americans are sedentary during leisure time as well; Americans watch an average of 2.7 hours of television per day, about half of all available leisure time.[50] At the same time, many schools are cutting funding for physical education; 36% of surveyed K–12 physical education teachers said their budgets had been cut between 2006 and 2009.[51] Addressing these impediments to physical activity will be important for obesity prevention.

Physical and social aspects of neighborhoods also seem to be critical in inhibiting or promoting physical activity. Most of those who report exercising say that they do so on neighborhood streets.[52] Neighborhood characteristics that are associated with physical activity include the presence of sidewalks, streetlights, access to trails, and enjoyable scenery.[52–53] Another study found that social aspects of the neighborhood such as the perceived safety of the neighborhood and the degree of interaction between neighbors were related to children's levels of physical activity.[54]

When efforts are made to change the environment, lifestyles change. A pilot intervention in New Orleans measured children's physical activity levels in two comparable neighborhoods, one with a new safe schoolyard for children and one without. The number of children who were physically active and outdoors was 84%

higher among children with access to the safe play space than in the control neighborhood. Children with the safe schoolyard also spent less time watching television and playing video games than children in the control neighborhood.[55] Physical activity interventions can take place on an even smaller scale. Several studies have shown that simply putting up a sign about stair use increases their use in the short term.[56] As with diet, the physical and social environment can push people toward or away from healthy physical activity behaviors.

WHAT MUST BE DONE?

It is time to be courageous. Ramping up existing approaches will be insufficient; hence, creative approaches to making food environments less toxic and activity environments more enabling are essential. Public health leaders and elected officials will face tremendous pressure from food companies, often in the same forms used by tobacco companies.[57] Public policy is the promising tool for creating such changes. In some cases, policy changes might occur at state or national levels, but they also might involve local institutions such as schools (eg, banning soft drinks and snack foods) or community organizations (eg, sponsoring trails for walking and cycling).

Box 1 outlines possible actions that could be taken to address the obesity issue on a number of levels. These changes require participation by a wide range of actors including governments, school officials, parents, and industry. These changes also require a strong collective will and a recognition that a systemic problem like obesity necessitates systemic solutions.

The following section gives examples of recent public health measures taken to prevent or reduce obesity.

LEGISLATIVE EFFORTS

Legislation is one means for making the environment healthier. Until recently, the use of legislation to change the food environment was seen as a radical and unrealistic proposal. In 1994, for instance, Brownell[58] wrote an opinion/editorial about the obesity epidemic in the *New York Times.* This piece recommended changes in the food environment by decreasing children's exposure to food advertising and, if needed, taxing unhealthy foods. The response at that time was negative and blistering, especially from the political right and from groups funded by the food industry.[11]

However, in recent years the public has become more receptive to legislative approaches to improving food environments. Each year more states pass laws to improve food environments in schools,[59] and even controversial policies like food and beverage taxes are gaining interest; excise taxes on sugar-sweetened beverages were proposed in 10 states in 2011.[60] A recent example of the use of legislation to improve food environments has been the Child Nutrition Reauthorization Act of 2010, also known as the Healthy, Hunger-Free Kids Act. The bill included several obesity prevention measures in its updates to federal nutrition programs, especially the National School Lunch Program (NSLP). Key among these measures is that the law gives the USDA the authority to regulate the availability and quality of "competitive foods," non-NSLP foods sold in à la carte programs, vending machines, and school stores. (Currently, the snacks and beverages most commonly offered à la carte are baked goods, juices, juice drinks, ice cream, and chips.[61] Only 4% of à la carte foods are fruits and vegetables.[62]) The law also offers additional funding to schools whose lunch programs meet stricter nutritional standards than the NSLP minimum, providing an incentive to improve nutritional quality for all students. Other

Box 1
Summary of recommended actions to prevent obesity

Thinking differently

Appreciate that a changing environment has caused the obesity epidemic and that the environment is a logical place to intervene.

Recognize that personal resources (responsibility) can be overwhelmed when the environment is toxic, that culture already places heavy emphasis on personal responsibility, and that further emphasis will have limited impact on the obesity epidemic.

Move beyond the "there are no good foods or bad foods" stance into a public perspective that identifies the types of food people should consume less or more of.

Recognize that treating obesity is difficult and can be costly, meaning that prevention must be a national priority.

Appreciate that investing in children will likely produce the first victories in the fight against poor diet and inactivity.

Encourage political leaders to be bold and innovative in addressing the obesity crisis and to remove political barriers to taking action.

Mobilize parents to demand a healthy environment for their children.

Prevent weight bias, stigma, and discrimination in individuals and institutions.

Physical activity

Earmark transportation funding to increase activity (eg, bike and walking paths, buses with bike racks, traffic calming).

Design activity-friendly communities.

Promote walking and biking to school and improve physical education.

Offer incentives for physical activity and strive to decrease sedentary behavior.

Promote activity through work sites and physician practices.

Commercialization of childhood

Object to thinking of children as market objects.

Protest to companies that offer up their characters to sell unhealthy foods.

Encourage celebrities not to promote unhealthy food and to help promote healthy eating and physical activity.

Encourage entertainment executives to stop using product placements in programming with large numbers of child viewers.

Level the playing field so that healthy foods are promoted at least as much as unhealthy foods.

Mandate equal time for nutrition and activity messages to counter promotion of unhealthy foods.

Create a superfund to promote healthy eating, perhaps from assessments placed on food advertisements.

Increase awareness of new media food marketing practices such as advergaming.

Promote media literacy among children.

Food and soft drinks in schools

Determine how healthy eating and activity are connected to academic performance.

Permit commercial television in schools only if it is free of advertising for unhealthy foods.

If food is used as an academic incentive, use healthy foods.

Have nonfood or healthy food fundraisers.

Do not allow food company logos or advertisements on school property, including buses.

Improve school lunch programs, and use the cafeteria as a learning laboratory.

Find alternatives to snack foods, soft drinks, and fast foods in schools, with the goal of eliminating unhealthy foods entirely.

Support programs that teach children about nutrition and activity.

Have only healthy foods and beverages in vending machines. If this is impossible, use pricing to encourage purchase of healthy items.

Require schools to be open and clear about industry contacts and connections.

Challenge industry claims that they are helping education.

Portions

Help make health professionals, the public, and government leaders aware that larger portion sizes lead to increased consumption and that people tend not to compensate for the additional calories at later meals.

Educate people on appropriate serving sizes.

Encourage food companies to show reasonable portions in advertisements and avoid pushing consumers to eat larger amounts.

Require food packaging to have the number of servings in a container accompany weight or volume figures on the front of containers.

Economic issues

Help make the public aware of the economic forces that contribute to obesity, noting how the imbalance of incentives to eat unhealthy foods versus healthy foods would itself predict an epidemic of obesity.

Increase the awareness of social inequities that predispose the poor to obesity, and increase access to healthy foods and opportunities to be active for those living in poverty.

Engage federal food programs as allies in the fight against obesity.

Consider changing the price structure of food by lowering the cost of healthy foods and increasing the cost of unhealthy foods.

Think of food taxes not as a means for punishing people for bad choices but as a means for raising revenues for programs aimed at improving the nation's diet.

Sensitize consumers to financial inducements to buy large amounts of unhealthy foods.

Interacting with the food industry

Celebrate positive changes the industry makes in its products and the support it provides for programs aimed at improving diet and activity.

Make transparent the impact of the industry on national nutrition policy.

Increase awareness of industry tactics in responding to criticism; reinforce reasonable tactics and fight those that will impede progress.

Challenge the industry regarding funding provided to shadow groups like the Center for Consumer Freedom that fight efforts to curtail smoking or to change practices of the food industry.

obesity-related measures in the law include support for farm-to-school programs and the establishment of standards for nutrition education and physical activity clauses in school wellness policies.[63]

Legislation ultimately could address many issues, including the prices of various food items, marketing of foods and beverages, and more. A wide range of obesity prevention bills are considered in state and federal legislatures every year. The Rudd

Center for Food Policy and Obesity maintains a searchable database of legislative efforts related to food policy and obesity in the United States and nationwide (http://yaleruddcenter.org/legislation/). The Centers for Disease Control and Prevention's Division of Nutrition and Physical Activity also tracks nutrition and physical activity legislation (http://apps.nccd.cdc.gov/DNPALeg/). Additional information on legislative and policy changes can be found at the Center for Science in the Public Interest (http://cspinet.org/nutritionpolicy/index.html).

PRIORITIES AND SUGGESTIONS

Obesity prevention priorities should center on prevention and children. Schools are a key venue for obesity prevention in that they affect 95% of American children and also serve as a place where children can develop healthy habits.[64] Policies and interventions aimed at modifying the school environment should improve the nutritional quality of the foods served, restrict access to unhealthy snacks and beverages, remove food company logos and advertisements from school property, find alternative sources of funding for schools than from marketing unhealthy foods to children, and do everything possible to increase physical activity.[62,64] School-level policies can be affected at the federal, state, or district level and are also an arena in which parents and community members can play a role in improving children's health.

Because obesity has such a complex set of causes, changing schools alone will not be sufficient to prevent obesity among children. Children's home and community environments can also promote or prevent weight gain. For example, a study in Philadelphia documented the role that neighborhood corner stores play in children's food intake: children purchase an average of 350 kcal worth of snacks and beverages with each visit to the store. New programs have been designed to increase access and consumption of healthy foods among young children by improving nutrition education in schools and working with local corner store owners to provide and advertise affordable and healthy snacks and beverages to children.[65]

Another obesity prevention policy tool is to change the relative prices of unhealthy and healthy foods, either by subsidizing healthy foods or taxing unhealthy ones. French and colleagues[66] conducted several studies in the community to measure the impact of cost on consumption of healthy foods. In one study conducted at work sites and schools,[67] they found that lowering the cost of lower fat snack foods by 10%, 25%, and 50% increased sales by 9%, 39% and 93%, respectively, compared with sales of the same snacks with their usual prices. The investigators found that price reductions of fresh fruit and carrots yielded similar sales increases. Subsidizing healthy foods would increase consumption.

In turn, policymakers can also reduce consumption of unhealthy foods by increasing the price to consumers. A key example of this type of policy, excise taxes on sugar-sweetened beverages, has been gaining interest: the taxes have been proposed in major cities as well as at the state level.[68–69] Although taxes have been met with considerable resistance from the beverage industry, they appeal to policymakers not only because they would reduce consumption of unhealthy beverages but also because of the revenue they would generate. Given that sugar-sweetened beverages contain no healthy nutrients and are the source of over half the added sugars in the American diet,[70] they are a reasonable target of a pricing intervention like a tax.

Other policies geared toward prevention should focus on the physical environment. Communities can be built with healthy lifestyles in mind by incorporating sidewalks and shared outdoor space (eg, parks and trails), building crosswalks at traffic intersections, and perhaps building bike lanes if the shared roads would otherwise be too dangerous for bikers.

NOTE: THE FOOD INDUSTRY AND PUBLIC HEALTH

The appropriate role of the food industry in obesity prevention efforts is a contentious issue. Many food and beverage manufacturers including Kraft, Tyson, PepsiCo, Coca-Cola, and Nestlé have announced their commitment to the health, nutrition, and wellness of their consumers, but few have addressed allegations that their products have contributed to high rates of obesity. Although many companies are introducing healthier options, they still maintain the position that there are no good foods or bad foods and that the key to obesity prevention is achieving energy balance by increasing physical activity. PepsiCo's product portfolio classifications of "good-for-you," "better-for-you," and "fun-for-you" are an example of the complex strategies food companies have manufactured as they attempt to deflect criticism about the unhealthfulness of their foods while still continuing to sell unhealthy products.[71–72] The Healthy Weight Commitment Foundation, a health and wellness nonprofit funded by over 40 major food and beverage corporations, typifies the response of the food and beverage industry to the challenge of obesity. The approach, summed up by the tagline "fighting obesity by balancing calories in with calories out," focuses on the importance of physical activity and, predictably, makes no mention of environmental determinants of obesity.[73]

In addition to promoting physical activity programs, food companies have also implemented several widely publicized self-regulatory programs to reduce food marketing to children and limit access to sugary drinks in schools. These pledges have met with varying degrees of success. The 2007 Children's Food and Beverage Advertising Initiative (CFBAI), sponsored by the Council of Better Business Bureaus, commits companies to reduce or eliminate marketing of unhealthy food to children. A second pledge, the School Beverage Guidelines, was developed by the trade association of the beverage industry, the American Beverage Association, in con-junction with the Alliance for a Healthier Generation (a partnership between the Clinton Foundation and the American Heart Association). Beverage companies pledged to remove full-calorie soft drinks from schools and to sell healthy beverages in appropriate portion sizes.

Although these programs commit to important public health goals, their implementation leaves much to be desired. Vague definitions of "advertising primarily directed at children" and "healthier food" have allowed CFBAI compa-nies to continue to market unhealthy products to children, especially on the Internet.[74–75] The School Beverage Guidelines have been slightly more effective; the American Beverage Association's self-evaluation has indicated some progress in reducing access to unhealthy beverages in schools.[76] However, the pledge leaves other calorie-dense drinks such as sports drinks unregulated and does nothing to reduce branding effects because companies are still permitted to sell other drinks in schools.[77]

Food industry contributions to obesity prevention, through sponsorship of nutrition and physical activity programs and through self-regulation, could be a welcome contribution to efforts to improve the nation's health. However, policymakers and the public must be careful not to let these contributions take the place of policy or sway commitment to building effective, evidence-based policy that will reduce the preva-lence of obesity.

FEASIBILITY AND FUNDING

Necessary funding for obesity prevention measures varies widely, both in turns of how much preventive measures cost and in terms of which entity is expected to fund the measure. Currently, there is no doubt that obesity and attending health problems are generating costs for individuals, for businesses, and for governments.[78] Thus, even though some interventions may require initial investments, if they effectively reduce obesity they could ultimately be cost-saving. Certain measures such as limiting advertising of unhealthy foods to children are anticipated to be cost-saving,[79] or, in the case of a tax on sugared beverages, could actually generate funds for further prevention.[69] The Assessing Cost Effectiveness–Obesity project is a valuable research program working to systematically evaluate the cost-effectiveness of a wide range of obesity programs by comparing the strength of evidence to support each measure, the estimated cost of each measure, and anticipated health benefits.[80-81]

Some interventions such as nutrition education or physical activity promotion are politically benign and likely to receive widespread support. However, other measures such as limiting marketing to children and removing soft drinks from schools are likely to meet resistance from industry. Policymakers and the public will need to be courageous in standing up to these powerful interests and implementing policies that will benefit the health of current and future generations.

SUMMARY

Obesity is an epidemic that likely will worsen without substantive changes to the current environment. Although treatment of the individual has conventionally been the focus of the obesity field, prevention using a public health model will be essential for making progress on a population level. There are encouraging signs that communities across the country are acknowledging the complex causes of obesity and making impressive reforms to improve their health and that of their children. Public policy changes long have been used to combat infectious and chronic diseases and will be vital in the attempt to reduce the toll of poor diet, physical inactivity, and obesity.

REFERENCES

1. Finucane MM, Stevens GA, Cowan MJ, et al. National, regional, and global trends in body-mass index since 1980: systematic analysis of health examination surveys and epidemiological studies with 960 country-years and 9.1 million participants. Lancet 2011;377:557–67.
2. Flegal KM, Carroll MD, Ogden CL, et al. Prevalence and trends in obesity among US adults, 1999–2008. JAMA 2010;303,235–41.
3. Lavie CJ, Milani RV, Ventura HO. Obesity and cardiovascular disease: risk factor, paradox, and impact of weight loss. J Am Coll Cardiol 2009;53:1925–32.
4. Mokdad AH, Ford ES, Bowman BA, et al. Prevalence of obesity, diabetes, and obesity-related health risk factors, 2001. JAMA 2003;289:76–9.
5. Young T, Skatrud J, Peppard PE. Risk factors for obstructive sleep apnea in adults. JAMA 2004;291:2013–6.
6. Calle EE, Kaaks R. Overweight, obesity and cancer: epidemiological evidence and proposed mechanisms. Nat Rev Cancer 2004;4:579–91.
7. Finkelstein EA, Ruhm CJ, Kosa KM. Economic causes and consequences of obesity. Annu Rev Public Health 2005;26:239–57.
8. Ebbeling CB, Pawlak DB, Ludwig DS. Childhood obesity: public-health crisis, common sense cure. Lancet 2002;360:473–82.

9. Yach D, Stuckler D, Brownell KD. Epidemiologic and economic consequences of the global epidemics of obesity and diabetes. Nat Med 2006;12:62–6.
10. Brownell KD, Schwartz MB, Puhl RM, et al. The need for bold action to prevent adolescent obesity. J Adolesc Health 2009;45:S8–17.
11. Brownell KD, Horgen KB. Food fight: the inside story of the food industry, America's obesity crisis, and what we can do about it. New York: McGraw-Hill, Contemporary Books; 2004.
12. Nestle M. Food politics: how the food industry influences nutrition and health. Berkeley (CA): University of California Press; 2002.
13. Brownell KD, Nestle M. The sweet and lowdown on sugar. New York Times. January 23, 2004:1.
14. Wing RR. Behavioral weight control. In: Wadden TA, Stunkard AJ, editors. Handbook for obesity treatment. New York: Guilford Press; 2002. p. 301–16.
15. Wing RR, Phelan S. Long-term weight loss maintenance. Am J Clin Nutr 2005;82: 222S–5S.
16. Doyle YG, Furey A, Flowers J. Sick individuals and sick populations: 20 years later. J Epidemiol Community Health 2006;60:396–398.
17. Friedman KE, Ashmore JA, Applegate KL. Recent experiences of weight-based stigmatization in a weight loss surgery population: psychological and behavioral correlates. Obesity (Silver Spring) 2008;16:S69–74.
18. Drury CAA, Louis M. Exploring the association between body weight, stigma of obesity, and health care avoidance. J Am Acad Nurse Pract 2002;14:554–60.
19. Griffin AW. Women and weight-based employment discrimination. Cardozo Journal of Law and Gender 2007;13:631–62.
20. Puhl RM, Brownell KD. Bias, discrimination, and obesity. Obes Res 2001;9:788–905.
21. Puhl RM, Heuer CA. The stigma of obesity: a review and update. Obesity (Silver Spring) 2009;17:941–64.
22. Simon M. Appetite for profit: how the food industry undermines our health and how to fight back. New York: Nation Books; 2006.
23. Brownell KD, Kersh R, Ludwig DS, et al. Personal responsibility and obesity: a constructive approach to a controversial issue. Health Aff (Millwood) 2010;29: 379–87.
24. Gale SK, Van Itallie TB, Faust IM. Effects of palatable diets on body weight and adipose tissue cellularity in the adult obese female Zucker rat (fa/fa). Metabolism 1981;30:105–10.
25. Bates LM, Acevedo-Garcia D, Alegria M, et al. Immigration and generational trends in body mass index and obesity in the United States: results of the National Latino and Asian American Survey, 2002–2003. Am J Public Health 2008;98:70–7.
26. Cairney J, Ostbye T. Time since immigration and excess body weight. Can J Public Health 1999;90:120–4.
27. Lauderdale DS, Rathouz PJ. Body mass index in a US national sample of Asian Americans: effects of nativity, years since immigration and socioeconomic status. Int J Obes Relat Metab Disord 2000;24:1188–94.
28. Lillioja S, Bogardus C. Obesity and insulin resistance: lessons learned from the Pima Indians. Diabetes Metab Rev 1988;4:517–40.
29. Saad MF, Knowler WC, Pettitt DJ, et al. The natural history of impaired glucose tolerance in the Pima Indians. N Engl J Med 1988;319:1500–6.
30. Ravussin E, Valencia ME, Esparza J, et al. Effects of a traditional lifestyle on obesity in Pima Indians. Diabetes Care 1994;17:1067–74.
31. Wilks R, Bennett F, Forrester T, et al. Chronic diseases: the new epidemic. West Indian Med J 1998;47:40–4.

32. Martorell R, Khan LK, Hughes ML, et al. Obesity in Latin American women and children. J Nutr 1998;128:1464–73.
33. Lizarzaburu JL, Palinkas LA. Immigration, acculturation, and risk factors for obesity and cardiovascular disease: a comparison between Latinos of Peruvian descent in Peru and in the United States. Ethn Dis 2002;12:342–52.
34. McKeigue PM. Metabolic consequences of obesity and body fat pattern: lessons from migrant studies. Ciba Found Symp 1996;201:54–64 [discussion: 64–57, 188–93].
35. US Department of Agriculture Economic Research Service. Table 10. Food CPI and expenditures. Washington, DC: United States Department of Agriculture Economic Research Service; 2010. Available at: http://www.ers.usda.gov/briefing/cpifoodand expenditures/data/Expenditures_tables/table10.htm. Accessed June 3, 2011.
36. Todd JE, Mancino L, Lin BH. The impact of food away from home on adult diet quality. Washington, DC: Economic Research Service; 2010. ERR–90.
37. Nielsen SJ, Popkin BM. Patterns and trends in food portion sizes, 1977–1998. JAMA 2003;289:450–3.
38. Diliberti N, Bordi PL, Conklin MT, et al. Increased portion size leads to increased energy intake in a restaurant meal. Obes Res 2004;12:562–8.
39. Holt DJ, Ippolito PM, Desrochers DM, et al. Children's exposure to TV advertising in 1977 and 2004: information for the obesity debate. Washington, DC: Federal Trade Commission; 2007.
40. Marketer Trees 2011. Advertising Age. Available at: http://adage.com/datacenter/market ertrees2011/. Accessed June 1, 2011.
41. Neuman W. Nutrition plate unveiled, replacing food pyramid. New York Times. June 3, 2011; section B:3.
42. Harris JL, Pomeranz JL, Lobstein T, et al. A crisis in the marketplace: how food marketing contributes to childhood obesity and what can be done. Annu Rev Public Health 2009;30:211–25.
43. Drewnowski A, Darmon N. Food choices and diet costs: an economic analysis. J Nutr 2005;135:900–4.
44. Drewnowski A. Obesity and the food environment: dietary energy density and diet costs. Am J Prev Med 2004;27:154–62.
45. Ludwig DS, Nestle M. Can the food industry play a constructive role in the obesity epidemic? JAMA 2008;300:1808–11.
46. Wansink B, Sobal J. Mindless eating: the 200 daily food decisions we overlook. Environ Behav 2007;39:106–23.
47. Pleis J, Ward B, Lucas J. Summary health statistics for US adults: National Health Interview Survey, 2009. In: National Center for Health Statistics. Vital health stat 10(249). Washington, DC: US Government Printing Office; 2010.
48. Church TS, Thomas DM, Tudor-Locke C, et al. Trends over 5 decades in US occupation-related physical activity and their associations with obesity. PLoS One 2011;6:e19657.
49. McDonald NC. Active transportation to school: trends among US schoolchildren, 1969–2001. Am J Prev Med 2007;32:509–16.
50. American Time Use Survey—2010 results. Washington, DC: Bureau of Labor Statistics; 2011.
51. Roslow Research Group. Physical education trends in our nation's schools: a survey of practicing K–12 physical education teachers. Port Washington (NY): National Association for Sport and Physical Education; 2009.
52. Brownson RC, Baker EA, Housemann RA, et al. Environmental and policy determinants of physical activity in the United States. Am J Public Health 2001;91:1995–2003.

53. Huston SL, Evenson KR, Bors P, et al. Neighborhood environment, access to places for activity, and leisure-time physical activity in a diverse North Carolina population. Am J Health Promot 2003;18:58–69.

54. Franzini L, Elliott MN, Cuccaro P, et al. Influences of physical and social neighborhood environments on children's physical activity and obesity. Am J Public Health 2009; 99:271–78.

55. Farley TA, Meriwether RA, Baker ET, et al. Safe play spaces to promote physical activity in inner-city children: results from a pilot study of an environmental intervention. Am J Public Health 2007;97:1625–31.

56. Kahn EB, Ramsey LT, Brownson RC, et al. The effectiveness of interventions to increase physical activity. A systematic review. Am J Prev Med 2002;22:73–107.

57. Brownell KD, Warner KE. The perils of ignoring history: Big Tobacco played dirty and millions died. How similar is Big Food? Milbank Q 2009;87:259–94.

58. Brownell K. Get slim with higher taxes [editorial]. New York Times. December 15, 1994; section A:29.

59. Levi J, Vinter S, St. Laurent R, et al. F as in fat: how obesity threatens America's future. Washington, DC: Trust for America's Health; 2010.

60. Yale Rudd Center for Food Policy & Obesity. Sugar-sweetened beverage tax legislation: 15 states filed as of May 2011. Available at: http://www.yaleruddcenter.org/resources/upload/docs/what/policy/SSBtaxes/SSBTaxMap_2011.pdf. Accessed June 3, 2011.

61. Lytle LA, Kubik MY, Perry C, et al. Influencing healthful food choices in school and home environments: results from the TEENS study. Prev Med 2006;43:8–13.

62. Story M, Kaphingst KM, French S. The role of schools in obesity prevention. Fut Child 2006;16:109–42.

63. Child nutrition reauthorization. Healthy, hunger-free kids act of 2010. Available at: http://www.whitehouse.gov/sites/default/files/Child_Nutrition_Fact_Sheet_12_10_10.pdf. Accessed May 12, 2011.

64. Story M, Nanney MS, Schwartz MB. Schools and obesity prevention: creating school environments and policies to promote healthy eating and physical activity. Milbank Q 2009;87:71–100.

65. The Food Trust. Healthy corner stores: issue brief. Healthy Corner Stores Network 2011. Available at: http://www.thefoodtrust.org/php/programs/Winter2011issue brief.pdf. Accessed June 3, 2011.

66. French SA. Pricing effects on food choices. J Nutr 2003;133:841S–3S.

67. French SA, Jeffery RW, Story M, et al. Pricing and promotion effects on low-fat vending snack purchases: the CHIPS Study. Am J Public Health 2001;91:112–7.

68. Kamerow D. The case of the sugar sweetened beverage tax. BMJ 2010;341:c3719.

69. Brownell KD, Farley T, Willett WC, et al. The public health and economic benefits of taxing sugar-sweetened beverages. N Engl J Med 2009;361:1599–605.

70. US Department of Agriculture and US Department of Health and Human Services. Dietary guidelines for Americans, 2010. 7th edition. Washington, DC: US Government Printing Office; 2010.

71. PepsiCo 2010 Annual Report. Purchase (NY): PepsiCo, Inc; 2010.

72. Seabrook J. Snacks for a fat planet. The New Yorker 2011;87:8p.

73. Overview: fighting obesity by balancing calories in with calories out. Healthy Weight Commitment Foundation 2011. Available at: http://www.healthyweightcommit.org/about/overview/. Accessed May 12, 2011.

74. Schwartz MB, Ross C, Harris JL, et al. Breakfast cereal industry pledges to self-regulate advertising to youth: will they improve the marketing landscape? J Public Health Policy 2010;31:59–73.

75. Harris J, Schwartz M, Brownell K, et al. Fast food FACTS: evaluating fast food nutrition and marketing to youth. New Haven (CT): Rudd Center for Food Policy & Obesity; December 2010.
76. American Beverage Association. Alliance school beverage guidelines: final progress report: American Beverage Association; 2010. Available at: http://www.foodpolitics. com/wp-content/uploads/School-Beverage-Guidelines-Final-Progress-Report-Executive-Summary.pdf. Accessed June 5, 2011.
77. Sharma LL, Teret SP, Brownell KD. The food industry and self-regulation: standards to promote success and to avoid public health failures. Am J Public Health 2010;100:240–6.
78. Finkelstein EA, Trogdon JG, Brown DS, et al. The lifetime medical cost burden of overweight and obesity: implications for obesity prevention. Obesity (Silver Spring) 2008;16:1843–8.
79. Magnus A, Haby MM, Carter R, et al. The cost-effectiveness of removing television advertising of high-fat and/or high-sugar food and beverages to Australian children. Int J Obes (Lond) 2009;33:1094–102.
80. Carter R, Moodie M, Markwick A, et al. Assessing cost-effectiveness in obesity (ACE-obesity): an overview of the ACE approach, economic methods and cost results. BMC Public Health 2009;9:419.
81. Haby MM, Vos T, Carter R, et al. A new approach to assessing the health benefit from obesity interventions in children and adolescents: the assessing cost-effectiveness in obesity project. Int J Obes (Lond) 2006;30:1463–75.

Index

Note: Page numbers of article titles are in **boldface** type.

Psychiatr Clin N Am 34 (2011) 911–919
doi:10.1016/S0193-953X(11)00101-8
0193-953X/11/$ – see front matter © 2011 Elsevier Inc. All rights reserved.

1. Publication Title	2. Publication Number	3. Filing Date
Psychiatric Clinics of North America	0 0 0 - 7 0 3	9/16/11

4. Issue Frequency	5. Number of Issues Published Annually	6. Annual Subscription Price
Mar, Jun, Sep, Dec	4	$265.00

7. Complete Mailing Address of Known Office of Publication (Not printer) (Street, city, county, state, and ZIP+4®)

Elsevier Inc.
360 Park Avenue South
New York, NY 10010-1710

Contact Person
Stephen Bushing
Telephone (Include area code)
215-239-3688

8. Complete Mailing Address of Headquarters or General Business Office of Publisher (Not printer)

Elsevier Inc., 360 Park Avenue South, New York, NY 10010-1710

9. Full Names and Complete Mailing Addresses of Publisher, Editor, and Managing Editor (Do not leave blank)
Publisher (Name and complete mailing address)

Kim Murphy, Elsevier, Inc., 1600 John F. Kennedy Blvd. Suite 1800, Philadelphia, PA 19103-2899

Editor (Name and complete mailing address)

Sarah Barth, Elsevier, Inc., 1600 John F. Kennedy Blvd. Suite 1800, Philadelphia, PA 19103-2899

Managing Editor (Name and complete mailing address)

Sarah Barth, Elsevier, Inc., 1600 John F. Kennedy Blvd. Suite 1800, Philadelphia, PA 19103-2899

10. Owner (Do not leave blank. If the publication is owned by a corporation, give the name and address of the corporation immediately followed by the names and addresses of all stockholders owning or holding 1 percent or more of the total amount of stock. If not owned by a corporation, give the names and addresses of the individual owners. If owned by a partnership or other unincorporated firm, give its name and address as well as those of each individual owner. If the publication is published by a nonprofit organization, give its name and address.)

Full Name	Complete Mailing Address
Wholly owned subsidiary of	4520 East-West Highway
Reed/Elsevier, US holdings	Bethesda, MD 20814

11. Known Bondholders, Mortgagees, and Other Security Holders Owning or Holding 1 Percent or More of Total Amount of Bonds, Mortgages, or Other Securities. If none, check box ☐ None

Full Name	Complete Mailing Address
N/A	

12. Tax Status (For completion by nonprofit organizations authorized to mail at nonprofit rates) (Check one)
The purpose, function, and nonprofit status of this organization and the exempt status for federal income tax purposes:
☐ Has Not Changed During Preceding 12 Months
☐ Has Changed During Preceding 12 Months (Publisher must submit explanation of change with this statement)

PS Form 3526, September 2007 (Page 1 of 3 (Instructions Page 3)) PSN 7530-01-000-9931 PRIVACY NOTICE: See our Privacy policy in www.usps.com

---

13. Publication Title			14. Issue Date for Circulation Data Below
Psychiatric Clinics of North America			September 2011

15. Extent and Nature of Circulation			Average No. Copies Each Issue During Preceding 12 Months	No. Copies of Single Issue Published Nearest to Filing Date
a. Total Number of Copies (Net press run)			1228	1000
b. Paid Circulation (By Mail and Outside the Mail)	(1)	Mailed Outside-County Paid Subscriptions Stated on PS Form 3541. (Include paid distribution above nominal rate, advertiser's proof copies, and exchange copies)	602	541
	(2)	Mailed In-County Paid Subscriptions Stated on PS Form 3541 (Include paid distribution above nominal rate, advertiser's proof copies, and exchange copies)		
	(3)	Paid Distribution Outside the Mails Including Sales Through Dealers and Carriers, Street Vendors, Counter Sales, and Other Paid Distribution Outside USPS®	230	243
	(4)	Paid Distribution by Other Classes Mailed Through the USPS (e.g. First-Class Mail®)		
c. Total Paid Distribution (Sum of 15b (1), (2), (3), and (4))		▲	832	784
d. Free or Nominal Rate Distribution (By Mail and Outside the Mail)	(1)	Free or Nominal Rate Outside-County Copies Included on PS Form 3541	65	49
	(2)	Free or Nominal Rate In-County Copies Included on PS Form 3541		
	(3)	Free or Nominal Rate Copies Mailed at Other Classes Through the USPS (e.g. First-Class Mail)		
	(4)	Free or Nominal Rate Distribution Outside the Mail (Carriers or other means)		
e. Total Free or Nominal Rate Distribution (Sum of 15d (1), (2), (3) and (4))		▲	65	49
f. Total Distribution (Sum of 15c and 15e)		▲	897	833
g. Copies not Distributed (See instructions to publishers #4 (page #3))			331	167
h. Total (Sum of 15f and g)		▲	1228	1000
i. Percent Paid (15c divided by 15f times 100)			92.75%	94.12%

16. Publication of Statement of Ownership

☐ If the publication is a general publication, publication of this statement is required. Will be printed in the **December 2011** issue of this publication.   Publication not required.

17. Signature and Title of Editor, Publisher, Business Manager, or Owner   Date

Stephen R. Bushing   September 16, 2011

Stephen R. Bushing –Inventory Distribution Coordinator

I certify that all information furnished on this form is true and complete. I understand that anyone who furnishes false or misleading information on this form or who omits material or information requested on the form may be subject to criminal sanctions (including fines and imprisonment) and/or civil sanctions (including civil penalties).

PS Form 3526, September 2007 (Page 2 of 3)

Printed and bound by CPI Group (UK) Ltd, Croydon, CR0 4YY

03/10/2024

01040455-0002